Visual arts and medicine in early modern Europe and beyond

Manchester University Press

Visual arts and medicine in early modern Europe and beyond

A collection of essays and sources

Edited by

Robert Brennan, Fabian Jonietz, and Romana Sammern

Manchester University Press

Published with the support of the Austrian Science Fund (FWF): 10.55776/PUB1176

FWF Austrian Science Fund

Published by Manchester University Press
Oxford Road, Manchester, M13 9PL

www.manchesteruniversitypress.co.uk

British Library Cataloguing-in-Publication Data
A catalogue record for this book is available from the British Library

ISBN 978 1 5261 8287 6 hardback

First published 2026

EU authorised representative for GPSR:
Easy Access System Europe, Mustamäe tee 50, 10621 Tallinn, Estonia
gpsr.requests@easproject.com

Typeset
by Deanta Global Publishing Services, Chennai, India

Contents

Figures

Contributors

Carly B. Boxer is Assistant Professor of Art History at Bucknell University, Lewisburg, PA. She is a historian of medieval art whose work centres on the connections between medieval image-making practices and period ideas about vision, knowledge, and the capacity of images to structure and guide thought. Her current book project explores medical manuscripts in late medieval England, analysing their role as pedagogical tools.

Robert Brennan is Lecturer in Italian Art, c. 1300–1500, at the Courtauld Institute of Art, London. He is the author of *Painting as a Modern Art in Early Renaissance Italy* (London, 2019), as well as articles in journals such as *The Art Bulletin*, *Oxford Art Journal*, and *Res: Anthropology and Aesthetics*.

Julia Czapla is an art historian and Adjunct Professor at the Pontifical University of John Paul II, Cracow. She received her PhD at the Jagiellonian University in 2019. Since then, she has published extensively on early modern scientific illustrations of animals, plants, and herbs.

Fabrizio Federici studied art history at the University of Pisa and the Scuola Normale Superiore. From 2008 to 2012 he was team leader of the project *Osservatorio Mostre e Musei* of the Scuola Normale, while from 2016 to 2019 he was post-doc fellow at the Bibliotheca Hertziana in Rome. His interests include art patronage and collecting in the seventeenth century, the history of antiquarianism, and the reception of medieval art in the early modern period.

Frances Gage, Associate Professor at Buffalo State, SUNY, specialises in sixteenth- and seventeenth-century Italian art, criticism, and collecting. She authored *Painting as Medicine in Early Modern Rome* and numerous journal articles. Her work has been supported by major institutions. Currently, she is writing a cultural biography of Annibale Carracci.

Jana Graul is currently holding a professorship in art history at Hamburg University. She earned her doctorate in 2020 with the multi-awarded dissertation *Invidia als Künstlerlaster. Neid in Kunst und Kunstliteratur der Frühen Neuzeit*. Her research has been supported by institutions including the Kunsthistorisches Institut in Florenz, the Gerda Henkel Stiftung, the Istituto Nazionale di Studi sul Rinascimento in Florence, and the Deutsches Studienzentrum in Venice.

Fabian Jonietz is a scholar at the Zentralinstitut für Kunstgeschichte in Munich, where he leads a research project on the premodern commemoration of animals. Since receiving his PhD in Art History, he has been awarded numerous fellowships and held research and teaching positions in Germany, Italy, Switzerland, and the United States. He has published extensively on early modern art and art theory.

Catherine Lawless is an art historian who works on gender, piety, and representation in late medieval Florence. She is the Director of the Centre for Gender and Women's Studies in Trinity College Dublin. Before her present post she was Course Director of the MA in History of Art and Architecture at the University of Limerick. She is presently completing a book on the representation of female saints.

Ariella Minden is scientific assistant at the Bibliotheca Hertziana, Rome. She completed her doctoral dissertation *In Dialogue: Medial Thinking in Bolognese Printmaking, 1500–1530* at the University of Toronto in 2024. Minden's current research evaluates Bologna's role as a centre of printmaking by using media theory as a lens through which to explore the emergence of new artistic technologies.

Katharina Sabernig, MD/PhD, is a researcher at the Medical University of Vienna and the Austrian Academy of Sciences. She specialises in Tibetan medical illustrations, anatomical terminology, and pharmacology. Her projects include a Tibetan medical terms database and a textile anatomy project, exploring the history of anatomical depiction.

Romana Sammern is an art historian and permanent research scholar at the University of Salzburg. She researches and teaches at the intersection of the body, art, cosmetics, and medicine in the early modern period, with relevance to the present. She received her PhD from the Humboldt University in Berlin (*Hurenbilder*, published by Böhlau in 2014). In October

2024, she completed her habilitation project *Beauty, Art, and the Body in the Early Modern Perio*d at the University of Passau.

Paolo Sanvito studied art history in Rome, Freiburg, and Frankfurt, earning his PhD in 1995. He held research and teaching positions at Notre Dame, USA, Rome (2004–2008), Naples, and at the Austrian Academy of Science, Vienna.

Katharine Stahlbuhk was trained as a conservator for wall paintings before obtaining her PhD in art history. She has held positions at the Kunsthistorisches Institut in Florenz and the Bibliotheca Hertziana. She received fellowships at Villa I Tatti, the Harvard University Center for Italian Renaissance Studies, the University of Padua, and the Italian Academy at Columbia University. Her book *Oltre il colore. Die farbreduzierte Wandmalerei zwischen Humilitas und Observanzreformen* was published in 2021.

Introduction: *Ut pictura medicina*?

Robert Brennan, Fabian Jonietz, and Romana Sammern

Ut pictura poesis, 'as in painting, so in poetry'. Few phrases have done as much to catalyse the development of European art theory as this famous verse, written in the first century by the Roman poet Horace.[1] In the Renaissance, Horace's dictum led many artists and writers to explore programmatic similarities between painting, poetry, and a wide variety of other 'liberal' and 'mechanical' arts.[2] By the Enlightenment, it had stimulated extensive reflection on the incommensurability of text and image, a central principle within emergent theories of aesthetic autonomy.[3]

The doctrine of autonomy did not put an end to comparisons between painting, poetry, and other disciplines, but in the long term, it did tend to subordinate such comparisons to broader teleological narratives, in which each individual art was seen to progress toward its own distinctive ends. In the historiography of Renaissance art, for example, connections continued to be recognised between painterly naturalism and medical sciences, such as optics and anatomy. However, the impact of such connections was constrained by the assumed trajectory of each discipline: painting, it was thought, may well have assisted the medical sciences in their turn toward nature, and vice versa, but in the long term, the link between them would have to dissolve in order for each field to assume its proper function in modern society.[4]

In recent decades, as the authority of such teleologies has begun to wane, art historians have begun to recuperate the *ut pictura* principle as a leitmotif of current methodology.[5] Early modern painting has been put back into productive dialogue with liberal arts like rhetoric and music, as well as mechanical arts like alchemy and textile production, to name just a few of many examples.[6] In the case of medical science, however, the imprint of the older, teleological framework remains in large part intact. Although a great deal of pathbreaking research has been done on the relationship between painting and medicine in recent years, the focus has remained fixed on the traditional nexus of painting, anatomy, and optics, centred predominantly in sixteenth- and seventeenth-century Italy.[7] An anachronistic depiction of *Michelangelo teaching anatomy* evokes this approach (Figure 0.1).[8] Surrounded by renowned fellow painters such as Andrea del Sarto, Sebastiano del Piombo, Baccio Bandinelli, Raphael, and others, Michelangelo sits in the centre between the legs of an already flayed corpse and performs a dissection. The subject may originate in Ascanio Condivi's biography of Michelangelo.[9] Ascanio describes how, as

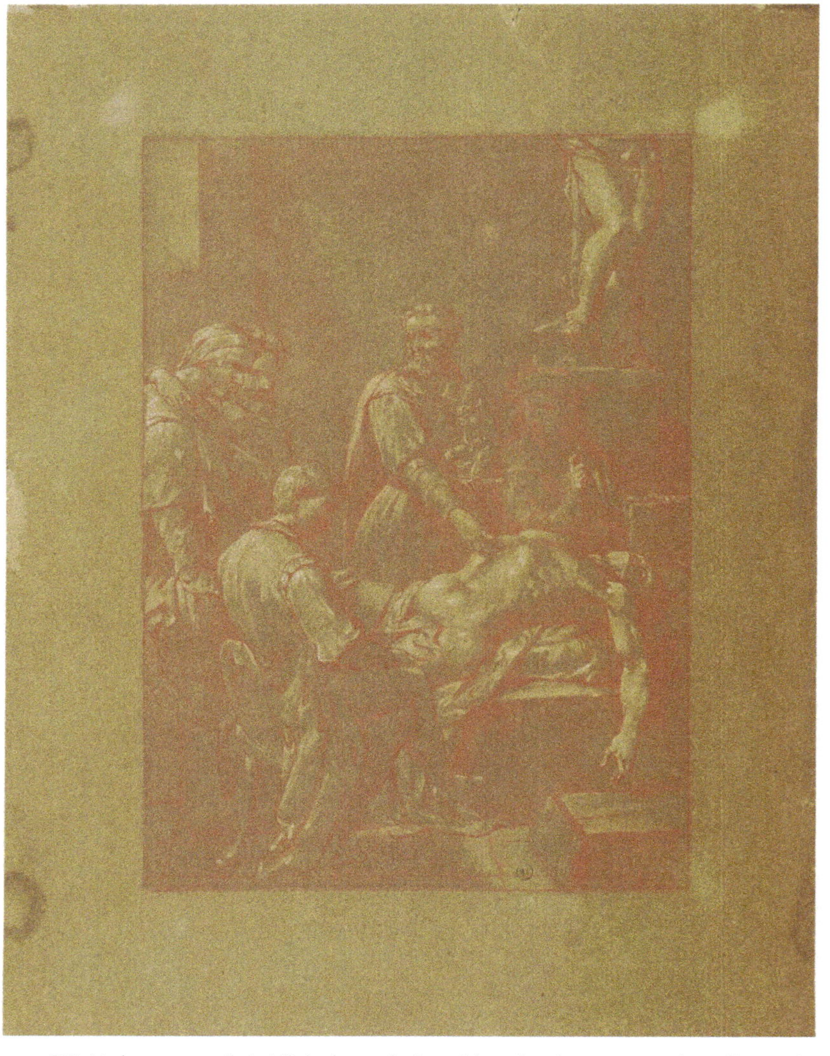

Figure 0.1 Unknown artist, *Michelangelo teaching Anatomy*, seventeenth-century, drawing, 38 × 29 cm. Montpellier, Musée Fabre, inv. 895.7.118. Image credit: Musée Fabre de Montpellier Méditerranée Métropole.

a student of Michelangelo, he received anatomical instructions during a dissection from his master.[10] Accordingly, in the drawing, Michelangelo imparts to his peers a profound understanding of the human body that altered the practice of painting and art education: by the second half of the seventeenth century, anatomy was considered an integral element of artistic education and, as such, was part of allegories of both *disegno* and the newly founded art academies.[11] In a print depicting Simone Pignoni's (1611–1698) self-portrait in a private collection (Figure 0.2), for instance, the artist is shown painting a female nude. Pignoni has already painted a skeleton on the canvas, which he now covers with the visible surface of

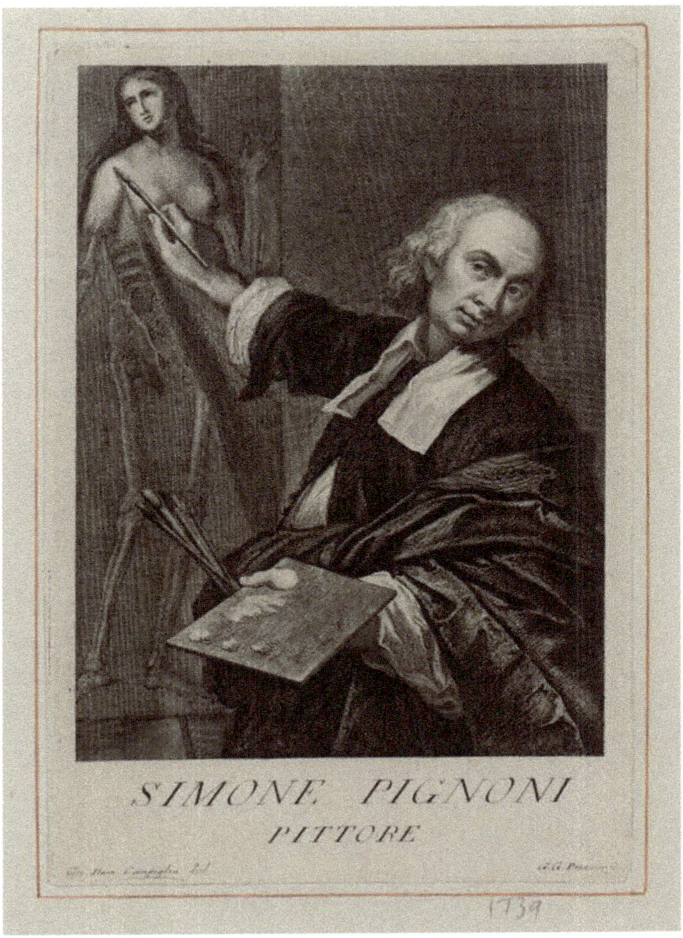

Figure 0.2 Giovanni Domenico Campiglia (draftsman) and Georg Caspar von Prenner (etcher) after Simone Pignoni, self-portrait of Simone Pignoni, c. 1752/62, drypoint and etching, 231 × 172 mm. Private collection. Image credit: The Courtauld, London (Samuel Courtauld Trust)

the human body from top to bottom: the hair, the face, and the chest are already finished. This layered understanding of the human body, which starts from its internal structure (the skeleton) and progresses through the addition of muscles and ultimately skin, required anatomical knowledge that had been standard in Italian painting from the second half of the sixteenth century. In the fifteenth century, Leon Battista Alberti introduced this procedure as an example of good compositional practice in his treatise on painting.[12]

This book seeks to move beyond this established grouping, and the teleologically circumscribed interests that stand behind it. The aim is not to write a visual history of the medical profession, nor to chronicle the role that medical illustration has played in art history.[13] Rather, it is to rethink the relationship between the two professions from the ground up, in pursuit of entirely new points of departure for future study. To this end, we foreground types of connection that have remained marginal or overlooked in previous scholarship: for example, collaborations between painters and doctors on colour charts, handwork skills common to sculptors, engravers and surgeons, the transmission of art theory through medical texts long before the emergence of art writing itself as an independent genre, and the kinship of medical diagnosis with early modes of analytical connoisseurship. In many cases, we will argue, these types of connection bear an intrinsic relation to one another. Painting and medicine were bound by a complex network of affiliations that cuts across material, institutional, and theoretical modes of analysis, and can help us rethink the broader social and epistemological standing of each discipline.

On one level, then, the book proposes that visual art and medicine enjoyed a special degree of intertwinement, beyond the typical range of connections that bound the arts together in premodernity. On another level, we also aim to demonstrate the relevance of this intertwinement to a number of pressing methodological concerns in current humanities scholarship. The affiliation of art and medicine encompasses the kinds of relationship that have long occupied scholarship on the *ut pictura* principle, such as the relation of text and image, or the relation between senses (e.g., visuality and aurality). But it also brings into play a much wider range of material, technical, and institutional factors, which converge around shared modes of embodied knowledge that have only recently begun to attract scholarly attention.[14] Given the centrality of the human body as a principle object of knowledge and representation for each discipline, this common grounding in embodied knowledge holds great potential for broader histories of the body. It is also emerging as a crucial methodological platform for global histories of both art and medicine – a relationship that is all the more urgent in light of the role that these two disciplines played as key nodes of transcultural exchange, as well as their centrality in the formation of colonial, and in particular racialised, ideologies.[15] Much work remains to be done in connecting these lines of inquiry, which have thus far tended to run parallel along established disciplinary lines.[16]

Charting connections

To introduce the network of interdisciplinary connections that stand at the heart of this volume, we begin with one of the most canonical early invocations of the *ut pictura poesis* principle in European art theory: the opening chapters of Cennino Cennini's *Libro dell'arte*, a handbook on painting written near the end of the fourteenth century or first quarter of the fifteenth century. Cennini starts the book with a series of broad reflections concerning the origin and status of his art:

> And for good reason [painting] deserves to sit in second rung to science (*scienza*) and to be coronated with poetry. The reason is this: that the poet, with science, though he has [just] one, it makes him worthy and free, able to compose and lay together [words] in one way or another as he wishes, according to his desire. Likewise, liberty has been given to the painter, the ability to compose a figure standing, seated, half-man half-horse, as he wishes, according to his imagination (*fantasia*).[17]

Comparable allusions to artistic licence recur several times subsequently in Cennini's text.[18] While the precise implications of this statement have long been a matter of debate among art historians, Cennini clearly mobilises the Horatian affinity between painting and poetry to establish a distinctive place for painting within the broader hierarchy of arts and sciences. In his view, the affinity is grounded by the role that 'fantasy' (*fantasia*) plays in painting – a concept also central to poetic theory in this era.[19]

This affinity can easily be taken for granted today, given the tendency in our own time to classify painting and poetry together as 'creative' arts. In the fifteenth century, however, such a category did not yet exist.[20] As Martin Kemp shows, moreover, *fantasia* was not yet conceived in opposition to 'reason', but rather was seen to work in conjunction with it.[21] Alongside its association with creative invention in arts such as poetry or rhetoric, *fantasia* performed an important analytical function in the selection and processing of all sensory data, and was thus relevant to broader scientific and epistemological questions. As Wolf-Dietrich Löhr points out, it was also a physiological concept, which medical writers of the period linked to the activity of a specific ventricle within the brain (Figure 0.3).[22] Against this background, it comes as little surprise that a similar invocation of 'fantasy' turns up about a hundred years later in an early Florentine pharmacological handbook, known as the *Ricettario Fiorentino*.[23] Here too, in the final paragraph of the second book on antidotes, the text informs the reader about the necessity of *phantasia* for the crafting of medical remedies.[24]

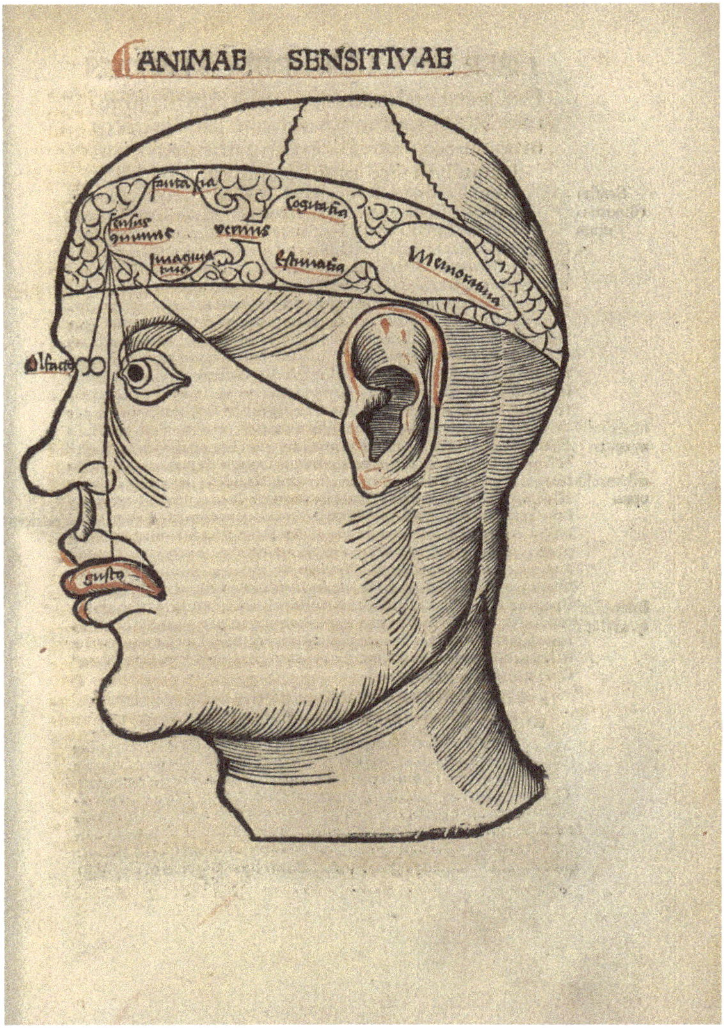

Figure 0.3 *Fantasia*, as labelled in the upper portion of the brain's first ventricle: Urs Graf (?) in Gregorius Reisch, *Margarita Philosophica*, 1503. Image credit: Library of Congress, Rare Book and Special Collections Division

In both of these cases, then, the necessity of *fantasia* is asserted within what modern readers have often regarded as mere 'recipe books'. Both the *Ricettario Fiorentino* and Cennini's *Libro dell'arte* consist in large part of detailed, practical instructions for the sourcing and preparation of materials, followed by straightforward, step-by-step instructions for their use. In fact, some of these materials and procedures are shared between the two treatises. A good example can be seen in the use that the two treatises make of lapis lazuli, a stone that typically came to Italy from Central Asia throughout this period, as indicated by its name (*lazuli*), which derives from a Persian word for 'sky' or 'heaven'.[25] The *Ricettario* includes a recipe for 'pills of lapis lazuli by Mesue', referring to the physician Yūḥannā ibn Māsawayh (777–857 CE).[26] The instructions for these pills begin with a refined, 'washed' version of the mineral (*lapis lazuli lavato*), which corresponds with a method of preparation that can be traced back to a work attributed to Jābir ibn Ḥayyān (c. 721–816 CE; known in Latin as 'Geber'). Cennini provides detailed instructions for precisely this same method of washing lapis lazuli, and openly acknowledges its use in contemporary medicine, repeatedly characterising his procedures with phrases such as 'in the method of the pharmacists' (*a modo [de] gli speziali*).[27]

In this light, there is not only a direct overlap in the material and technical contents of Cennini's *Libro* and the *Ricettario*; this overlap also reveals common paths of transmission from Arabic medical writings. The phenomenon is by no means unique to the case of lapis lazuli. The material culture of Florentine pharmacies testifies to many links with the Islamic world (Figure 0.4),[28] and in fact, the vast majority of the *Ricettario*'s recipes derive from Arabic sources composed between the ninth and twelfth centuries: in particular, works by the aforementioned Mesue, as well as Avicenna (Ibn Sīnā) and Rhazes (Abū Bakr Muḥammad ibn Zakarīyyā' al-Rāzī).[29] Similar sources were prized by the generation of Tuscan artists to which Cennini's book is addressed. Lorenzo Ghiberti, for example, who trained in a Florentine painter's workshop around 1400, went on to compile an extensive series of passages transcribed from Italian vernacular translations of Avicenna's and Averroes's (Ibn Rušd) works on medicine.[30] In fact, the physiologically inflected concept of *fantasia* that Cennini invokes was itself shaped to a large degree by Arabic medical discourse.[31] As Gülru Necipoğlu points out, Avicenna himself explicitly links the concept of 'fantasy' (*al-muḥāqā*) with that of 'mimesis' (*al-takhyīl*) – a connection that would go on to play a central role not only in early modern European art theory, but also in art theory across the Islamic world during the same period.[32]

This deep discursive intertwinement between painting, medical theory, and pharmacology can be explained in part by the closely related social position of these disciplines. The *Ricettario Fiorentino* was produced by the *Collegio degli eximii doctori della arte et medicina*, an institution that organised disputations, public dissections, and medical examinations in conjunction with the University of Florence. The *Collegio* was in turn governed by the guild of the *Arte dei Medici e Speziali* (i.e., doctors and pharmacists), which also included painters, alongside representatives of other manual arts, such as barbers and saddlers.[33] During his training in Florence, Cennini was without question intimately familiar with this same guild: his teacher, Agnolo Gaddi, served as a 'counsellor' (*consigliere*) of the *Arte dei Medici e Speziali*, and his forebear, Giotto, was the first artist listed for enrolment when painters were first formally incorporated into the guild around 1320.[34]

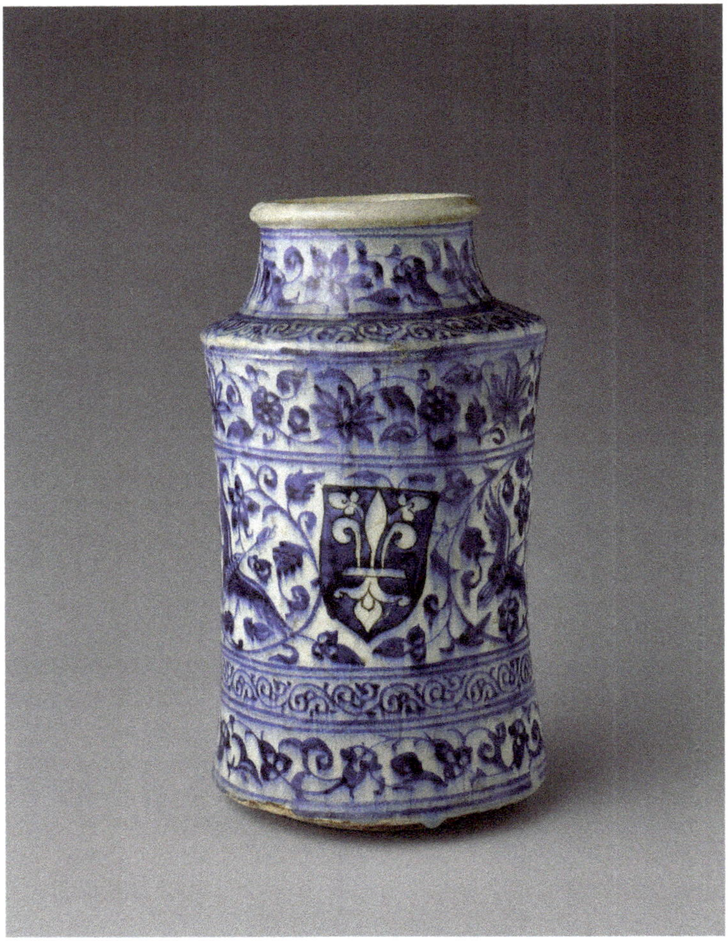

Figure 0.4 Drug Jar (*albarello*) with Florentine emblem, made in Damascus (?), Syria, c. 1400–1450. Paris, Musée du Louvre, inv. AD 4288. Image credit: Musée du Louvre, Dist. GrandPalaisRmn / Chipault – Soligny

What these two texts share, then, is not only a multifaceted technical and discursive connection, but also a more or less direct institutional affiliation. The *Ricettario Fiorentino* represents an authoritative collaboration between doctors and pharmacists, created under the auspices of the *Collegio*, which was intended to serve as a standard for pharmacological practice.[35] Cennini exhibits a comparable concern to ground the authority of his text, and many scholars have hypothesised a direct link between the *Libro* and the contemporary guild system.[36] The invocation of 'fantasy' in both sources should thus be analysed in terms of a common social predicament. The struggle of painters to achieve recognition as practitioners of a 'noble' or 'liberal' art is well known to art historians, but physicians and pharmacists engaged in similar debates throughout the same period.[37] Petrarch, for example, criticised the claims of both painting and medicine to noble status.[38] The invocation of 'fantasy' that opens both the *Libro* and the *Ricettario* can thus be seen to reflect not only the common epistemological predicament of each discipline, perched as they were between scientific knowledge, handwork, and the observation of nature. It also represents a common effort to mobilise this predicament as part of a broader project of social advancement, utilising precisely the same institutional affiliations and genres of writing.

This particular network of connections is perhaps easier to imagine for the fourteenth and fifteenth centuries, when the transformations entailed by Europe's fabled 'scientific revolution' were still a long way off. However, a glance forward in time confirms that connections of this kind persisted well into later centuries, despite drastically changing social and intellectual conditions. As Michael Stolberg demonstrates, the adoption of humanistic practices among physicians was driven in large part by a need to distinguish themselves from non-academic competitors, such as unlearned healers, barbers, and charlatans.[39] This process, which itself recalls the efforts of learned artists to distinguish themselves from uneducated labourers, had the corollary effect of introducing drawing and other artistic skills into medical education. As Craig A. Hanson demonstrates for England around 1600, doctors such as Richard Haydocke, Théodore de Mayerne, and William Harvey all actively cultivated practices of art making, antiquarianism, and connoisseurship as a part of their professionalisation; indeed, as he observes, it is possible to think of a broader process of social differentiation that encompassed the division not only of doctors from charlatans, but also artists from craftsmen.[40] In the long term, such distinctions left a deeply patriarchal imprint on both art and medicine, despite the extensive roles that early modern women played in both fields.[41]

Signs of this same long-term process of social distinction and intellectual exchange are discernible in Italy as well, not only in the art historical writings of physicians like Paolo Giovio or Giulio Mancini in the early sixteenth and seventeenth centuries, but also in so late a figure as Giovanni Morelli, who would radically reorient the practice of connoisseurship through the scientific methodology in which he had been trained as a physician in the mid-nineteenth century.[42] However, this European story is also part of a wider process that unfolded in complex interaction with the emerging colonial world. Across the Atlantic, for example, hierarchical distinctions between learned and unlearned medical practitioners enabled colonial authorities to associate the practices of Black and Indigenous healers with witchcraft or 'sorcery' (in Portuguese, *feitiçaria*), even though such practitioners often drew upon empirical knowledge of natural remedies that would stand up to modern pharmacological explanation, as careful archival work by James Sweet, Pablo Gómez, Kalle Kananoja, and others has recently shown.[43] Again, there is a direct overlap here with a simultaneous tendency to associate African and Indigenous artifacts with craft, idolatry, and 'fetishism' (in Portuguese, *feitiçaria*) as opposed to 'art'.[44] In such colonial contexts art and medicine converged around a common discourse of exclusion and repression, despite their entanglement in ongoing processes of transcultural exchange.

A crucial background for this exclusionary process is the delicate, and at times rather conflicted relationship between art, medicine, and religion within the European tradition – a relationship inextricably bound up with the institutional affiliations outlined above. The sense of belonging that situated painters and physicians in the same guild was reinforced by the fact that they shared a common patron saint: Saint Luke the Evangelist. A longstanding tradition, whose roots can be traced back to biblical sources, imagines Saint Luke as both a doctor and a painter who made portraits of the Madonna and Child.[45] This legendary connection has nurtured a host of relations between art and Christian healing practices, which flourished alongside the professionalisation of medical discourse. Just as King Agbar of Edessa's leprosy was thought to have been cured by the sight of the Mandylion (a miraculous imprint of Christ's face), so too healing legends came to circulate around the images attributed to Saint Luke.[46] For example, Jacobus de Voragine, the widely read medieval hagiographer, reports how Pope Gregory the Great drove the plague out of Rome by carrying an image painted by St Luke in procession from the Church of Santa Maria Maggiore. The icon, he writes, transformed the city's plague-ridden stench into pure, clean air.[47]

This is yet another connection between art and medicine that tends to be phased out of the modern history of each discipline, due to the demands of teleology. Karl Möseneder has shown how images retained healing power (*kraft und tugent*) in the art theoretical writings of the sixteenth-century physician Paracelsus, despite the fact that he was a follower of the Reformed churches.[48] There is also ample evidence of the continuing vitality of such traditions in Europe throughout the seventeenth century and beyond. One particularly revealing example can be seen in a painting by Lanfranco that depicts Saint Luke's dual professional status (Figure 0.5). The Evangelist appears in the act of healing a waterlogged child, whose illness is clearly evident from his skin colour, distended stomach, and languished eyes. At this moment, Saint Luke has interrupted his work on a portrait of the Madonna in order to take the child's pulse. Lanfranco is careful to show that Saint Luke places his trust in theoretical medicine as well as divine healing, for a copy of Hippocrates lies on the table in the lower-right foreground. At the same time, the picture itself testifies to the relevance of sacred art to the healing process, insofar as it may have functioned as a votive image: an offering of thanks for the fulfilment of a promise made to the deity.[49]

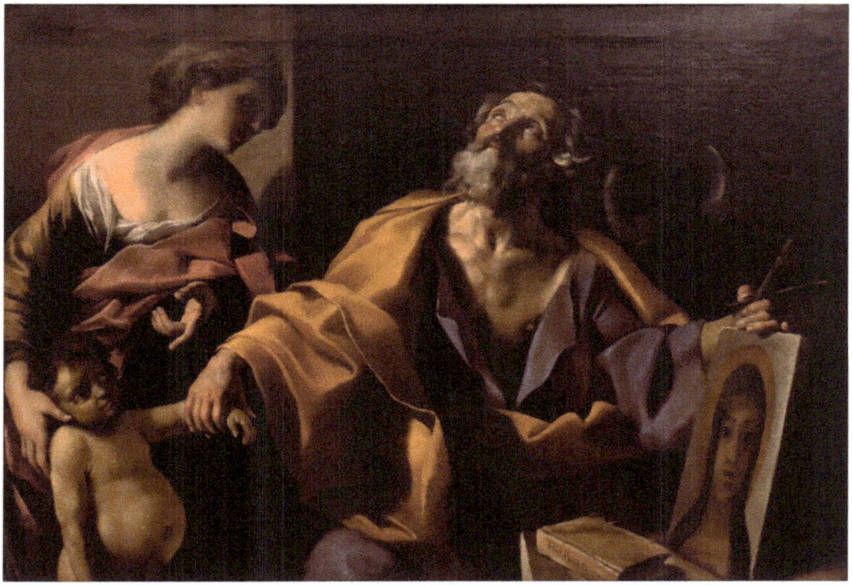

Figure 0.5 Giovanni Lanfranco, St Luke healing the hydropic child, c. 1620. Rome, Palazzo Barberini, Galleria Nazionale d'Arte Antica. Image credit: Wikipedia Commons

This intricate intermeshing of artistic, cultic, and scientific perspectives on healing, which the first chapters in the present volume address, persisted in Europe well into the modern period and beyond, as the ongoing practice of offering votive images in Catholic cults demonstrates. These practices are best understood in connection with the materiality of objects and the affective reactions of embodied observers – dynamics that become fully apparent in early modern depictions of Christ as a pharmacist, weighing his 'medicine' just like contemporary apothecaries.[50] In Figure 0.6, the suffering devotees not only reach out metaphorically toward the Redeemer's medicine, as in the case of the crippled man with a crutch under his arm, but also to printed broadsheets and cheap engravings with religious scenes: relatively inexpensive images that could be attached as ephemeral votives to cult images, brought into homes to aid prayers for the recovery of health, or even swallowed to increase their medicinal effect.[51]

Mapping the volume

By placing this religious connection into dialogue with the broader array of material, technical, discursive, and institutional connections described above, this volume aims to outline a richer, more complex, multilateral, and transcultural picture of the relationship between art and medicine in early modern Europe. Many of the book's nine chapters engage with case

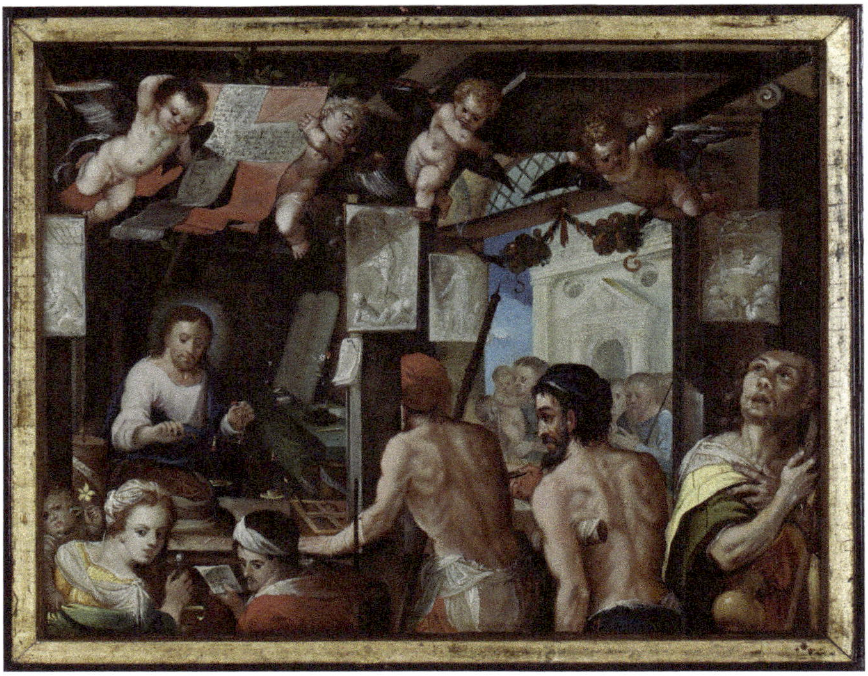

Figure 0.6 Michael Herr, Christ as Pharmacist, 1619, oil on copper, 26.6 × 35 cm. Marburg, Museum für Kunst und Kulturgeschichte der Philipps-Universität Marburg, inv. 7040. Image credit: Bildarchiv Foto Marburg/ Horst Fenchel

studies from late medieval and early modern Italy, where scholarship has traditionally tended to locate the emergence of the figure of the artist, as well as canonical modes of collaboration between artists and physicians, revolving around optics and anatomy. By shifting attention to other modes of collaboration, these essays demonstrate Italy's entanglement with a wider range of transcultural and interdisciplinary developments. Chapters on England and Tibet compliment this shift of perspective by taking up a view from regions that have traditionally been deemed 'peripheral', but can in fact be recognised as crucial nodes within the wider networks of exchange between art and medicine that constitute the central concern of this book.

The volume opens with two chapters on crucial aspects of the link between religious imagery and therapeutic efficacy at the dawn of the early modern period. Departing from Jacques Le Goff's observation that in the Middle Ages the body did not exist unless co-penetrated with the soul, the first chapter by Catherine Lawless looks at relations of imagery, sanctity, and healing, starting with the objectification – and externalisation – of the suffering body or body part in the form of ex votos, usually in wax, of the supplicant, and proceeding to the image of the saint in which *virtus* was located, and which also served the function of popularising their thaumaturgic properties. Lawless examines co-existing systems of medicine and spirituality demonstrating how both hagiography and iconography maintained the superiority of spiritual medicine, while nevertheless acknowledging medical and surgical procedures. Particular attention is given to the relationship between physical and mental health, as well as the gendered dynamics at play in 'diseases' such as demonic possession. Similarly, Carly B. Boxer's essay on wax votive offerings in England investigates the relationship between wax ex votos, medical practice, and broader economies of healing in late medieval England. Analysing extant wax ex votos from Exeter Cathedral alongside visual and textual descriptions of votive offerings from the region, the essay draws comparisons with other instances of wax sculpture from the period, such as death masks and anatomical models used by physicians. These connections complicate the modes of reference that bind the ex voto to the votary and foreground the materiality and modes of production particular to wax: for example, its connection with the cultivation of bees, as well as its propensity toward quasi-mechanical modes of reproduction. In these ways, the chapter sheds light on economies of representation that span medical and cultic approaches to healing.

The following two chapters take up the question of materiality and connect it to the complex field of colour. Robert Brennan investigates the role of skin colour in Italian painting and medicine in the era of Cimabue and Giotto, engaging with recent scholarship on premodern discourses of race. His chapter begins by demonstrating the relevance of medical discourse to the rendering of soft-tissue anatomy in the work of Florentine painters in the late thirteenth and early fourteenth century, and then turns to little-studied writings of contemporary Florentine physicians, who explicitly connect techniques of painting and sculpture with Galenic theories of white skin as a sign of ideal complexion (*complexio aequalis*). Based on this connection, the essay argues that the establishment of whiteness as an authoritative, anatomically rationalised standard of beauty was the product of active exchange between painters and physicians in this period, and ultimately reflects social – and specifically, gendered – interests common to both professions. In the following chapter, Katharine Stahlbuhk begins from Marsilio Ficino's Neoplatonic remarks on the favourable effect of the colour green and investigates the theory and practice of 'chromotherapy' in fifteenth-century Italy – in particular, the conviction that exposure to green walls (sometimes containing figurative decoration) could serve as therapy for the eyes. Drawing on ancient sources, such as Aristotle, who regarded green pigment as 'a drug for the eyes', Renaissance artists and intellectuals situated the colour green within a complex array of medical, scientific, religious, and aesthetic forms of inquiry. Drawing upon recent restoration campaigns that have reconstructed the colour of a wide variety of spaces, including libraries, bedchambers, and cloisters, the chapter excavates period-specific notions of well-being that straddle intellectual and material culture, nature and artifice, metaphorics and physiology. In doing so, it demonstrates the intertwinement of colour perception with broader aesthetic, epistemic, ethical, and political questions.

The reception of ancient knowledge and the question of colour serve also as starting points for two chapters discussing collaboration and shared skills between artists and physicians in central Italy. Fabian Jonietz investigates the role of urine in discursive exchanges between early modern artists and physicians, taking as its point of departure an overlooked collaboration between the physician Dominicus de Ragusa and the painter Gentile da Fabriano, who was tasked with the colouring of a uroscopic treatise in the early fifteenth century. The idea that painters were particularly well-suited to such a task can be traced back to a passage attributed to Galen but written by the ancient medical authority Quintus (Κοίντος). On the one hand, the essay shows that the chemical properties of urine were integral to the workshop traditions of painters as well as a range of other artisans who worked with colour. On the other hand, it shows that physicians had a greater stake in systematising the classification of colours than has been recognised in previous research. The investigation of these issues reveals that the ideal of mimetically accurate, lifelike representation led early modern artists to investigate the forms and functions of the body from a medical, as opposed to merely anatomical perspective. Ariella Minden's chapter then examines the language used in three medical texts written between 1518 and 1522 by the professor and surgeon Jacopo Berengario da Carpi in order to consider how he employed a shared vocabulary common across craft practice to define surgical expertise. As a figure who started his career as an apprentice to his barber-surgeon father and subsequently gained a university education and held a professorship at the University of Bologna, Berengario premises his work on the impossibility of translating experience into language, a direct jab at the theoretical medicine privileged in the university environment. To further these claims of the necessity of hands-on training, Berengario fashions himself as an *artifex* and *operator*, a craftsman and labourer, to present himself to a literate audience as an expert whose professional capabilities are predicated on his handiwork. Minden argues that in doing so, the surgeon also sets the terms of engagement and achievement, in particular the concepts of difficulty and judgement, in close alignment to how they were being simultaneously mobilised in an emergent art theory.

The final chapters move forward into the seventeenth and eighteenth centuries. Frances Gage takes up issues raised in the previous chapter on the manual exercise of the artist by investigating the relationship between the occupational health of artists and theoretical reflections on the status of the arts. Her essay shows how the emergence of a genre of vernacular health manuals in the sixteenth century led artists to incorporate medical principles and regimens of self-care into their professional practice. Within this medical framework, artistic labour was theorised in relation to a surprising yet revealing range of professions. The trials of the artists could at times be compared to the heroic self-sacrifice of military professionals (*condottieri*), but also to the working conditions of enslaved people. In this latter respect, the Roman painter Girolamo Muziano went so far as to shave his head in the style of an enslaved galley oarsman, in order to concretise his youthful pledge of devotion to painting.

Fabrizio Federici, in the following chapter, investigates the role of medical knowledge in the making of early modern connoisseurship, focusing on the seventeenth-century physician Giulio Mancini and his student, Sebastiano Vannini. The relationship between Mancini's medical practice and connoisseurship has been a widespread topic of scholarly debate, but little attention has been devoted to Vannini's development of the connection. This chapter situates both Mancini and Vannini's approach to art writing within broader trends in the history of medicine, such as Paduan Aristotelianism, which provided a model for their efforts to explain cultic, putatively supernatural images in secular, art historical terms. In Vannini, this line of thought culminates in a curious mix of resolutely empirical, yet patently fantastical interpretation, attentive to the embodied experience of painting, while simultaneously offering physiological explanations for the symbolic gestures of medieval art.

Katharina Sabernig's essay closes the volume by demonstrating that the societal and scientific upheaval of the seventeenth century was not confined to Europe but represents a globally interconnected phenomenon. Following the anatomical atlases of the Renaissance, centres for anatomical research and corresponding conventions of representation were established not only throughout Europe, but across Asia as well. Sabernig's chapter traces these connections by following four anatomists with different religious, scientific, and artistic backgrounds, all of whom were born in 1638. Providing a broad, comparative overview of their heterogenous work and biographies, the chapter charts life stories where success and failure were closely interwoven, highlighting similarities and differences of circumstances which enabled anatomical discussions and achievements in a period of intellectual change and transfer of knowledge. The possibility of a direct link becomes discernible between developments spanning across Eurasia, mediated in large part by the French Jesuit China Mission and the *Manchu Anatomy* sent by King Louis XIV – a figure who also happens to have been born in 1638. By charting these connected histories, Sabernig's contribution counters traditional Eurocentric accounts of the Scientific Revolution, in which the seventeenth century is seen as a moment of definitive rupture between Europe and the wider world.[52]

The chapters of this book are framed by a series of shorter commentaries on primary sources that highlight lesser-known, yet crucially important windows onto the themes of the volume (and beyond). The aim of these six texts is to indicate the wide range of primary sources that remain to be analysed, while also making a diverse range of sources in languages such as Latin, Italian, Polish, and Tibetan – all offered here for the first time in English translation – available for use in the classroom. While in some cases these sources relate closely to the content of the surrounding chapters, others suggest how a related cluster of themes could be traced out into new geographic or chronological contexts, ranging from the late Middle Ages to the seventeenth century, connecting continental Europe with regions across the Mediterranean and Asia, and demonstrating the benefits of a diachronic approach to the relation of visual culture and medicine.

The sources section opens with a classic source on the diseases of painters, published in 1700 by the physician Bernardino Ramazzini and introduced by Jana Graul. Julia Czapla and Robert Brennan then provide two examples of the transmission of medical and artistic knowledge. Czapla demonstrates the diffusion of medical knowledge through printed medical texts in early modern Europe: in this case, a little-known treatise by the Polish physician Stefan Falimirz. Brennan traces Florentine medical writings on the Greek sculptor Polykleitos back to sources in Arabic medical theory. Fabian Jonietz's commentary on a Tuscan physician's treatise on painting, deriving from the first quarter of the seventeenth century, parallels famous treatises by physicians such as Giulio Mancini or Michelangelo Biondo and once again proves the close exchange between medicine and the visual arts for the understanding of the human body. Paolo Sanvito highlights the exchange between Central Europe and South Asia in the drawings of the Jesuit physician and pharmacist Georgius Josephus Camel at the turn of the eighteenth century, while Katharina Sabernig brings the series to a close with an overview of illustrated Tibetan Materia Medica.

The present volume originated in a conference organised by the three editors on 11–13 November 2021 at the University of Salzburg and at Frohnburg Castle, Salzburg. Its realisation would not have been possible without the endorsement and generous financial support provided by the focus area *Figurations of Transition* of the Inter-University Organization *Science and Arts* of the University of Salzburg and Mozarteum University, the Austrian Science Funds (FWF, V822-GBL), and the State of Salzburg. We express our sincere gratitude to Anna Arabindan-Kesson, Mechthild Fend, Christiane J. Hessler, Jasmin Mersmann, Diana Policarpo, and Bernhard Seidler for enriching our discussions and for numerous important insights offered at the conference. The event was supported by the help of Franz Jäger, Vivian Nattrodt, and Sabrina Jocher. We thank Sabrina for her assistance with the preparation of the edited volume as well. The publication was made possible with the support of the Austrian Science Fund (FWF, PUB 1176-P).

Notes

1 Horace, *Ars poetica*, line 316, cf. 1–23.
2 Classic accounts include Lee, *Ut pictura poesis*, 1967; Chastel, 'Le dictum Horatii', 1977. More recently, see Locher, 'Ut pictura poesis', 2003; Hessler, *Zum Paragone*, 2014.
3 Mitchell, *Iconology*, 1986, esp. Chapter 4; Kohle, *Ut pictura poesis non erit*, 1989.
4 For a classic statement of this thesis, see Panofsky, 'Artist, Scientist, Genius', 1962.
5 For example, Campbell, 'On Renaissance Nonmodernity', 2017; *Ut pictura poesis*, 2020; cf. also Locher, 'Ut pictura poesis', 2003, p. 364.
6 For rhetoric, see, e.g., Baxandall, *Giotto and the Orators*, 1971; recently, Hoare, 'Salvator Rosa's Allegory of "Philosophy" as "ut pictura rhetorica"', 2013. For music, see *Ut musica pictura*, 2010; *Intermedialität von Bild und Musik*, 2017; Weissert, 'Ut pictura musica', 2018; *Music in the Art of Renaissance Italy*, 2020. For alchemy, see Elkins, *What Painting Is*, 1999; Bucklow, *The Alchemy of Paint*, 2009; Leonhard, *The Fertile Ground of Painting*, 2020. For textiles, see recently, e.g., *Kleider machen Bilder*, 2012; Schulz, 'Bild, Ding, Material', 2016.
7 Excellent recent works on early modern art and anatomy include *L'anatomia tra arte e medicina*, 2010; *Michelangelo, Anatomy as Architecture*, 2010; *Leonardo da Vinci's Anatomical World*, 2011; *Le corps transparent*, 2013; *Art of Vesalius*, 2014 Kleinbub, *Michelangelo's Inner Anatomies*, 2020. For optics, see Kemp, *The Science of Art*, 1990; Raynaud, *Studies on Binocular Vision*, 2016. For a recent reassessment of anatomical studies before the era of the Renaissance, see McCall, *The Art of Anatomy*, 2023.
8 There are several variants of the drawing and a painting from Passarotti's circle in the Galleria Borghese in Rome. The Louvre drawing is attributed to Bartolomeo Passarotti (1529–1592).
9 Olson, 'Caravaggio's Coroner', 2005, p. 92.
10 Bull (ed.), *Michelangelo*, 1999, p. 64.
11 Cf. Jacobs, '(Dis)assembling', 2002.
12 Alberti, On Painting, p. 56. For the corresponding practice in sixteenth-century and later painting, see Barr, 'Alessandro Allori', 2019.
13 For visual histories of medicine and the human body in the early modern period, see recently e.g. Cowen and Helfand, *Pharmacy*, 1990; *Hot Dry Men*, 1997; *The Physician's Art*, 1999; Wheeler, *Five Hundred Years of Medicine in Art*, 2001; *L'arte nella medicina e la medicina nell'arte*, 2008; *The Body Within*, 2009; Koos, *Haut, Farbe und Medialität*, 2014; Klemm, *Bildphysiologie*, 2013; Il *corpo e le arti*, 2016; Cuir, *Renaissance de l'anatomie*, 2016; Minni, *Arte e chirurgia*, 2019; *Representing Infirmity*, 2021; *Take Care*, 2022; *Flesh and Bone*, 2022; *Ars medica nelle Gallerie degli Uffizi*, 2022. Another related approach, which differs from our own, is to use modern medicine as a diagnostic lens for the interpretation of premodern art: e.g., Nelson, 'Cancer in Michelangelo's *Night*', 2021; *Disease and Disability*, 2021.
14 Duden, *The Woman Beneath the Skin*, 1991; Smith, *The Body of the Artisan*, 2004; Rankin, *Panaceia's Daughters*, 2013; Gómez, *The Experiential Caribbean*, 2017; Beyer, *Künstler, Leib und Eigensinn*, 2022.
15 On transcultural exchange, see Sweet, *Domingos Álvares*, 2011; Gómez, *The Experiential Caribbean*, 2017; *Drugs on the Page*, 2019. On racialisation in medicine, see the recent excellent overview by Murphy, 'Re-writing race in early modern European medicine', 2021. For recent arguments that early modern art and visual culture served as key agents of racialisation, see, e.g., Bindman and Gates, *The Image of the Black in Western Art*, 2010–14; Stoichita, *Darker Shades*, 2019; Bindman, *'Race Is Everything'*, 2023.
16 Two recent projects that aim to bridge this divide are Anna Arabindon-Kesson's *Art Hx: Visual and Medical Legacies of British Colonialism* https://artandcolonialm

edicine.com/ (accessed 14 January 2025) and Hannah Murphy's *Medicine and the Making of Race, 1440–1720* https://www.mmor.co.uk/ (accessed 6 August 2025).

17 Cennini, *Il libro dell'arte*, 2003, p. 63 [ch. I].

18 Cf. Löhr, 'Dantes Täfelchen', 2008, p. 169.

19 For example, Dante, *Purgatorio*, XVII, lines 13–27; Mocan, *La trasparenza e il riflesso*, 2005.

20 On the inconceivability of the 'creative arts' as category in premodernity, see Panofsky, 'Artist, Scientist, Genius', 1962, pp. 171–173.

21 Kemp, 'From "Mimesis" to "Fantasia"', 1977.

22 Löhr, 'Dantes Täfelchen', 2008; Löhr, '"Disegnia sechondo che huoi"', 2008.

23 The text describes itself as a *nuovo ricettario*, indicating a pre-existing tradition that must stretch further back at least into the fifteenth century, if not further. See Shaw and Welch, *Making and Marketing Medicine in Renaissance Florence*, 2011.

24 'Et nota che molte confectioni et lactouari cordiali si possono comporre secondo laphantasia [*sic*] del medico arrogendo & leuando a sua discretione & secondo lanecessita del patiente per chi si ordina [...] che non acchade a porle qui perla uarieta delli operanti & loro phantasie: [...]'. *Nuovo Ricettario*, 1498, fols 78v–79r (here and throughout, references are to the handwritten foliation on the copy in the Wellcome Collection: https://wellcomecollection.org/works/f7h5wv75).

25 Dunlop, 'On the Origins of European Painting Materials, Real and Imagined', 2014, p. 78. The stone was otherwise known as 'ultramarine': i.e., 'beyond the sea'.

26 *Nuovo Ricettario*, 1498, fol. 57r.

27 Cennini, *Il libro dell'arte*, 2003, p. 104 [ch. LXII]; see Dunlop, 'On the Origins of European Painting Materials, Real and Imagined', 2014, p. 80, with note 50 for further bibliography on the method and its provenance; cf. Dunlop, 'On the Origins of European Painting Materials, Real and Imagined', 2014, p. 84, on the crossover between pharmaceutical and painterly uses of the stone.

28 See Clark, '*Objets croisés*: *Albarelli* as Vessels of Mediation Within and Beyond the *Spezieria*', 2019.

29 *Nuovo Ricettario*, 1498, preface, fol. Aii (6r); *Le prime farmacopee*, 1887, p. 6. See Beck, 'Authority, Authorship, and Copying', 2019, p. 45.

30 Cf. *Der dritte Kommentar Lorenzo Ghibertis*, 1988, and Ghiberti, *I commentarii*, 1998, both *ad indicem*; for a recent summary of Ghiberti's sources see *Ghiberti teorico*, 2019.

31 Löhr, 'Dantes Täfelchen', 2008.

32 Necipoğlu, 'The Scrutinizing Gaze in the Aesthetics of Islamic Visual Cultures', 2015, p. 33.

33 Ciuti, 'Il Collegio dei fisici', 2012, p. 5; for the guild, see *Statuti dell'Arte dei medici e speziali*, 1922.

34 *Giottus Pictor*, 2004, pp. 235–239; doc. I c 4. For Giotto's involvement in the guild, see Skaug, *Giotto and the Flood of Florence*, 2013.

35 See Colapinto, 'The Beginning of the Pharmacopoeia', 1993, p. 44.

36 See Cennini, *Il libro dell'arte*, 2003, pp. 11–54, with bibliography. We do not necessarily adopt the thesis that the book was written for a guild, but much of this same evidence would support a broader affinity with a guild-oriented mentality.

37 *La disputa delle arti nel Quattrocento*, 1947; Salutati, *Vom Vorrang der Jurisprudenz oder der Medizin*, 1990.

38 Petrarca, *De remediis utriusque fortunae*, 204 (I.40); *Invective contra medicum*, 2005; see Buck, 'Die Medizin im Verständnis des Renaissancehumanismus', 1984; Bergdolt, *Arzt, Krankheit und Therapie bei Petrarca*, 1992.

39 Stolberg, *Learned Physicians*, 2022, here, e.g., pp. 47, 83, 91, 121.

40 Hanson, *The English Virtuoso*, 2008, p. 53.

41 Snook, *Women, Beauty and Power*, 2011, pp. 28–36. On women and medicine in early modern Europe, see Broomhall, *Women's Medical Work*, 2004; Cavallo, *Artisans of the Body*, 2007; Cavallo and Storey, *Healthy Living*, 2013; *Conserving*

Health, 2017; *Gender, Health, and Healing*, 2020; Strocchia, *Forgotten Healers*, 2020. On female artists, see recently, e.g., Bohn, *Women Artists, their Patrons, and their Publics in Early Modern Bologna*, 2021; Spies-Gans, 'Why Do We Think There Have Been No Great Women Artists?', 2022. Studies which take into account women in the interplay of medicine and art are still strikingly absent: cf. e.g. *Conserving Health*, 2017; Strocchia, *Forgotten Healers*, 2020, pp. 98–99.

42 On Giovio, see Agosti, *Paolo Giovio*, 2008; on Mancini, see Gage, *Painting as Medicine*, 2016; on Morelli, see Ginzburg, 'Spie', 1979. Giovio and Mancini are of course not unique cases in the early modern period but should be considered alongside medically trained art theorists such as Michelangelo Biondo or Francesco Scannelli, in addition to figures such as Samuel Quiccheberg, the author of the first printed treatise on collections.

43 Sweet, *Domingos Álvares*, 2011; Gómez, *The Experiential Caribbean*, 2017; Kalle Kananoja, *Healing Knowledge in Atlantic Africa*, 2021.

44 Pietz, 'The Problem of the Fetish, II', 1987; Preston Blier, 'Capricious Arts', 2009; Cummins, 'The Golden Calf in America', 2009.

45 The Biblical connection lies in Colossians 4:14. For the Byzantine background of the tradition, see Bacci, *Il pennello dell'Evangelista*, 1998; more generally the contributions in the volume *San Luca Evangelista*, 2003–2004.

46 On the Agbar legend, see *The Holy Face*, 1998.

47 *Legenda Aurea*, life of Gregorius. On the image and procession, see Wolf, *Salus populi romani*, 1990.

48 In his *Liber de imaginibus* (1572): Möseneder, *Paracelsus und die Bilder*, 2009, pp. 72–73.

49 For the painting, see Crispo, 'Un inedito San Luca', 2008–2009, and on this possible function, see Jacobs, 'Infirmity in Votive Culture', 2021, p. 191. For an opposing view, however, see note 15 in Fabian Jonietz's essay in this volume.

50 For this iconography, see Krafft, *Christus ruft in die Himmelsapotheke*, 2002.

51 Cf. Koering, *Les iconophages*, 2021.

52 On this tendency in the history of science, see recently Fancy (et al.), 'Current Debates and Emerging Trends in the History of Science in Premodern Islamicate Societies', 2023.

Source 1

Bernardino Ramazzini, *De morbis artificum diatriba*, 1700

Jana Graul

The Italian artist and intellectual Bernardino Ramazzini (Capri 1633 – Padua 1711) ranks among the pioneers of occupational medicine for his work, *De morbis artificum diatriba*.[1] After studying philosophy and medicine in Parma and Rome, as well as a formative experience working as a physician for a predominately poor, rural population in the Duchy of Castro (present-day Latium), Ramazzini first set up a practice in his hometown of Carpi, before moving to Modena in 1676 and finally to Padua in 1700. Alongside his activity as a physician, he also occupied the chair of medicine at universities first in Modena and later in Padua. With his foundational publications on preventative medicine as well as climatic and occupational pathologies, among other topics, he made a name for himself well beyond the borders of Italy. He maintained a friendly exchange with Gottfried Wilhelm Leibniz, on whose recommendation he became a member of the Accademia Leopoldina in Halle and the Societas Regia Scientiarum, the precursor of the Berlin-Brandenburg Academy of Sciences in Germany.

In the treatise *De morbis*, Ramazzini summarised ancient and contemporary knowledge of occupational diseases, while also systematising it in a variety of ways, such as by devoting an individual chapter to every profession. The first edition of 1700, published in Latin, was followed by an English translation published in London, and a German translation published in Leipzig, both appearing in 1705. This first iteration contains forty-one chapters, whereas the expanded edition of 1713 has fifty-four. Each section elucidates the pathologies, therapies, and preventative measures relevant to a given profession. At the center of the analysis stands the causes of diseases, which forms another central ordering principle of the book. As a matter of principal, Ramazzini distinguishes between diseases brought about by poisonous substances that are produced or utilised as part of the profession, and those that are conditioned by monotonous or harmful movements and postures during work.

The following excerpt is from the chapter that Ramazzini dedicates to the occupational diseases of painters. The text relativises the influence of humoral pathology on the health of this occupational group and instead lays emphasis on the dangers involved in the painter's use of mineral pigments such as quicksilver and lead. In the text, Ramazzini presents himself first and foremost as a practicing physician, who knows the relevant pathologies first-hand, as when he determines that the harmful, and at times poisonous smells of pigments can lead to a loss of smell, which was clearly a widespread phenomenon among painters of his time, as well as to severe stomach problems, which could at times even be deadly. In this regard, he advises a medical treatment analogous to that of miners, tailored to the harms caused by minerals.

That Ramazzini's procedures correspond with what was then the current state of medical knowledge, which had itself been transformed by the increasingly widespread normalisation of autopsies over the seventeenth century, is proved by comparison with the case of Elisabetta Sirani, the famous Bolognese artist.[2] Sirani passed away unexpectedly in 1665 at the age of just twenty-six and was subjected to autopsy on a court order, due to the suspicion of poison. Two autopsies performed on the corpse of the artist demonstrated that she had died of natural causes. Sirani suffered from a stomach ulcer, whose cause was already attributed to her daily handling of poisonous colorants by some of the doctors who participated.[3] Ramazzini's writing makes the harmful effects of such substances on artists' health starkly apparent:

> [...] ac perraro contingit, ut Pictores, qui aliorum imagines elegantiores, & coloratiores, plus quam par est, solent effingere, ipsi colorati sint ac boni habitus. Ego quidem quotquot novi Pictores, & in hac in aliis Urbibus, omnes fere semper valetudinarios observavi, & si Pictorum historiae evolvantur, non admodum longaevos fuisse constabit, ac praecipue, qui inter eos praestantiores fuerint. Raphaelem Urbinatem, Pictorem celeberrimum, in ipso juventae flore e vivis ereptum fuisse legimus, cujus immaturam mortem Balthassar Castilioneus eleganti carmine deflevit. Culpari quidem posset illorum Vita sedentaria, ac genius melancholicus, dum ab hominum fere commercio sejuncti mentem in phantasticis suis Idaeis semper involutam habent; ast alia potior causa subet, quae Pictores morbis obnoxios reddit, colorum nempe materia, quam semper prae manibus habent ac sub ipsis naribus, ut Minitum, Cinnabaris, Cerussa, Vernix, Oleum nucum, lini, quibus utuntur ad colores temperandos, multaque ex variis fossilibus pigmenta. Hinc in illorum Officinis latrinalis odor percipitur, qui satis gravis e Vernice, & praedictis Oleis exspirat, & capiti valde insenus est, unde forsan odoratus abolitio deducenda. Ipsique quoque Pictores in ipso opere sordidas, ac pigmentatas vestes solent induere, quare fieri nequit quin ore, ac naribus pravos halitus excipiant, qui ad spirituum animalium sedem perreptando, ac per vias spiritales sanguinis domicilia subeundo, naturalium functionum oeconomiam perturbent, & superius memoratos affectus excitent. Cinnabarim sobolem esse Mercurii, Cerussam ex Plumbo parari, Aes viride ex

Cupro, colorem ultramarinum ex Argento (cum metallici colores vegetabilibus longe durabiliores sint, & hanc ob causam a Pictoribus magis expetantur) sicque omnem sere colorum materiam, e mineralium classe desumi, nemo non novit, & propter hanc causam satis graves noxas subsequi.[4]

[...] For it seldom happens that the Painters who use to draw the Pictures of others handsomer and better Complexion'd than the Originals, are themselves either handsome or well Complexion'd. For my part I have always observ'd that all the Painters I know either in this or other Towns, are a'most always sickly; and if we consult the Histories of Painters, we'll find they were not long-liv'd; especially if we confine our view to such as made a distinguishing Figure. History informs us that Raphael Urbinas, a very famous Painter was snatch'd away in the very Flower of his Age; & Baltasar Castilioneus condol'd his untimely Death in a very pretty Poem. 'Tis true, the Diseases of this sort of men may be imputed to their sedentary Life, and the Melancholy that seeds upon'em, while they retire from human Society and bend all their Thoughts upon their Phantastick Idæa's. But the principal Cause of their sicklyness is the Matter of the Colors that's always among their Hands, and unter their Nose; I mean the red Lead, Cinnabar, Cerus, Varnish, Oil of Wallnuts, and Oil of Linseed, with which they temper their Colours, and several other Paints made of various Minerals. Hence 'tis that their Shops have such a nasty stinking Smell, which is chiefly owing to the Varnish and foresaid Oils, and is very offensive to the Head; and perhaps the loss of Smell usual among Painters flows from no other Cause. Besides, when the Painters are about their Work, they have nasty daub'd Cloaths upon 'em; so that they can't avoid taking in at Mouth & Nostrils the offensive Exhalations; which, by invading the Seat of the Animal Spirits, and accompanying the Spirits to the Blood, disturb the Oeconomy of the natural Functions, and give rise to the above-mention'd Disorders. All the World knows that Cinnabar is the offspring of Mercury, Cerus is made of Lead, Verdigrise of Copper, and the Ultramarine colour of Silver; for the Metallick Colours are much more durable than those of a vegetable Extraction, and for that reason the Painters value 'em more: In fine, 'tis plain that a'most all the Ingredients of Colors are taken from the Mineral Family, upon which score they can't choose but do harm, and by Consequence Painters must be liable to the same Distempers (tho not in so flaming a Degree) with the Workmen that work in Mettal.[5]

Notes

1 Cf. on this, also in the following, Baldasseroni and Carnevale, *Malati di lavoro*, 2015, pp. 35–211; *Bernardino Ramazzini, primo medico di lavoro*, 2020. On Ramazzini's life and work, cf. Marinozzi, 'Ramazzini, Bernardino', 2016.

2 On this case cf. Graul, 'Intrigues, Punches, and a Poisoned Salad', 2022. For further reading on artistic illnesses in the early modern period cf. Beyer, *Künstler, Leib und Eigensinn*, 2022; Graul, 'Wenn der frühneuzeitliche Künstler erkrankt', 2024.

3 In the autopsy report, the phrase is 'la continua applicazione della sua professione', as cited in Manaresi, *Il processo di avvelenamento*, 1904, p. 79.

4 Ramazzini, *De morbis artificum diatriba*, 1700, pp. 53–56.

5 Ramazzini, *A Treatise*, 1705, pp. 40–41.

1

Saintly systems of healing: images, devotion, and cures

Catherine Lawless

Jacques Le Goff notes that in the Middle Ages the body did not exist in itself but was always co-penetrated with the soul.[1] The experiences of illness and therapeutic regimes, involving prayer, imagery, magico-religious regimens or practices as well as medico-surgical ones should therefore be considered symbiotically as overlapping, although sometimes competing, systems. The relationship between sanctity, healing, and images in the late Middle Ages was complex.

A saint's thaumaturgic power was shown during his or her lifetime through miracles, usually following the biblical model of healing the blind, the crippled, the lame, lepers, and the obsessed. Post-mortem, these powers were retained, or usually increased, where contact with the relics produced miraculous cures. The image played a dynamic role both in the process of healing and in the propagation of the cult. Ex votos were the outcomes of a vow made privately by an individual to their patron, but which publicly acknowledged the grace received and established or reinforced the power of the cult.[2] In the anthropomorphic ex voto, a projection of self was made concrete, which may have had a therapeutic function in displacing the illness or casting it out into another materiality. In the case of an ex voto painting, the miracle and the recipient were memorialised, and the power of the saint demonstrated.

In the later Middle Ages images played an increasing role in spreading the cult of the saint by illustrating the miracles enacted and substituting in part, but also reinforcing and overlapping the role played by relics. A locus for the *virtus* of the saint was thus to be found in their image. In the case of these images, the gaze is captured, while the image is also frequently touched, rubbed, kissed, and embraced. The relics and images of the saint worked in a network of cult involving the needs of the devotee, the management of the shrine, the manufacture and sale of ex votos, and the popularity of the saint and the promotion of their cult. A further, and neglected, role of the image of the saint was that of comfort and consolation.

Ex votos, imagery, and healing

The ex voto, often anthropomorphic, consisted of a model or image of the afflicted body part or even the whole figure. These were usually made out of wax but other materials used include rich ones, such as gold or silver, or poor ones, such as gesso and even bread.[3] Giorgio Vasari, writing in 1568, states that the ex votos were first of all made in silver, or small painted panels, or crudely modelled in wax, until Orsino Benintendi perfected the technique of modelling whole bodies in the fifteenth century.[4] The ex voto could also be symbolic, with an offering in wax or other materials equal in height, weight, or girth of either the devotee or the body part in question. Both types of ex voto could have the performative function (among many others) of realising the cure, and the commemorative function of recording the efficacy of the saint. The ex voto makes concrete the invisible, spiritual relationship between the devotee and the saint. It represents, or, as Daniel Arasse notes, it 're-presents', makes what is absent, present.[5]

Anthropological studies of modern ex votos attest to the continuity of the symbolic exchange between the sufferer and the patron, made concrete in the production of the image, whether a simulacrum of the body part or the entire individual, most often in wax, or other commemorative images.[6] As Michele Bacci notes, wax symbolised the light of the Resurrection, but also had practical use in liturgy, prayers, and illumination.[7] Further, as Cardini comments, wax could be easily worked, it was malleable, received imprints, and changed forms, and even more importantly, it resembled human skin, as Carly B. Boxer states in her essay in this volume.[8] Christopher Wood goes further, showing how the medium itself could resemble the ebb and flow of the experience of the devotee: 'The medium of wax symbolises both the flow of experience – the disease, all the passions accompanying it – and the stilling of that flow'.[9]

The types of ex voto varied as to part of body and type of illness, but there was a kind of mass production of them from moulds.[10] Noël Coulet's study examines how apothecaries, involved in producing ex votos, commissioned moulds in hard wax or wood by analysing a 1459 contract with the Provençal apothecary Gilles Calhon. He also demonstrates in the study that an individualisation of types took place with different head coverings and garment types.[11] Giordana Charuty, in her study of modern ex votos in Portugal, highlights the pilgrims' careful, precise selection of rented wax objects, emphasising its importance despite their manufacture using identical moulds.[12] The canonisation process discussed by André Vauchez of Thomas of Hereford (d. 1282) and by Boxer in her essay in this volume report that pilgrims laid at his tomb 170 silver ships, 41 wax ships, 129 images of a person or body part in silver, 1,424 images of a person or body part in wax, 108 crutches, and 3 little cards in wood.[13]

The displacement of illness onto a wax image, of oneself or the afflicted body part, must surely have had some psychological therapeutic value. Belief in its efficacy can be seen by its inverse use, when it was used to cause illness or harms. The mimetic qualities of wax alluded to above also, as shown by Bisogni, made it a perfect medium for *maleficium*, with the fears for its use expressed by Pope John XXII, revealing his suspicions that people made wax figures of their enemies in order to stick pins in them and cause them harm or death.[14] In Florence, Vieri di Michele Rondinelli accused a woman named Caterina of bewitching his brother Paolo through means of placing a wax image of him in her bed and casting a spell. Caterina, condemned in contumacy to be burned at the stake, ultimately had her sentence cancelled three years later.[15]

The famous shrine in Florence, the church of SS Annunziata, was built up around a miraculous image of the Annunciate Virgin, in the thirteenth century.[16] The Florentine writer Franco Sacchetti noted in the late fourteenth century that so many wax figures had been hung there that if the walls had not been reinforced they would have been in danger of collapsing.[17] Vasari gave a detailed account of how full-size figures were made and described how Orsino Benintendi had been told to make three images of Lorenzo de' Medici, wounded in the Pazzi conspiracy of 1478 in an attack which killed his brother, Giuliano. The first was placed in SS Annunziata, having become renowned as much for the ex votos of full-size figures placed there as for the miraculous image which inspired them.[18] Another Lorenzo, the young exile Lorenzo di Matteo Strozzi (1432–1479), working in Bruges, asked his mother, Alessandra, to have a wax image offered to the miraculous image in SS Annunziata. The unknown reason may be related to his breaking an arm a month before in a ball game.[19] The second wax figure of Lorenzo de' Medici had been placed in the church of St Maria Regina Coeli, opposite a miracle-working crucifix, and the third was placed in St Maria degli Angeli in Assisi.[20]

Images of the saints can possibly offer us some examples of the ways in which pilgrims approached the tomb and ex votos were hung or placed, but must be used with caution, as the representation of the curative powers of the saint, rather than being illustrative, belongs to the same realm as the ex votos themselves, that is, of the miraculous, and the need to promote the *virtus* of the saint (Figure 1.1). The fresco of the tomb of St Peter Martyr by Andrea Boniauti, c. 1366, in the chapter house of St Maria Novella in Florence shows us (and the audience of Dominican friars) some of the processes at work at a shrine, similar to the stained-glass panel at York Minster, shown by Carly B. Boxer. The tomb is raised as an *arca*, supported on piers allowing pilgrims to go underneath it, and the sick can be seen raising their hands to the edges of the tomb in the hope of

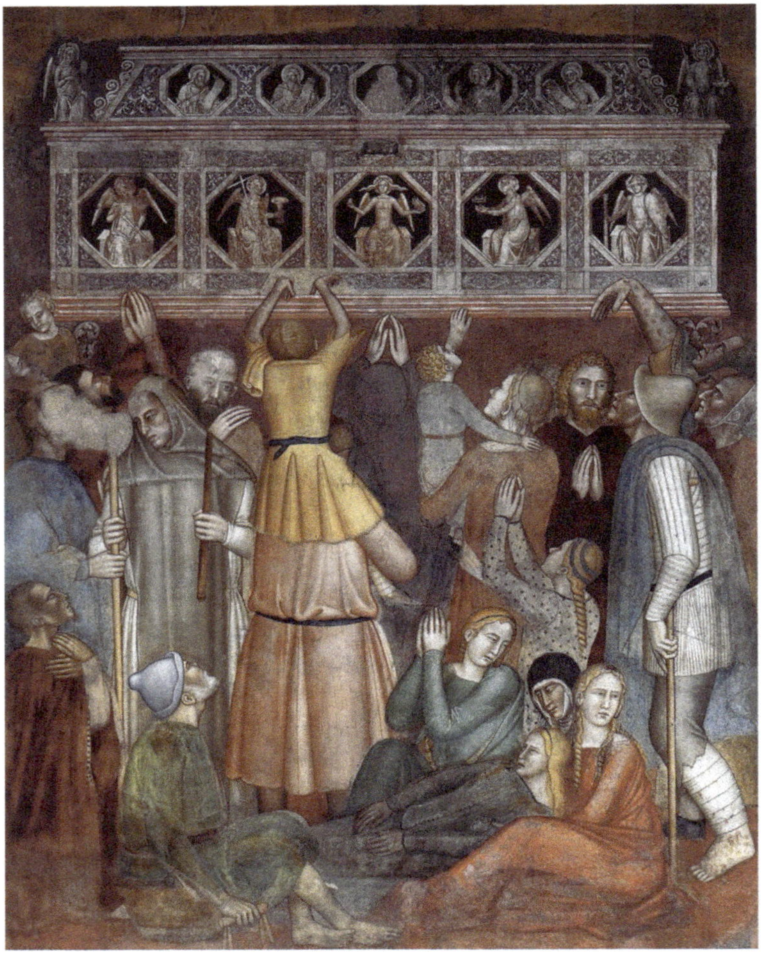

Figure 1.1 Andrea Bonaiuti, Triumph of the Dominican Order, including scenes from the lives of SS Peter Martyr, Thomas Aquinas, fresco, c. 1366–1368. Florence, St Maria Novella, Spanish chapel. Image credit: Wikipedia Commons

acquiring some of the holy oil being secreted by the body within, like the figures of pilgrims catching the liquid coming from the tomb of St William in York. In the foreground we see a woman laid out on the ground, helped by other women, in a miracle possibly related to childbirth, of which Peter was an unlikely patron.[21] We also see the interesting social detail of the sacristan selling candles. The kneeling figure may be Mico Guidalotti, who bequeathed 325 florins in his testament of 1355 for the decoration of the chapel and named the Dominican friar Jacopo Passavanti (who probably conceived the iconological programme) as his testamentary executor.[22] It must be noted that the frescoes were in a part of the church not usually open to the laity, and that the friars themselves were their principal audience, which may have provided food for contemplation and material for preaching. The presence of the scene, in a scheme showing the importance of the Dominican order in the role of salvation, could indicate that the thaumaturgic powers of the martyred Peter, who had defeated heretics in the city of Florence from the site of St Maria Novella itself, contributed to the charisma of the order and its ability to heal both body and soul.[23]

A *vita* panel of St Margaret of Antioch (c. 1400), now in the Vatican, shows St Margaret with a donor, one that we could assume has benefitted, or hopes to benefit, from the intercession of his patron (Figure 1.2). Like other *vita* panels the narrative scenes take place around the side, beginning in the lower left and moving up to the top, crossing over to the top right, and then moving downwards, culminating in a scene at her shrine. The torture of the saint is vividly rendered, showing her with her arms outstretched in a position echoing the Crucifixion, and naked from the waist up. The torture and martyrdom of the saint show her passion and suffering in *imitatio Christi*, evoking the compassion of the viewer, but may also have allowed a viewer suffering with physical pain to contemplate the vulnerability of the flesh while still praying for a cure. In the top right the saint gains her victory over the dragon and is then shown naked, again, in a boiling cauldron, followed by her decapitation. In the final scene we are shown her shrine, with pilgrims at her tomb, in front of wax ex votos hung on a beam. A woman, fainting behind the tomb is probably seeking the intercession of the saint for safe childbirth, as the saint had famously recommended to women to pray to her for safe delivery.[24] The inclusion of the scene with the shrine and the ex votos has led Larson to suggest that the panel came from the shrine of St Margaret at Montefascione.[25] Bisogni also notes the emphasis and points out that only one in all of the ten Italian cycles dedicated to St Margaret by the end of the fifteenth century depict the thaumaturgic powers of the saint at the tomb. He, however, more cautiously attributes its provenance to Montefiascone.[26]

The lives of the saints are filled with details of the various types of wax offerings given to them.[27] Raymond of Capua in his biography of Agnese da Montepulciano (d. 1317) writes that there were so many images and ex votos at her tomb that he could not relate all the miracles, a motif he repeats in his life of St Catherine of Siena (d. 1380).[28] The examples are multiple, a few will suffice here, taken from the lives of some female saints of the fourteenth century. They are not remarkable, instead, they are typical of the hagiographic literature relating to cures. A deaf noblewoman with crippled feet was cured after St Margaret of Hungary (d. 1270) appeared to her, telling her to bring wax feet to her tomb.[29] A woman with incurable tumours on her breast vowed to offer wax breasts to the blind Umbrian saint, Margherita of Città di Castello (d. 1320). As soon as she had done so, the saint appeared in a vision, touched her on the breast and she was

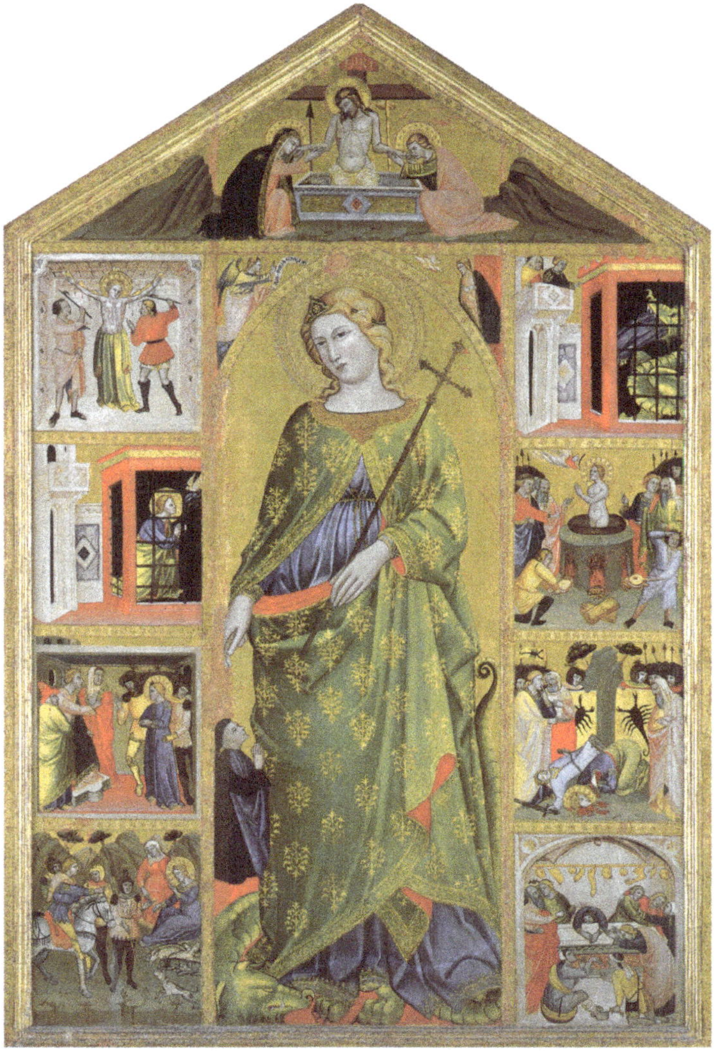

Figure 1.2 Turino Vanni?, Vita Panel of St Margaret of Antioch, panel, 166 × 106.8 cm, c. 1400. Vatican, Pinacoteca Vaticana, no. 7 (4). Image credit: Wikipedia Commons

healed. It seems that the hagiographer may have had hopes of making this a speciality of Margherita, as another woman was healed of the same illness in a similar way, except without the vision: she went to bed, made the vow of the wax breasts and woke up healed.[30] Lucia, wife of Jacopo, was bitten by a serpent and her leg became infected. Although she prayed to St Zita of Lucca (d. 1272), her condition worsened, and she lost the power of speech. Fortunately, her husband and his friend vowed a wax leg to

St Zita, and she was cured.[31] In Rome, a woman in Castel Sant'Angelo had intolerable pain in her limbs, head, and breast. She vowed to make a pilgrimage to the tomb of St Birgitta of Sweden (d. 1371) (then in Rome) and have a wax image made, and was cured.[32] In Linköping, Birgitta restored to life a stillborn child after his mother, Elbynara, promised a wax image of the saint for her tomb in Vadstena.[33] Another woman who had given birth a child who died before baptism brought him to the tomb of Birgitta in Vadstena, with an ex voto of him in silver, and the child was revived.[34] Instead of visiting her relics, when Domina Joanna, in Italy, fell from a staircase and broke her arm, a vision of Birgitta told her to bring a wax ex voto of her arm to her image in Rome and she would be healed.[35] The healing of Domina Johanna's arm was activated through the vision of Birgitta, the wax ex voto of the arm, and the image of Birgitta itself.

Ex votos and painting

A miracle drawn from the *Treatise on the Miracles of St Francis* (chapter XIII) written by Tommaso da Celano in preparation for the saint's canonisation shows in an exemplary manner the harshness and difficulties of illness and the coming together of ritual, saint, time, place, and image in the effecting of a cure. The son of a man of Cisterna in Marittima had a terrible laceration in his genital parts, with the result that the output of the intestines could not be contained. The usual remedy, according to Celano, a belt, was of no use, indeed, it only procured worse pain and lesions. The parents made a vow to St Francis, brought the child to the new church dedicated to the saint in Velletri on the day of the saint's feast, laying him in front of the saint's image. While the Gospel was being sung, at the words of Matthew chapter 11 verse 25, 'That which was hidden to the wise is revealed to children', the belt broke, the wound was healed and the child was saved.[36] The child in the miracle was healed by the saint, but the efficacy of the saint was activated by the image.

The panel by Bonaventura Berlinghieri, painted around 1235 for the church of St Francesco in Pescia is the first 'vita panel' of St Francis, and thus one which occupies an important position in iconography of St Francis and the development of narrative iconography more generally (Figure 1.3).[37] The panel combines what Charles Hope called the iconic or devotional and the narrative, with the central figure of St Francis surrounded by scenes from his life and miracles after his death.[38] Four of the scenes are posthumous miracles. Below two scenes which were to become iconic, the Stigmatisation of St Francis and the Preaching to the Birds, is the miracle of the crippled girl, an early miracle which happened at the tomb of St Francis. The child had suffered the loss of all her members for a year and was brought by her nurse to the tomb of St Francis, with a wax figure. The cure itself is represented and the painting becomes testimony

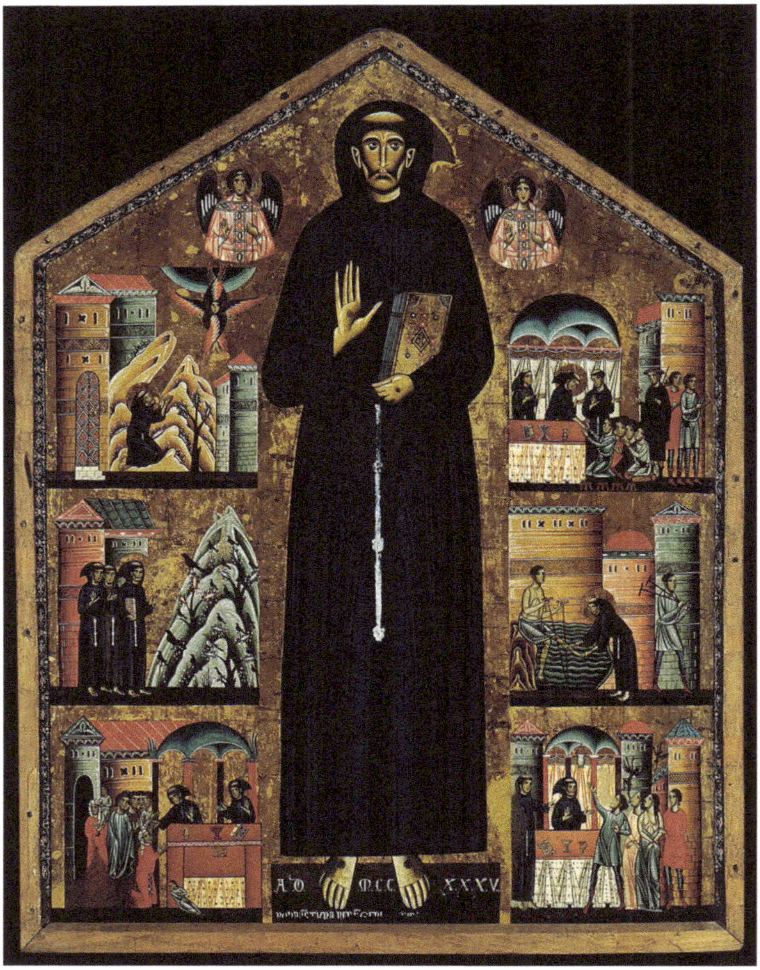

Figure 1.3 Bonaventura Berlinghieri, St Francis, with scenes from his life and miracles, panel, 160 × 123 cm, c. 1235. Pescia, S. Francesco. Image credit: Wikipedia Commons

of the healing power of the saint. This is followed on the right by the healing of cripples at the tomb, then the healing of Bartolomeo of Narni of gout through a vision of St Francis who tells him to go to the baths, which he does, and the saint heals him.[39] At the bottom is the exorcism of three people possessed by the devil at the tomb, which I shall return to later.

Jérôme Baschet, referring to a term coined by Jean-Claude Bonne, uses the word 'image-object' in discussing medieval images, pointing out their relational importance between people, and also between people and the supernatural.[40] Arguably the religious image has its origin in ritual, and with the cult of the saints, ritual, memory, and performativity are incorporated: the image is used in the celebration of the sacred, it sometimes becomes the sacred itself, it records the power of the saint as a healer, and as such provides a dynamic relationship between the sacred, those who received miraculous cures and those who seek them.[41] The relics in the tomb of the saint are, in Berlinghieri's image, made iconic as the agents of healing and by being depicted they function as advertisement of the power of the saint. The image, as noted by Frugoni, can also function as replacement for the relics, acting as a *locus* itself for the power of the saint.[42] This is evident in a sermon Archbishop Federico Visconti delivered in Pisa in 1264, when he pronounced that those who looked at the image of the saint were blessed, like those who had seen the saint and his miracles.[43]

Hagiography provides many examples of the importance of the image as an agent of healing and as transmitter of cult. Sometimes the hagiographer provides evidence of an existing cult to a saint with reference to an existing image. In the case of the Pisan Saint Bona (d. 1207), the story tells of Mornetto and Julia, citizens of Lucca, whose child, aged nine, appeared to be dying. Julia prayed in front of an image of St Bona in a church in Pisa, and promised that if her child was cured, she would feed six paupers every feast day of St Bona.[44] In the late fourteenth century, the life of St Birgitta of Sweden is particularly rich with cures provided through images, or the promise to have images made, of the holy woman. Eliana Cibo, from Genoa, sister of Villano and Luchino Cibo, lived in Naples. Luchino, having returned from Damascus was gravely ill. Eliana made a vow to St Birgitta that if he was cured, she would take an image of St Birgitta to Genoa, and have her image painted there from it.[45] Candolus, a merchant of Naples, who suffered a severe pain in his toe was cured after promising to have an image painted of St Birgitta in St Gregorio Maggiore in that city.[46] In an another miracle, Palmieri of Trebizond was healed by a vision of St Birgitta after his wife, who had known her when she was alive, went to St Maria del Carmine in Naples where there was an image of the saint, and offered wax there.[47]

The relationship between image and healing is also strong in the life of B. Andrea Corsini (d. 1373), Carmelite saint and Bishop of Fiesole. Andrea's very conception was owed, according to his biographer, to the miraculous image of the Madonna del Popolo in St Maria del Carmine.[48] His parents lived for a long time without issue and in despair went to the miraculous image of the Virgin in the Carmine, the 'icon or panel', where the author informs us many women prayed in hopes of conception, promising to dedicate their first-born child to religion.[49] Their vow was granted and they conceived Andrea. In another instance a relative of Andrea Corsini suffers from rotting flesh, described in the text as lupus, after being told by the saint to abstain from games for a week and to fast for six days, pray a Pater Noster, Ave Maria, and a Salve Regina. Though he is cured for a while, his permanent cure comes only after he and the saint go to the Madonna del Popolo.[50] His own image, then, after death, effected cures. An English Carmelite, Nicholas Kenton, Provincial of England, while in Florence was struck with a severe fever. He heard bells ringing and asked why and was told that there was a new saint in his order. He entered the church and saw a crowd of sick people, touching an image and rubbing their faces afterwards, and being healed. He then prayed in front of the same icon 'in which was painted the image of B. Andrea' and was healed. When he returned to England, he had the image of the saint painted there.[51]

Medica sum

The coexistence of medical systems is also shown in the saints' lives, with the saint triumphant where physicians and surgeons have failed. Images depict the superior power of the saint over physicians. In the upper church frescoes at St Francesco in Assisi, attributed to Giotto or his school, the scene depicts the saint healing the sick man from Lerida, while the physicians stand by, shrugging helplessly. Pietro Lorenzetti's altarpiece of St Umiltà of Faenza (1226–1310), painted around 1332 for the Vallombrosan church of St Giovanni Evangelista in Florence, provides a typical representation of this process. The church housed the saint's burial site and was the centre of her cult.[52] We see a Vallombrosan monk of Faenza, whose gangrenous leg the doctor wishes to amputate. Instead, in a subsequent scene, St Umiltà heals him (Figure 1.4).[53] We also see the posthumous miracle, in Florence, of St Umiltà healing a nun of a haemorrhage that doctors had failed to stop, like the doctors depicted in the frescoes of Assisi, the doctor is shown outside the room, shrugging (Figure 1.5).[54] The message powerfully asserts that the saint is the superior physician, a point made explicit in several saints' lives, where the saint is either described or describes themselves, through reported speech, as a physician or occasionally as a surgeon. For example, a woman of Lucca having fallen from her horse and broken her arm, sees a woman approach her as she lies in bed, dressed in white, who states that she is a 'medica' from San Martino and proceeds to heal her arm. The woman sent to San Martino to find out who she was, and was told that she was St Bona (d. 1207); she then went on pilgrimage to her tomb, and every vigil of her feast spent the night in front of her altar.[55] St Fina of San Gimignano (d. 1253) was described by her biographer as a surgeon: 'In healing also the wounds of men the admirable Virgin of God exercised surgery'.[56]

Mental health, possession, and images

I want to return now to the panel by Bonaventura Berlinghieri and discuss the last scene, and semantically, the most difficult: the exorcism of devils. A possessed person could rarely invoke the saint themselves, being usually

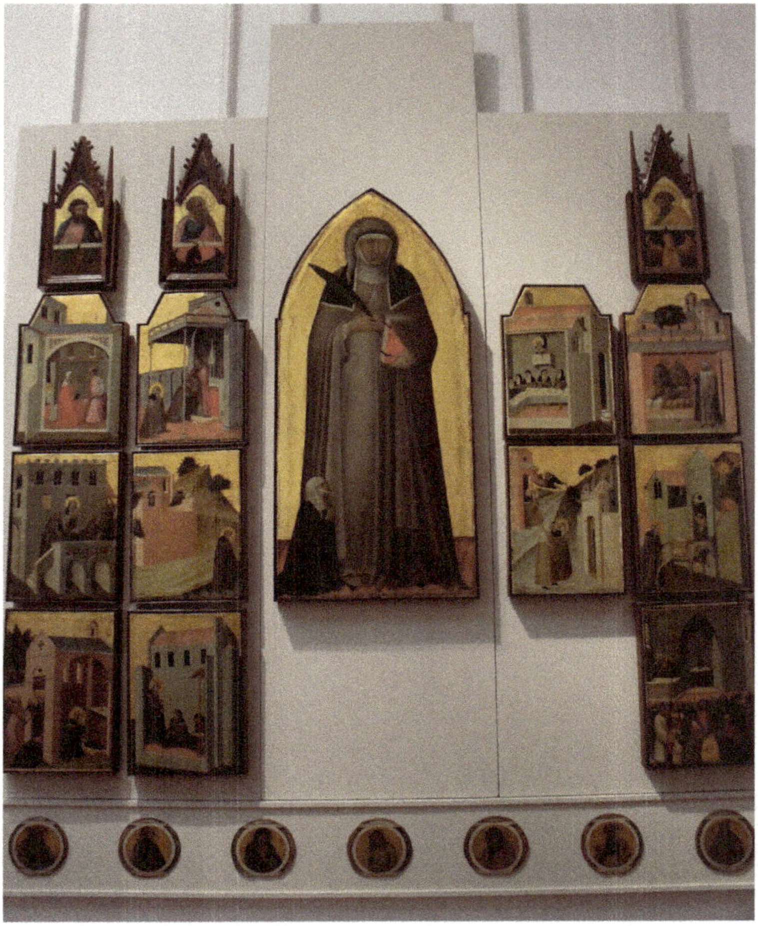

Figure 1.4 Pietro Lorenzetti, St Umiltà polyptych, c. 1332. Florence, Uffizi, no. 8347 (some panels in Berlin). Image credit: Wikipedia Commons

dependent on others to force them to the shrine. Nor is it readily imaginable what kind of ex voto could be made in such circumstances. Tommaso da Celano's chapter in his *Treatise on Miracles* (chapter xvi) deals with the insane and the possessed together, and Vauchez, in an attempt to categorise the types of miracle, groups as a separate category mental illnesses, comprised of 'demoniacs', epileptics, and the 'mad'.[57] In the case of Jacopa di Bartolo, a young servant aged eight in the employment of Bernardo Machiavelli in 1483, 'came out of herself' (*era uscita di sé*) and 'was saying and doing mad things and could not serve us' (*e diceva e facea cose paze e non ci potea servire*). Machiavelli and his wife immediately took her, not to a doctor, but to the cathedral and then the Cistercian abbey of San Salvi. The child was not cured and was sent back to her parents.[58] In

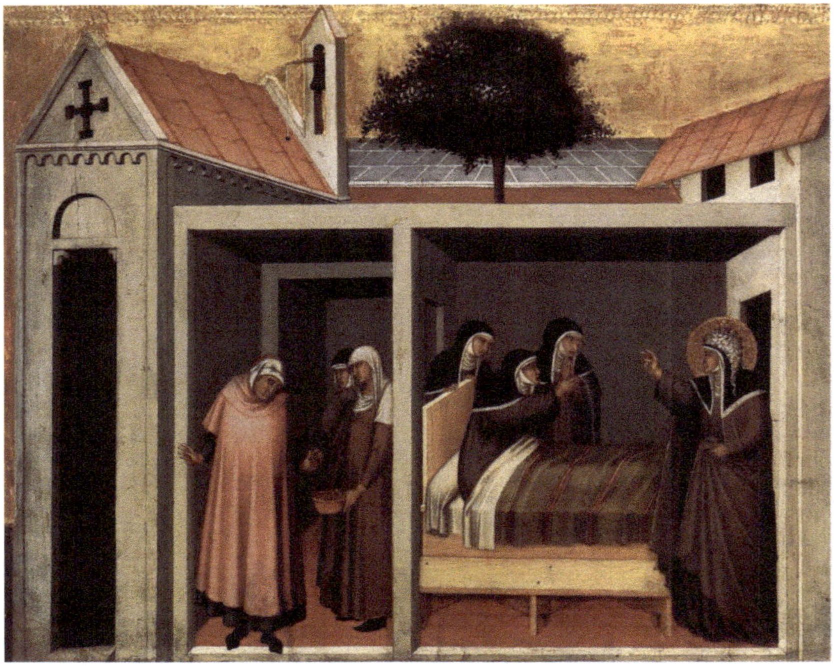

Figure 1.5 Pietro Lorenzetti, scene from the miracles of St Umiltà, from the St Umiltà (vita) Polyptych, c. 1332. Berlin, Staatliche Museen, Gemäldegalerie, no. 1077. Image credit: Wikipedia Commons

the Berlinghieri panel, we see the three possessed individuals: a man, a woman, with the exorcised devil coming out of her mouth, and a second woman, naked from the waist up, with the devil high in the air above her, her hands restrained in front of her, and held by another man. The exorcisms occur in the context of the tomb of St Francis, represented by the altar-like structure under the *baldacchino* and sign for the actual tomb in Assisi. As shown by Chiara Frugoni in her analysis of this panel, the possessed are shown in profile, indicating the two-faced nature of the malign.[59] The nudity of the woman is noticeable and quite deliberate, as the artist could have conveyed nudity yet still covered her breasts by any number of pictorial devices. Her nakedness in such a place shows her utter alienation and the breakdown of civilised values into an animal-like state of nature – a state from which women are never very far. The shocking behaviour, caused by her possession and referred to by Tommaso da Celano (*Vita Prima*, book III, chapter iii) is rendered thus by the painter in the nakedness of her torso.[60] Women were perceived as more likely to be susceptible to possession due to their more fragile nature, their colder temperament, their likelihood to be seduced by the devil, and the impressionability of their flesh. In liturgical exorcisms described by Nancy Caciola, a woman should be led to the right corner of the altar, undress completely and have her 'shameful parts' covered by linen. As Caciola points out, the removal of her clothing also removes her from social significance and recognition, as well as subjecting her to humiliation.[61]

In a panel by Giunta Pisano, for Pisa, St Francesco, the demonically possessed have been reduced to just one figure, the naked woman, with her hands restrained, here with even more of her chest exposed and her fully rounded breasts given prominence (Figure 1.6).[62] The binary between the possessed woman, vomiting the devil, and the clothed clerics surrounding her seems absolute, and the equation of the female body with sinfulness appears difficult to avoid. On the other side of the panel, another breast is seen, this one a sick one bearing a goitre, which is healed miraculously at the shrine of the saint (Tommaso da Celano, *Treatise on Miracles*, chapter xviii).[63] Horizontally therefore, there are two women, the physically sick, clothed woman, exposing only the putrid, ill breast, and the spiritually sick, possessed woman, naked, with perfect, but sinful breasts.

The obsessed frequently show their signs of possession by being unable to look at images of the divine. In the miracles of the Dominican saint Agnese of Montepulciano (d. 1317), written by Raymond of Capua, a man brought his obsessed son to the tomb of the saint. The boy, unable to look at any holy image or to stay in church during the divine office, was cured after contact with the relics.[64] A similar case is found in the life of Columba of Narni (1467–1501), where she made a pilgrimage to the image of the Virgin at Narni, bringing with her a possessed woman. The woman managed to enter the chapel, but the demon would not leave her, having dwelled within her for eighteen years. The Holy Spirit inspired Columba that the woman had some evil-working charms in her hair which bound the demon to her body. She and the nuns took them out of her hair, burnt them, then in front of the image of the Virgin the woman vomited, her teeth chattered, her mouth opened, the candles went out, and finally the demon left her in the form of a dragon.[65] As in the case of wax imagery, the divine and the demonic were intricately bound in the system of healing and images.

Images in the home: comfort for the sick and protection against illness

If wax ex votos or images helped the sick to externalise or transfer, in some way, their physical illness, then how much more may it have helped those suffering from some mental disorders to see the objectification of them in the form of little devils, able to be cast out through the power of prayer, acting within a network of signifiers with changing and variable dynamics such as saint, image, relic, site, and ritual. I want to conclude by examining images which could provide comfort and protection in the domestic sphere. A small folding triptych, attributed to Niccolò di Tommaso,

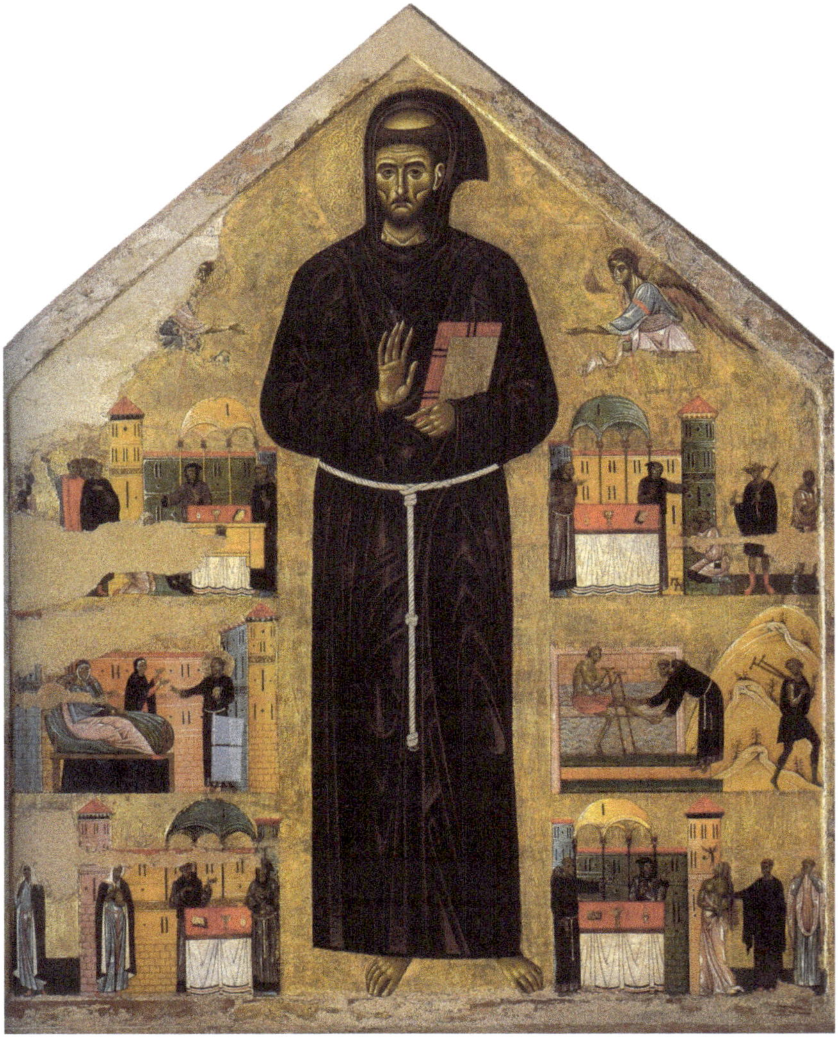

Figure 1.6 Giunta Pisano, St Francis and scenes from his life and miracles, 163 × 129 cm, c. 1250. Pisa, S. Francesco. Image credit: Wikipedia Commons

painted around 1370 and now in Baltimore shows, in the central panel, the Coronation of the Virgin, with below, St Anthony Abbot presenting a kneeling male donor, and a male, bearded saint, without attribute, presenting a female donor (Figure 1.7). On the wings are SS Nicholas of Bari, Peter, Paul, and Catherine. When the triptych was closed, the outer panels showed the standing figure of SS Anthony Abbot (again), and Christopher carrying the Christ Child, with inscriptions below.[66] Despite St Anthony's patronage of the illness known as St Anthony's fire and more generally as

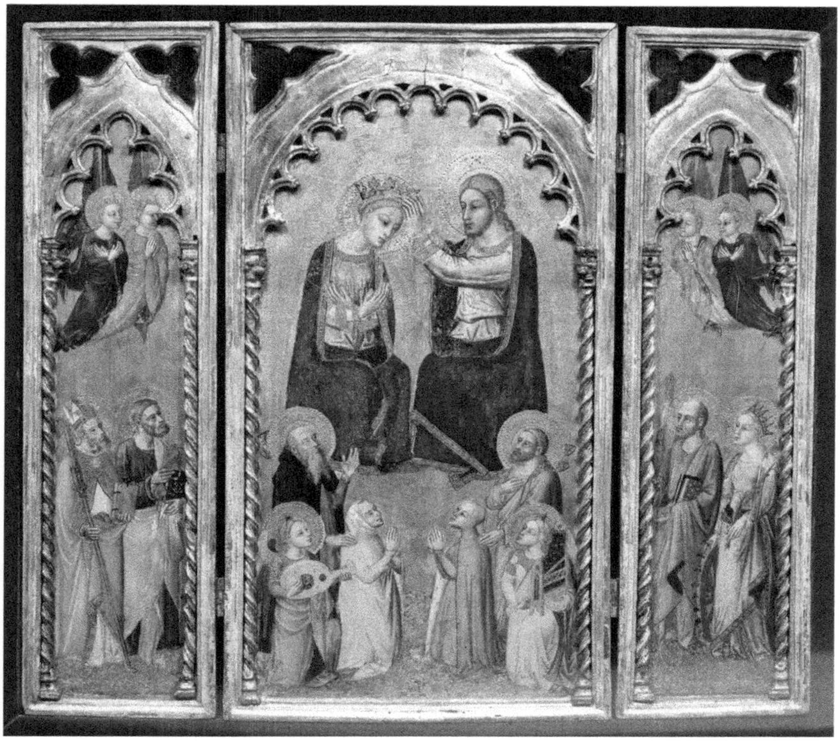

Figure 1.7 Niccolò di Tommaso, The Coronation of the Virgin, 66.8 × 73.5 cm, c. 1370. Baltimore, The Walters Art Museum. Image credit: The Walters Art Museum

a thaumaturge, the inscription below him refers to his exemplary qualities as a monk in Egypt: 'Lucerna veri luminis, doctor humilitatis, magister et viator mirae sinplicatatis; refulsit in Egitto' ('A lamp of the true light, a true master and traveller of admirable moral simplicity; he shone in Egypt'). Under St Christopher the inscription refers to his patronage against the much feared sudden death: 'Xpofori sancti spetiem quicumque tuetur, illo namque die nullo languor tenetur' ('Whoever looks at the image of St Christopher will not be taken by any illness during that day').[67] Saints such as Anthony, invoked against erysipelas, plague, and other illnesses, Christopher against sudden death, and Margaret for safe delivery in childbirth are found in many small tabernacles painted for domestic spaces.[68] The saints and their protections were thus made present in the home.

The comfort of images of the saints or the Virgin to the sick and dying must not be forgotten. The image of the Virgin that the Florentine *beata* Umiliana dei Cerchi (d. 1246) had in her room, forming a focal point of many of her devotions, played a role also in her death. Tormented by the devil at her death, her companion brought the panel, containing a relic of a lock of hair of the Virgin, and placed it, with blessed candles in the shape of a cross on her breast and sprinkled holy water on her head. The devil then left her at her command. 'And opening her eyes and seeing that portrait [of the Virgin] placed upon her breast, she placed [it] with honor in the silk cloth of her mantle and positioned it better upon her breast'. She died early the following day.[69] The Florentine merchant, Giovanni Morelli (1371–1444) wrote of the comfort provided by the image of the Virgin Mary when recording the heart-breaking death of his young son, Alberto, aged only ten, in 1406, and noted how the child had the panel of the Virgin brought to him, and embraced it with many prayers and vows, and then recommended himself to his family.[70]

The network of relations between the cure, the holy, and the image exemplifies Alessandra Foscati's consideration that illness cannot be seen as an event purely located in the field of medicine, but must be located culturally, in a historical and anthropological framework which takes into consideration Christian mentalities regarding sin, suffering, and the body.[71] The medico-surgical and magico-religious cannot be viewed in isolation, as they functioned in the same framework, because people engaged with both to heal bodies and minds. The image functioned at many levels as a place where the *virtus* of the saint could be accessed, a manifestation of the relationship between saint and devotee, a means of externalising illness and distress, a visual record in propagating cult and miracles, and as a source of comfort and consolation.

Notes

1 Le Goff, *Il Corpo nel Medioevo*, 2007, p. 101.
2 Antoine, 'Ex Voto', 1997, p. 564.
3 See, for example, the Sicilian ex votos discussed by Bronzini, 'Fenomenologia Dell'Ex Voto', 1978, p. 148.
4 Vasari, *Vite*, 1875–1885, vol. 3, pp. 374–375.
5 Arasse, 'Entre devotion et culture', 1981, p. 131.
6 Cousin, 'L'Ex-voto, Document d'Histoire', 1979, p. 107.
7 Bacci, *Lo Spazio*, 2005, pp. 102–103.
8 Cardini, *Le Mura di Firenze inargentate*, 1993, pp. 168–169.
9 Wood, 'The Votive Scenario', 2011, p. 209.
10 Holmes, 'Ex-votos', 2007, p. 161.
11 Noël Coulet, 'Pour l'histoire de l'ex-voto', 1993, pp. 401–404.
12 Charuty, 'Le vœu de vivre', 2007.
13 Vauchez, *Sainteté*, 1981, p. 535.
14 Bisogni, 'Ex-Voto e La Scultura', 2001, p. 5.
15 Brucker, 'Sorcery', 1963, pp. 9, 10.
16 Dameron, *Florence and Its Church*, 2005, p. 175.
17 Sacchetti, *Opere*, 1957, pp. 1113–1118; Lawless, 'Franco Sacchetti', 2009, p. 389.
18 Trexler, *Public Life*, 1980, p. 123; Panzanelli, 'Compelling Presence', 2008, pp. 13–39.
19 Strozzi, *Lettere*, 1877, pp. 127–130.
20 Vasari, *Vite*, 1875–1885, vol. 3, pp. 374–376.
21 Prudlo, 'Mothers and the Martyr', 2012, pp. 316–317.

22 Meiss, *Painting in Florence and Siena*, 1951, pp. 83, 94–95; Russo, 'Religion Civique', 1995, pp. 291–292.
23 *Acta Sanctorum, Aprilis, Tomus III*, 1866, pp. 700–702.
24 Voragine, *The Golden Legend*, 2012, p. 370.
25 Larson, 'St Margaret and St Marina', 2002, p. 31.
26 Bisogni, 'Ex voto', 2001, p. 73. Bisogni cites a number of other iconographical examples of ex voti at shrines.
27 For further Italian examples, see Lawless, 'Patienthood in Medieval Tuscany', 2016, pp. 76–80.
28 *Acta Sanctorum, Aprilis, Tomus II*, p. 808; *Acta Sanctorum, Aprilis, Tomus III*, 1866, p. 957.
29 *Acta Sanctorum, Januarius*, III, 1863, p. 521.
30 *Acta Sanctorum, Aprilis, Tomus II*, 1866, p. 195.
31 *Acta Sanctorum, Aprilis, Tomus III*, 1866, p. 530.
32 *Acta Sanctorum, Octobris, Tomus IV*, 1780, pp. 527–528, 537.
33 *Acta Sanctorum, Octobris, Tomus IV*, 1780, p. 471.
34 *Acta Sanctorum, Octobris, Tomus IV*, 1780, p. 525, and two similar miracles follow.
35 *Acta Sanctorum, Octobris, Tomus IV*, 1780, p. 539.
36 Armstrong (et al.) (eds), *The Founder. Vol. II of Francis of Assisi*, 2000, p. 446.
37 Schmidt, 'Tipologie e funzioni', 2003, p. 542.
38 Hope, 'Altarpieces and the Requirements of Patrons', 1990, pp. 535–571.
39 Tommaso da Celano, *Vita Prima*, book III, chapter 1; Armstrong (et al.) (eds), *The Saint. Vol. I of Francis of Assisi*, 1999, pp. 299–300.
40 Baschet, 'Introduction: L'Image-Objet', 1992, p. 23; Bonne, 'Répresentation médiévale', 1990.
41 Belting, *Likeness and Presence*, 1994, pp. 6–14.
42 Frugoni, *Francesco e L'Invenzione*, 1993, p. 323.
43 Frugoni, *Francesco e L'Invenzione*, 1993, p. 403.
44 *Acta Sanctorum, Maii, Tomus VII*, 1866, p. 157.
45 *Acta Sanctorum, Octobris, Tomus IV*, 1780, p. 537.
46 *Acta Sanctorum, Octobris, Tomus IV*, 1780, p. 527.
47 *Acta Sanctorum, Octobris, Tomus IV*, 1780.
48 *Acta Sanctorum, Januarius, Tomus III*, 1863, p. 680.
49 *Acta Sanctorum, Januarius, Tomus III*, 1863.
50 *Acta Sanctorum, Januarius, Tomus III*, 1863, p. 682.
51 *Acta Sanctorum, Januarius, Tomus III*, 1863, p. 687. He was provincial master of the English Carmelite province from 1444 to 1456, but according to Richard Copsey the recipient of the miracle was more probably an earlier provincial, John Keninghale (d. 1451). Copsey, 'Kenton, Nicholas', 2008.
52 Smith, 'Santa Umiltà', 2001, pp. 48–51; Schmidt, 'Tipologie e Funzioni', 2003, p. 567.
53 *Acta Sanctorum, Maii, Tomus V*, 1866, pp. 208–209.
54 *Acta Sanctorum, Maii, Tomus V*, 1866, p. 210.
55 *Acta Sanctorum, Maii, Tomus VII*, p. 157. Other examples of Bona acting as a surgeon, see *Acta Sanctorum, Maii, Tomus VII*, p. 254.
56 *Acta Sanctorum, Maii, Tomus II*, p. 241: 'In sanandis quoque vulneribus hominum admirabilem Virgo Dei exercuit chirurgiam'.
57 Armstrong (et al.), *The Founder: Vol. II of Francis of Assisi*, 2000, pp. 454–457; Vauchez, *Sainteté*, 1981, p. 457.
58 Machiavelli, *Libro di Ricordi*, 1954, par. 1483.
59 Frugoni, *Francesco e l'Invenzione delle Stimmate*, 1993, p. 325; Chave-Mahir, *L'Exorcisme*, 2011, p. 274.
60 Frugoni, *Francesco e l'Invenzione delle Stimmate*, 1993, pp. 335–336. Frugoni also points out that the devil being exorcised from Pietro da Foligno has been erased

by some devotee, but those of the women remain. For the miracles, Armstrong (et al.), *The Saint. Vol. I of Francis of Assisi*, 1999, p. 302.

61 Caciola, *Discerning Spirits*, 2003, pp. 129–130.

62 Gardner, *Giotto and His Publics*, 2011, p. 21, has noted that the protagonists of three out of six episodes are women. The iconography is repeated in a panel by an Umbrian painter, c. 1275–1299, in the Pinacoteca Vaticana.

63 Armstrong (et al.), *The Founder. Vol. II of Francis of Assisi*, 2000, pp. 466–467.

64 *Acta Sanctorum, Aprilis, Tomus II*, 1866, p. 808.

65 *Acta Sanctorum, Maii, tomus V*, 1866, p. 164.

66 Lawless, 'Domestic Devotions', 2020, pp. 15–16.

67 Schmidt, *Painted Piety*, 2005, p. 98. On St Christopher, see Rigaux, 'Un image', 1996, pp. 242–243.

68 Lawless, 'Domestic Devotions', 2020, p. 9.

69 Schuchman, 'Life of Umiliana de' Cerchi', 2009, p. 383.

70 Branca, *Mercanti Scrittori*, 1986, pp. 294–295.

71 Foscati, 'Il "Mal degli Ardenti"', 2010, p. 52.

2

Wax ex votos in late medieval England: bodies, health, and the problem of portraiture

Carly B. Boxer

Artificial limbs and organs crafted in wax hang above the pinnacles of a stone shrine in a stained glass scene at York Minster, painted c. 1414 (Figure 2.1).[1] The 78-foot-tall window in the cathedral's east end showing the life of St William (York's own Archbishop William Fitzherbert) depicts the saint's shrine as the setting for posthumous miracles in many of its ninety-five discrete narrative scenes.[2] In this depiction, a pilgrim approaches the shrine and offers a wax *ex voto*, a small gift given in exchange for divine favour, while other such gifts offered by previous visitors to the shrine hang from a rod in the background. The bearded pilgrim holds up a leg, complete with a delicately curving calf and differentiated toes, as if inserting the foot into the structure of the shrine. The leg, roughly to scale with the pilgrim's body, could very well be the pilgrim's own limb. It seems to poke out of his robes and has been painted in the same translucent white used to denote the man's flesh. The contrast of black lead outlining the major shapes of the pane creates the effect of a fracture – a clear break just below the knee – of the sort that could use a miraculous cure. Only the leg's position in the pilgrim's arms, held up awkwardly at chest level, and the presence of other votives at the shrine make clear its waxen composition.

Wax figurines like the leg this pilgrim holds were regularly given by donors at saints' shrines in late medieval England, usually with the hope that such a gift to a powerful saint would result in the miraculous restoration of the donor's health or fortune. Such gift-giving practices stemmed from ancient traditions and continue even today at religious sites.[3] The promise of miracles stimulated pious layfolk to make pilgrimages across England and to the Continent throughout the medieval period, but a growth in the cults of local saints in the late Middle Ages meant that miracles could happen closer to home, and at the behest of locally-venerated saints like William.[4] Not all miracles were bodily in nature, but written accounts

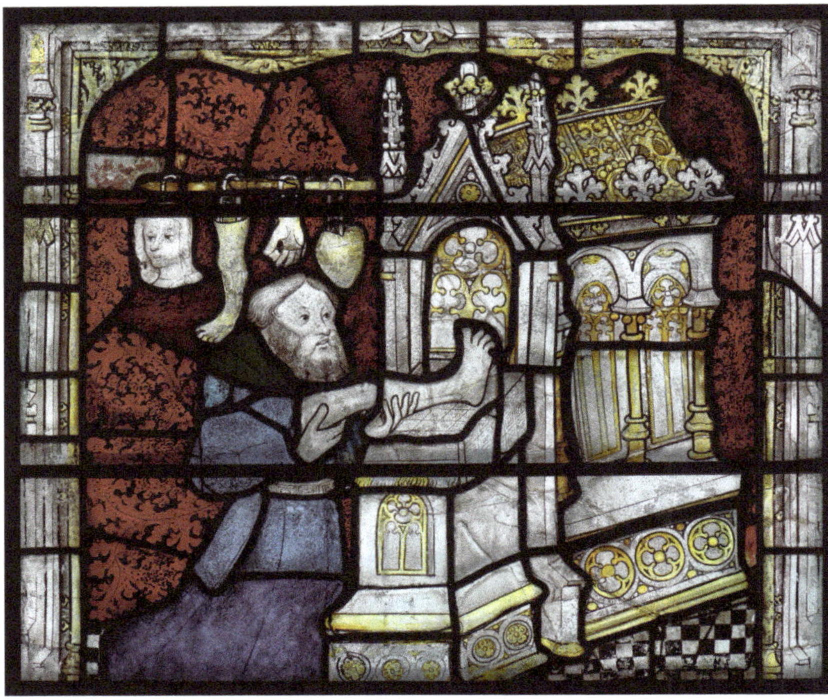

Figure 2.1 Ex votos at the shrine of St William, Life of St William Window, c. 1414. York Minster, East End. Image credit: Taken by The York Glaziers Trust, reproduced by kind permission of the Chapter of York

abound with stories of divine healing, and to escape illness in fifteenth-century England a miraculous cure was just as valid an approach as medical intervention.[5] A donor bringing an ex voto to a shrine would purchase (or perhaps fashion) a small object to give as a gift to the benevolent saint.[6] Leaving the gift at a shrine meant that the donor could maintain a physical presence in a space that worked most effectively when visitors stayed as close as possible for as long as possible. The material value of these gifts mattered to their donors and, presumably, to the holy figures who received them. But the shape of ex votos mattered too. Often votive gifts replicated the specific body part for which the donors sought or had recently received a miraculous cure; while it need not bear an exact visual likeness to the donor's own appearance, the votive could be considered more efficacious when it took the form of the ill, injured, or otherwise indisposed body part for which the donor sought help because it more accurately simulated the donor's physical presence through visual likeness.[7]

In the stained-glass scene from York Minster described above, the leg is one of five wax objects that has been brought to William's shrine to ensure a donor's health. Strung from a pole behind the pilgrim's head is a woman's face, complete with veil, another leg, a fist, and a heart.[8] All five ex votos have been depicted in the same translucent white glass with brown painted details; not only does the colouration of these figures look like particularly valuable clarified beeswax, but it also creates a parallel between the pilgrim and the gifts; the same milky white tone is used for both skin and ex votos.[9] The similarity between votive and votary in this scene of miraculous healing demonstrates the expectation that wax figures not only model the body parts of their donors, but also look like those donors' particular body parts, distinct from the bodies of other donors.[10] Comparing the wax leg held up by the pilgrim to a second leg strung up on the pole behind the shrine confirms the need for visual likeness in the votary's donation. The visible knees and differentiated toes on each of the two legs show that the pilgrim holds a right foot, while a left foot dangles behind him. Although both the pilgrim's bearded face and the wax woman's face behind him have been rendered in the same pale palette and wispy linework, the two are distinct from each other, but still resemble provisional subjects – two people who are visibly distinct, even if they are not attached to specific historical personages.[11] The pilgrim who donated that face donated a gift that bore her own resemblance. Whether through the specific part of the body depicted or the look of that body part, ex votos bore likeness to the specific votaries for whom they secured health.

Wax ex votos often replicate the look of the body of the votary by imitating a particularly meaningful body part, insisting on a relationship between the representation of a person or body part in wax and the person after whom that wax is modelled. This relationship is one of both physical surrogacy and visual likeness. Wax, unlike paint, could replicate a body or body part in addition to representing it: the parts of the body figured in wax were understood to be interchangeable with their corporeal referents – with the limbs and bodies they represented, at least in the economy of divine healing.[12] These representations nevertheless exist at a degree of remove from the look of the donor's actual body. They represent a single limb or organ, not the subject in full. Made serially by casting unworked wax in metal or wooden moulds, these objects complicate the expectation that a representation of oneself be a mimetic self-portrait.[13] While they may not portray their referents in the conventional sense, wax votive figurines make discernable physical qualities visible, draw their efficacy from the visual replication of their donors' distinctive features, and rely upon an identification of an individual donor with a sculpted wax figure. That is to say, as visual objects they work similarly to portraits and therefore offer insight into practices of self-representation in late medieval England. The complex ontological status of medieval wax ex votos as representations, body doubles, fragmented body parts, and serial objects offers a framework for understanding the convoluted and at times contradictory expectations for representing oneself and representing one's health in late medieval England.

Although few medieval wax ex votos survive, textual accounts and pictorial representations of votive objects – wax and otherwise – from late medieval England implicate not only the donor but also the donor's specific body in the process of healing. Often wax ex votos were produced serially for unspecified buyers, but the donors who left these objects at shrines saw a connection between small wax figures of body parts and that same part of their own bodies. This essay explores that connection. Votive giving played a significant role in the late medieval economy of health and healing; instead of, and often in addition to strictly medical cures, the ill and infirm sought well-being by making pilgrimages to shrines and offering gifts in exchange for a saint's curative touch. As well-attested votive gifts given in this period, replicative wax ex votos brought the particular form of a donor's body to bear on their own health. In the logic of votive giving, a gift that modelled the form of a broken limb or the dimensions of a donor's body promised a more effective cure for that same part on that individual's body.

The connection between the wax figure and the body it signified hinged on a careful balance between the generic form of the ex voto and its ability to reference its donor's body with sufficient specificity. This essay turns to a discourse in late medieval thought that grew alongside the tradition of the wax ex voto – that of portraiture – in order to better understand this apparent paradox of votive giving. Art historical literature on the early modern uses of wax as a portrait medium is robust, though few sources treat the medieval forerunners of wax effigies with the same eye toward the material's propensity for conveying visual likeness or its use in representations of the human body.[14] Wax ex votos functioned differently than portraits – this essay does not intend to claim votive figures as early portrait media – but their makers and donors thought about these objects as representations of individuals and of individual bodies in ways that benefit from comparison to portraiture. Wax ex votos confound modern (and early modern) expectations of what a portrait should be, but they also embody many of the qualities salient in fourteenth- and fifteenth-century portraiture. By considering wax ex votos alongside late medieval ideas about portraiture, the donor's place in making their own image becomes clear. Far from typical modern self-portraits, late medieval wax ex votos nevertheless enabled their donors to portray themselves and their bodies to gain access to a network of health and miraculous healing.

Divine medicine

A donor bringing a wax votive to a shrine would likely have purchased that miniature replica of the body part for which they sought a miracle from a shop just outside the holy site; while it need not bear an exact visual likeness to the donor's own appearance, the votive was more efficacious when it took the form of the ill, injured, or otherwise indisposed body part for which the donor sought a miraculous intervention.[15] This approach to health and healing persisted in parallel to the growth of the medical profession in late medieval England. Often as a complement, or perhaps an alternative, to the treatment offered by surgeons and itinerant practitioners, many patients turned to the Church to ensure their bodily and spiritual wellness.[16] For an ill or injured person seeking a cure, pilgrimage was just as viable a source of treatment as surgery or consultation with a physician.[17] Vibrant pilgrimage destinations in regional hubs like Canterbury, Hereford, Exeter, York, and London attracted pilgrims from throughout England; an association with a specific saint could make a given shrine an especially efficacious destination for certain types of illnesses and injuries.[18] Making the trip to a saint's shrine was one way of showing dedication to that saint and thereby appealing to divine power for an efficacious cure. Pilgrims' reasons for visiting shrines were varied, but often centred around healing. While some sought spiritual health, others travelled despite chronic sickness or debilitating injuries in order to find physical wellness.[19]

Ex votos were left at shrines, often at churches or sites associated with a specific saint, in fulfilment of a vow: in keeping with ancient traditions of votive giving, these objects serve as material remnants of the promise made by a votary to a deity in an act of supplication. In exchange for the health, luck, protection, or good fortune that might be divinely sanctioned in such a ritual, a votary could give only time, prayer, and material goods. Catherine Lawless examines the material dimensions of this relationship at length in her contribution to this volume. The variety of wax body parts left by pilgrims documented in church and canonisation records makes clear that specificity was crucial to the votary's donation. A wax arm would be of little help to a votary with a broken leg, for it could not act as a surrogate for the body part that needed healing. In several documented cases, votaries left the cause of the illness itself rather than a representation of it as a gift of thanks: for example, 'in 1332 the priest Henry has a lump from his throat mounted in silvers and suspended at the shrine of St Ethelreda, at Ely'.[20] Such gifts made literal the bodily presence that wax votives sought to imitate. Other cases record pilgrims with injured limbs crawling or crutching to churches, finding a cure at the shrine, then leaving their crutches as gifts to the saint who healed them.[21] Votaries saw the gifts they offered as closely tied to themselves and their experience of illness. A lump, crutch, or a man-made facsimile of a limb asserted the donor's identity and through it their presence, linking a specific person to one of the myriad gifts that populated the shrine.

Cathedral inventories, records from papal envoys, and surviving wax figures attest to the widespread donation of ex votos resembling bodies in late medieval England. In the course of renovations in the 1940s, a group of wax figures in the shape of different bodies and body parts were found on a ledge above the shrine of Bishop Edmund Lacey (d. 1455) at Exeter Cathedral (Figure 2.2). Surviving in this cache were hollow wax votives

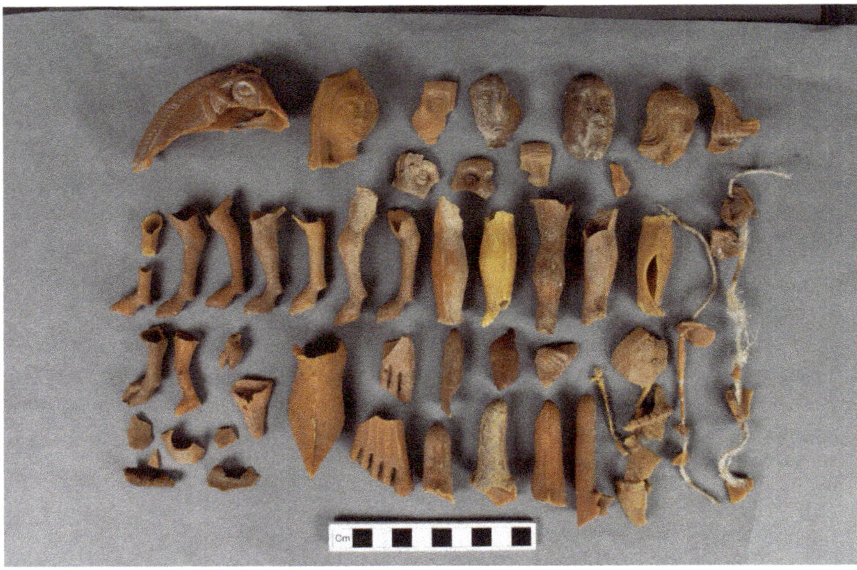

Figure 2.2 Wax votive fragments from the Shrine of Bishop Edmund Lacey, made after 1420. Exeter Cathedral, Archival Photograph by F. E. Norris, 1949. Image credit: Photograph courtesy of Dean & Chapter of Exeter Cathedral, Library & Archives

in the shape of limbs, fingers, feet, and one fully intact body of a woman (Figure 2.3).[22] 1,058 pieces were recovered from the hidden alcove above the shrine, some fragments of otherwise lost figures, others largely intact. Waxed threads poke out from some of these figures, indicating that they were made with the intention of being hung up near the shrine, as wax-votos are often pictured in prints and paintings from the period. Like the assortment of wax body parts behind the pilgrim in the York Minster window, these ex votos would have hung from any available surface, covering and ornamenting the shrine with the replicated forms of its visitors' bodies. Proximity was crucial to efficacy. A clear sightline or, even better, physical contact with the shrine ensured the efficacy of these objects.

Written records from Hereford Cathedral attest to a similar diversity of bodily ex votos offered in the century before the building of Lacey's shrine. In his discussion of pilgrimage sites as centres of healing, Ronald Finucane notes that

> A list of offerings was drawn up just twenty years after the first miracles were reported at the curative shrine of Thomas Cantilupe. Midway between his death (1282) and canonization (1320), papal commissioners went to Hereford where, early on Tuesday, 29 August 1307, they examined the dead bishop's shrine and found 170 silver ships, 41 wax ships, 129 silver images...diverse human limbs, 436 whole images of men in wax, 1200 wax images of parts of the body and limbs, 77 figures of horses, animals, and birds, an uncountable quantity of eyes, breasts, teeth, ears[.][23]

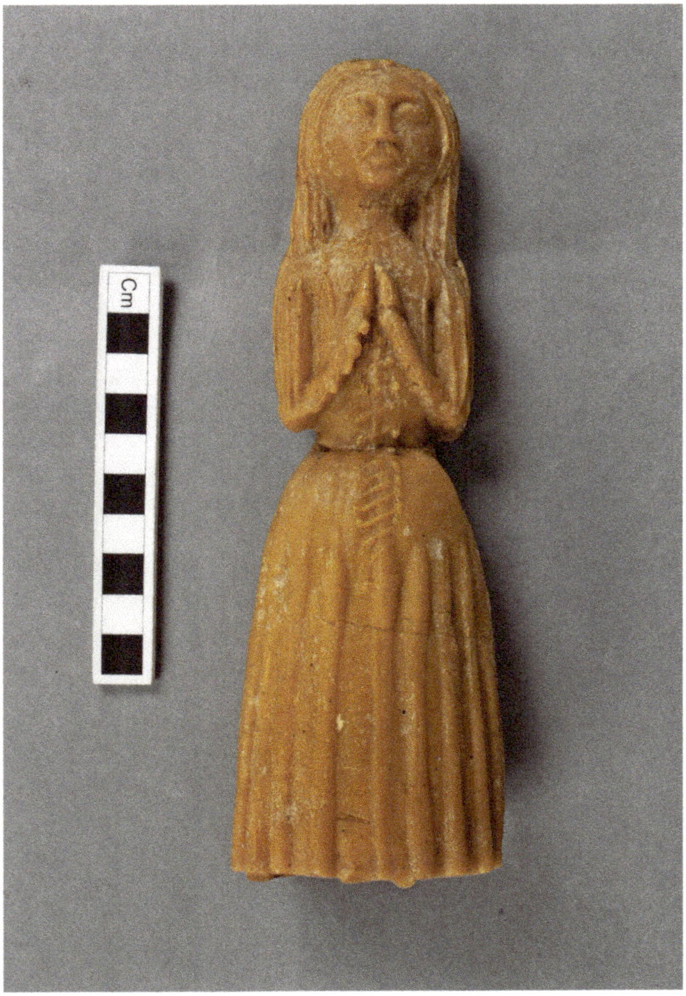

Figure 2.3 Wax votive figure from the Shrine of Bishop Edmund Lacey, made after 1420. Exeter Cathedral. Image credit: Photograph courtesy of Dean & Chapter of Exeter Cathedral, Library & Archives

The document produced by the papal commissioners contains an inventory of some 2,000 wax ex votos at Cantilupe's shrine in 1307 and another 100 wax figures that had appeared when the commissioners returned to the shrine several months later.[24] Of those 2,000 wax offerings, over 1,600 depicted either the bodies or body parts of those who offered them.

Leaving figurines of bodies and body parts enabled pilgrims to offer vows specific to their own infirmities. Eamon Duffy cites a similar array of ex votos left at the shrine of Richard Scrope in York in the sixteenth century: 'nine assorted images of men and women, two cows, sixteen eyes, thirteen legs, ten hearts, ten teeth, four breasts' in addition to several models of ships and sailing equipment.[25] Often a votary left a model of a previously-infirm body part that had already been cured as a gesture of thanks. Even while offering replicas that bore the specific curves and scars of their own bodies, though, votaries understood visual likeness to be just one aspect of producing an efficacious representation; efficacy could be enhanced through proximity, prayer, and multiple donations.

In another panel of the St William window in York, healing happens without the presence of votive offerings. Five men gather around the saint's shrine (Figure 2.4).[26] Rather than presenting ex votos, the men reach out with bowls and hands to catch the liquid that flows out of spouts in the pointed gables that surround the saint's tomb.[27] The pilgrims' physical contact with excretions from the saint have the power to heal, and incite the pilgrims to reach into the holes in the shrine, pressing their hands and eyes up against the spouts. The two panels from York reveal divergent approaches to healing at shrines that, through their divergence, indicate the perceived sameness of the bodies of votaries and the representation of those bodies in wax. In the second scene, the proximity and physical contact of the shrine's visitors with the bodily remains of St William heals ailments demonstrated by distinct outward signs: bandages on legs, a crippled limb, a cane. In contrast, the wax ex votos in the first scene supplant the physical contact of actual bodies, allowing for a longer duration of

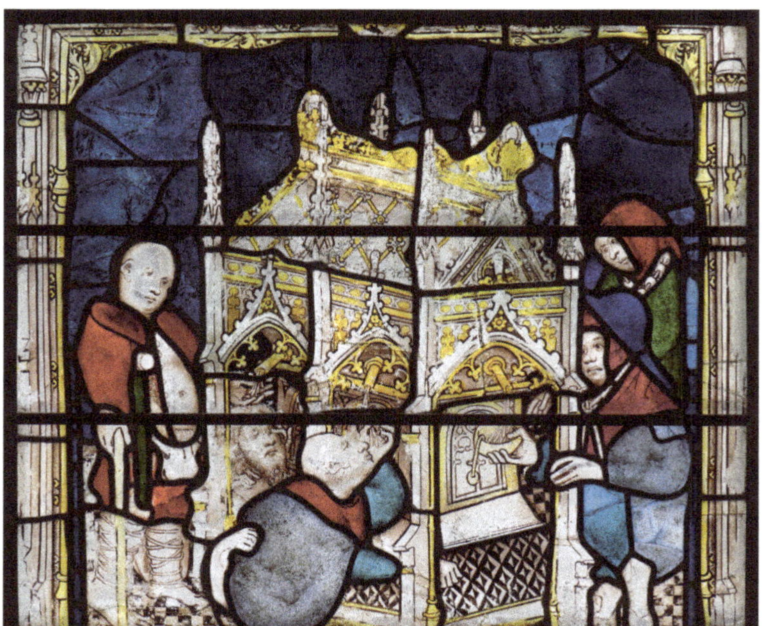

Figure 2.4 Pilgrims at the shrine of St William, Life of St William Window, c. 1414. York Minster, East End. Image credit: Taken by The York Glaziers Trust, reproduced by kind permission of the Chapter of York

contact through the continued presence of the ex voto at the shrine even after the votary had left. The two forms of contact – that of the pilgrim reaching out to touch the shrine and that of the wax ex voto – were both considered efficacious because the wax statuettes of visitors doubled the visitors' bodies.[28] Like charms and textual amulets that appear on manuscript rolls in this period, objects which promised their users effective cures in return for repeated looking, wax ex votos depended on an understanding that looking, representing, and healing were durational. Instead of frequently beholding an image on a roll as one might do with a charm, the ex voto made it possible for a votary to maintain their own presence by way of their image in a miraculous space over a long period of time in order to ensure their own miraculous healing.

Bodies in wax

By the fourteenth century, the same wax used for crafting ex votos was being put to use to represent the human body outside of the realm of miraculous healing. Italian wax-workers created lifelike models for anatomical demonstrations. The Italian anatomist Mondino de' Luzzi reportedly used wax figures created by Alessandra Giliani in his anatomy lessons.[29] In Michele Medici's nineteenth-century account, Giliani's skill came in her ability to

> clean most skillfully the smallest veins, the arteries, all ramifications of the vessels without lacerating or dividing them…she would fill them with various colored liquids which, after having been driven into the vessels, would harden without destroying the vessels, and she was also said to be a skillful modeler in wax.[30]

In Medici's recapitulation of these late medieval accounts, the ability to skilfully preserve a body is closely linked with the ability to replicate it (or its component parts) with wax simulacra. Indeed, Medici's mention of modelling wax in combination with postmortem surgical procedures employed for autopsies signals the similarity of working with wax and flesh in preparing a model for demonstration. Ariella Minden provides an account of similar overlaps in artistic and surgical craft knowledge later in this volume.

Although the account of Giliani's skilful elision of wax and corporeality has been mediated by nineteenth-century authors, medieval sources attest to a similar slippage between wax and human body parts in a sphere where the material's capacity for mimicking human appearance took on additional import: the making of wax portrait effigies for wealthy and royal clientele.[31] Records dating from the thirteenth century indicate the commissioning of lifelike votive figures, some intended for use in funerary contexts, others functioning as smaller votive figurines. These images deliberately served as portrait likenesses. Records survive for the making of such images in gold, including Henry III's donation to the shrine of Edward the Confessor a gold image of Eleanor of Provence, his bride, upon the occasion of their marriage.[32] While gold would certainly make for a more sumptuous donation, it lacked the uncanny verisimilitude wax afforded. Although the figures do not survive, wax votive portraits appear in written records. Sarah Blick notes the use of such images not only in royal ceremonies, but also in more routine actives of votive giving. When a votary could not physically attend a shrine to make a donation, wax likenesses could be given 'by devotees who could not make the journey themselves. In 1443, Margaret Paston sent her sick husband a costly "ymmage of wax" as a surrogate for himself to be presented to the shrine of Our Lady of Undercroft at Canterbury Cathedral'.[33] Wax served as the ideal medium for making votive portraits for reasons closely connected to its widespread use in making smaller ex votos: it gained authority from its traditional use in votive giving, it was a valuable, reusable commodity for the church to which it was given, and, unlike gold, it could imitate the physical appearance of its donor.

The ontological connection between the votary and their wax ex voto was emphasised by wax's unique capacity to mimic human likeness. David Freedberg notes that wax 'has the additional advantage of actually looking rather like flesh – especially if tinted'.[34] Wax, unlike small wood or metal statuettes and coins sometimes left at these same shrines, could take on the appearance of flesh because of its material properties. Julius von Schlosser, in his foundational work on the use of wax across historical periods, argues similarly that wax as a material made it uniquely possible to represent the bodies and bodily qualities of subjects. In his account, the use of wax votives in antiquity and the Middle Ages signals an investment in the particular appearance of the individual. According to Schlosser, the possibility of serial production in wax presented artists with the capacity for

> maximally individualized pictorial form in the cast taken from nature…where the observer's participation is reduced to a minimum; it is a development that one would be tempted to define as leading away from the most 'subjective' to the most 'objective' pictorial form, were these terms not so ambiguous.[35]

As a moulded material shaped by casting, wax suggested the objective accuracy of the image it produced; wax could mimic the look of a subject with precision, and perceptions of its capacity for likeness also benefited from a long association with death masks. Wax had long been the material used to create indexical images from individual models. As such, wax was celebrated for producing high quality portraits among its early twentieth-century exegetes precisely because it could be cast, without the mediation of an artist's hand. Roman waxworks embodied what von Schlosser characterises as a 'painstakingly naturalistic style of portraiture'.[36] This style was enabled in part by wax's propensity to 'look' human as well as the process of cast-making required to make a death mask with the material.[37] Wax, in short, could ensure visual likeness between votive and votary in a way that the use of other materials precluded, whether through its evocation of flesh tones or in its association with imprints.

Wax's long historiographic association with the development of portraiture is rooted in discussions of Roman waxworks, but scholarship regarding the material's reemergence in early modern portraiture more closely connects wax as a mimic of likeness to waxwork's uncanny presence. Aby Warburg understands the 'magical fetishism' of wax as crucial to the sudden appearance of portraiture in early modern religious settings.[38] In Warburg's formulation, the mimetic simulation of one's appearance in portrait painting was directly indebted to earlier Christian practices of leaving wax votives in proximity to altars and shrines. Even as painted illusionistic portraits of wealthy donors began to dot the walls of Florentine churches in the fifteenth century, votaries continually brought wax effigies into those same spaces, hanging them from chains and hooks alongside early portraits. Made to resemble their donors (Warburg gives the example of Lorenzo de' Medici commissioning three life-sized wax effigies to be installed in Florentine churches) these wax images held power not only because of their status as donations, but also because of the specific evocation they offered of their donor's physical presence in a holy space. Votive gifts did this precisely by resembling their donor – the look of their flesh, the size of their hands, the break in their legs, and other forms of visual difference.

The wax that comprised ex votos was loaded with metaphysical and generative meaning in the minds of its late medieval makers and donors. Albertus Magnus offered detailed theorisations of human cognition and reproduction using the metaphor of wax's ability to take on form through acts of imprinting.[39] Wax also shared a special connection to the crafting of individual identity in the high and late medieval periods that further links it to the capacity to convey information about oneself through images. The process of making symbolic objects out of wax using metal moulds was well established in making and circulating seals. Aden Kumler's discussion of the serial production of eucharistic wafers using stamping technology helps to clarify how a mass-produced wax figurine could, paradoxically, stand in for the body of a specific votary: through the process of impressing the wax into its new form, a stamp took on the identity of its referent. Making wax into body parts required similar techniques of moulding and stamping, resulting in figurines that carried with them the identities of the votaries who bought and donated them.[40] Using different colours of wax and metal seal matrices enabled medieval people to leave a personal mark, and the seal was taken as a personal emblem for the person it represented. Even the terminology for the device used to make a seal – the matrix – hints at the sign's status as the product of reproduction. Brigitte Bedos-Rezak has shown at length that seals could have functioned as a form of non-mimetic portraiture in the Middle Ages, giving specific, fixed, visual form to their subject despite the lack of mimetic likeness.[41] Wax as a medium was already deeply embedded in the semiotics of self-representation. In the case of seals, non-mimetic features like colour and symbol could be used as portraits of a sort – representational signs associated with a single subject despite their seeming obfuscation of mimetic convention.

Mimesis and measurement

Representing likeness in late medieval England did not necessarily require the depiction of visual similarity. Length and weight, rather than facial features or other outward signs, could assert the physical sameness of a votary and their donation.[42] Because the material value of wax came from its weight and quality as well as any workmanship that went into its form, donations in precise proportions suggested both a physical connection to the donor as well as the donor's desire to make a significant monetary investment in their own health. As Hugo Van Der Velden notes, wax could be given as a raw material or functional object instead of as a figure:

> Wax could be donated in any one of numerous ways, as unworked material, a candle or an image. All of these variants would be produced and supplied by the same craftsmen. In a decree passed by the English Parliament in 1423, it was laid down that the price charged by wax-chaundelers for 'Chaundelles, Images, Figures & autres overaigns de Cere, faitz pur oblations' should not exceed the price of unworked wax by more than a set amount.[43]

The wax donated was valuable regardless of the artisan's reworking of the raw material into a given form, even if body-part shaped ex votos improved the perceived efficacy of the donation. Sarah Blick elaborates on the role of other criteria to establish the likeness of the donated wax to the donor. She claims that

> A simple candle was effective, but many devotees wanted to make sure that their individual presence was sensed by the divinity through the donation of trindles or rotulas – coiled large candles made from lengthy wicks. Here personal interaction was crucial as the wicks, measured to the length of the afflicted person's body from fingertip to fingertip with the arms outstretched, or the circumference of the affected body part, became part of the candle.[44]

The likeness of the candle and its donor – established in these cases by criteria other than visual similarity – could ensure that a donor's plea for health could be fulfilled. In parallel to the way in which ex votos in the shapes of given body parts secured a cure for those afflicted parts, the mimetic repetition of a donor's weight or height in wax and wicks improved the efficacy of a cure for that donor.

The same English cathedrals that attracted pilgrims in the fourteenth and fifteenth centuries house iconographic programs that represent even earlier donations of ex votos as significant moments in healing narratives; in these representations mimesis is quantitative rather than visual.[45] At Canterbury Cathedral, a stained glass window from the first quarter of the thirteenth century depicts a woman who suffered through a difficult childbirth making an offering at Thomas Becket's shrine (Figures 2.5 and 2.6).[46] Two panes depict distinct moments in this healing narrative. First, the donor has a vision of Thomas Becket in the throes of her illness: Becket points to a candle burning atop his tomb. In the second panel, the woman donates an object at Becket's shrine. In this second pane, she is holding a trindle, a long, coiled candle with a continuous wick.[47] Despite lacking any obvious visual similarity to their votaries, such offerings explicitly invoked their donors' bodily presence through other physical means. Records attest to donors commissioning candles with wicks that match their own height, or with weights of wax that correspond proportionally to their own.[48] This correspondence was understood to improve the efficacy of the offering. Like late medieval prayer rolls that claim in text to represent the wounds of Christ at a reduced scale, wax could replicate a votary's bodily

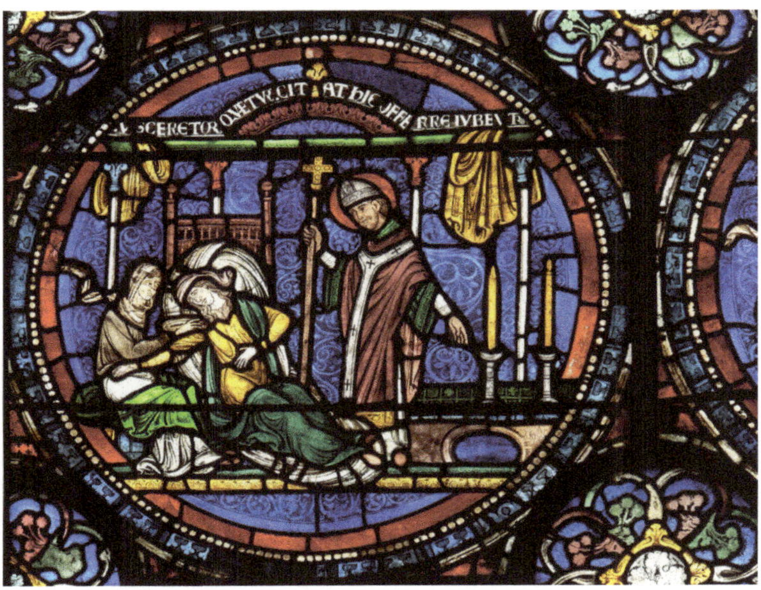

Figure 2.5 The vision of Thomas Becket, Stained glass, before 1220. Trinity Chapel, Canterbury Cathedral (Panel nIV 21). Image credit: Photograph by Painton Cowan, Reproduced with permission

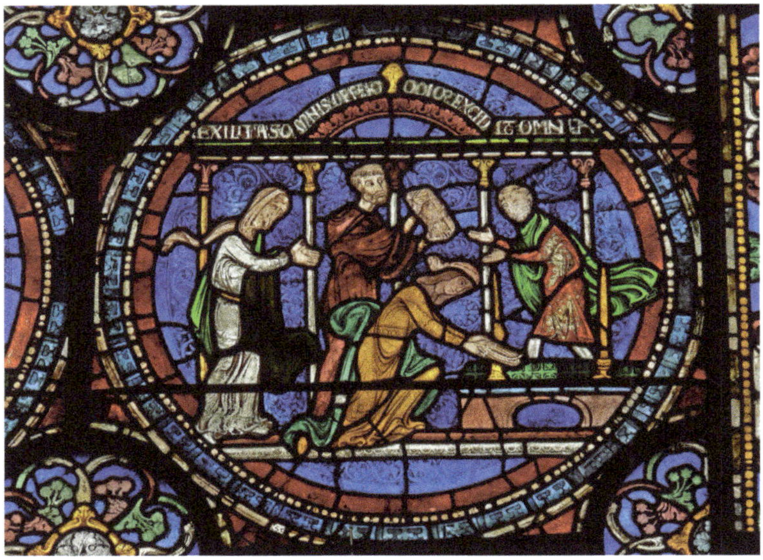

Figure 2.6 A woman donates a trindle at the tomb of Thomas Becket, Stained glass, before 1220. Trinity Chapel, Canterbury Cathedral (Panel nIV 22). Image credit: Photograph by Painton Cowan, Reproduced with permission

measurements.[49] Representing one's own body in wax through its weight or measure asserted an authenticity, or perhaps a mimetic presence, to the image. If a proportional rendering of Christ's measure could heal, and would be perceived to heal more effectively through the accuracy of its proportions, then a similar approach to signifying oneself could offer a similarly efficacious cure.

In many ways, these complex medieval functions of pictorial representation fall in line with medieval semiotics more generally. Hugo Van der Velden claims that because candles made with specific weights of wax and moulded wax figures were used simultaneously at many late medieval shrines 'a likeness forges exactly the same link between a portrait and the person depicted, sign and signified, as does the similarity in height between a votive candle and its donor'.[50] This correspondence proved fruitful for the woman depicted in the window from Canterbury, who purportedly, 'was cured after her nurse persuaded her husband to offer a candle as long and as wide as the lady's body'.[51] Her cure was attributed both to the donation itself, and to the fact that the donation mimicked the height and girth of the donor's body. This mathematical approach to likeness, while effective in its own right, did not exist in contrast to or isolation from visual likeness. While the weight of the candle or length of the wick insists on its connection to a specific donor through these non-visual, material similarities, those very same conceptions of material or quantitative similarity have a visual language all their own; the oversized scale and prominent coils of these candles – and the depiction of these objects in other media – always explicitly references the particularity of a donor's body, even if it does not mimetically replicate that donor's visible appearance.

Pilgrimage and/as portraiture

Horst Bredekamp writes of a fundamental tension in the production of images – both medieval and modern – that enables the substitution of images for bodies and bodies for images. 'The precondition for this phenomenon lies in a deep-seated tradition of conceiving of body and image as separate, and yet nonetheless identical'.[52] Wax ex votos from English pilgrim's shrines epitomise this conceptualisation of images and the bodies they represent as at once separate and identical. The relationship between ex voto and votary is more complex than a simple pictorial representation of a supplicant in wax would seem to suggest.[53] The ex voto stands in for the specific body part of the individual donor, despite being produced in serial, donated en masse, and not necessarily representing its donor's physical likeness with any readily recognisable outward signs. David Freedberg expands upon the need for likeness to make votive images work, and claims that 'with votive images of all kinds, one deals with the need to represent the event from which the devotee was saved (or the physical member saved), and to set up such representations as a form of lasting testimony and gratitude at a pilgrimage center or other shrine'.[54] In the case of English pilgrim shrines, the 'event' is condensed into an image of its outcome: illness, injury, or healing.[55] Representation is not limited to a past event from which the votary has been saved, but also includes figurations of body parts not-yet healed in order to bring about a miraculous cure. Freedberg continues by noting that

> in every case, manufacture and figuration is predicated on a strict concept of distinctiveness and accuracy. There may be cases where accuracy and distinctiveness seem to yield to a simpler idea of sufficient denotation, but even in such instances one has a sense of the diminished adequacy of the less true and the less precise.[56]

Accuracy comprised of non-visual, physical likeness to the donor required artisans to achieve a limited degree of distinctiveness in wax figures, but still made ex votos more efficacious. This tension – the need for likeness through physical form and simultaneous disregard for visual likeness – conforms to changing late medieval discourses around portraiture as a technique of pictorial representation.

By the fourteenth century, medieval artists had long-established conventions of representing particular people with heraldic symbols and other non-mimetic signs. Increasingly common in Northern European painting in the fourteenth century was a technology of representing the physical likeness of a subject. This occurs in luxurious royal commissions, however, not the fragments of wax infirmities left at English shrines.[57] In his discussion of early portrait painting in France, Stephen Perkinson uses the phrase 'physiognomic likeness' to describe the process through which 'images could represent particular people through the mimetic representation of facial features'.[58] Wax ex votos rely on a different sort of likeness, not entirely unlike the physiognomic likeness at hand in Perkinson's attempt to align medieval portraits with their early modern successors. Wax figurines made in late medieval England were made with the intention of reproducing a specific body part, even if the visible features of that body part ultimately fail to look like an identifiable individual. These images allowed donors to picture themselves; far from conventional self-portraits, wax ex votos nevertheless relied on their donor's understanding that these images were, in effect, both representations and replicas of their own bodies. Replication was predicated on likeness.

A single surviving copy of a woodcut print made c. 1415–1430 depicts King Henry VI as a saint with healing powers, surrounded by votaries with gruesome injuries that required saintly intervention (Figure 2.7).[59] The print, an uncoloured frontispiece pasted to the cover of a Wycliffite bible owned by Henry VI (now Oxford, Bodleian MS Bodley 277), shows men and women with their hands clasped in prayer kneeling at the King's feet. A woman in the right foreground has a knife through her throat; a man to the left holds a rope around his own neck; several men have been pierced by arrows; all the figures smile serenely, as if they feel no pain despite their visible injuries.[60] At the heavily-damaged top left corner of the image, the remnants of a shelf holding ex votos is visible. The lower body of one small ex voto faces toward the wall, his buttocks and bent elbows still visible despite heavy damage. Next to him, a horse raises one hoof mid trot. Two wax legs dangle from a now-destroyed rod. On the king's other side, crutches and chains hang from a rod – these are objects presumably left behind by pilgrims whose pleas were answered. Among them, a small tablet marked with a tally hangs on the wall; tables like this adorned late medieval shrines, enumerating in verse a saint's miracles.[61] While the injured, kneeling supplicants stay close to the king, the presence of those who have already benefitted from his miracles is equally visible in the image, even though these figures are physically absent from the image. Wax figurines ensure past votaries' continued proximity to Henry, while the tally on the wall makes the success of these past pleas visible both to the depicted petitioners as well as to the image's viewer. The perception of miraculous healing – like healing itself – depends upon the visible presence of surrogate body parts.

Wax ex votos left at tombs and shrines replicate the bodies of the votaries, offering an embodied form of *imitatio* that allowed donors to participate in their own healing.[62] Picturing one's body in wax would also

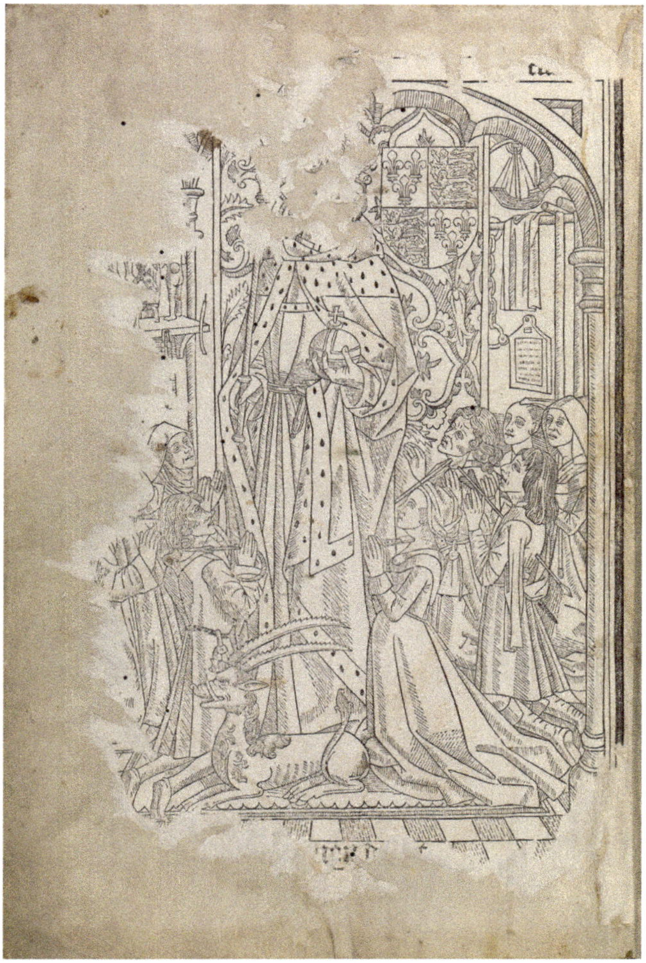

Figure 2.7 Large woodcut of Henry VI as a saint surrounded by petitioners, Oxford, Bodleian Library MS 277. Image credit: The Bodleian Libraries, University of Oxford

have brought to mind christological comparisons for medieval donors; wax ex votos therefore participated in the specific practice of *imitatio Christi*, the sometimes ascetic and often punitive effort to make oneself physically Christlike. Wax – and specifically wax candles – resonated with medieval churchgoers and exegetes as metaphors for Christ's divinity and his sacrifice. Medieval sources liken Christ to a candle: 'the wax his body, the wick his soul, and the flame the godhead'.[63] Popularly, the bees responsible for making the high-quality wax used in both liturgical candles and votive figures were compared to Christ. Because of the medieval belief that bees died in producing wax, the creatures were celebrated for making a sacrifice resonant of Christ's own.[64] Christopher Wood characterises votive giving as a form of semi-public performance, in which the act of donation forms a web of indebtedness and witness between the saint, votary, and onlookers. According to Wood, 'the ex voto registers an autobiographical impulse. The individual, encouraged to imitate Christ, performs his or her story in public'.[65] In Wood's words, the performance of giving a votive equates to an act of self-portraiture, in which 'individuals remain anonymous, but nonetheless they perform for others, and they deposit in the form of wax body parts, self-portraits'.[66] The portrait in question is not a traditional likeness of an individual; rather it is an evocation of spiritual and physical reality accomplished by equating one's own body with Christ's body. Crucially, in the case of late medieval miracle healing, this is done through an intermediary that emphasises those salvific metaphors and becomes efficacious through the act of giving: a manufactured wax image.

In the print of Henry VI as a saint, as in other depictions of wax ex votos and their donors from the late Middle Ages, the votaries' bodies are reflected in the fragmented wax body parts they offer to seek health and well-being. Here, both the King and his petitioners participate in embodied forms of *imitatio*; through his posture and his emblems (the orb, the crozier, the ermine cloak), Henry takes on the physical appearance of a saint, surrounded by supplicants in need of his help. These supplicants, meanwhile, perform their own *imitatio*. They are pierced by arrows and cut by knives, suffering, with Christ as their model. By donating wax ex votos in the forms of their own bodies, votaries added another layer to the paradigm of giving and imitation that yielded salvation and physical health. Donors gave material goods to secure a saint's favour, but the material goods they gave worked best when they pictured the donors themselves. Likeness made these ex votos work. The action that ultimately secured a donor's health was to represent oneself in an image – and the more obviously that image resembled its donor through weight, measure, or other physical and visual similarities, the more effective their plea would be. Votaries made and gave images of themselves. In donating images in wax, late medieval English votaries conflated their own bodies with their moulded wax images. These were not recognisable portraits, but nevertheless they posited a similarity between the image of the person they represented with that person's physical body, using surrogate, waxen body parts to reference the specific donors who gave them.

Notes

1 Rawcliffe, *Medicine & Society*, 1997, pp. 21–23; see also Townsend, 'Votive Offerings', 2003, p. 432.
2 Wilson, 'The Arts of the Great Church', 2003, pp. 356–357.
3 Weinryb, 'Votive Materials', 2018, pp. 33–59.

4 Christopher Wood notes that because records of votive giving are skewed toward those shrines recorded in saints' canonisation hearings, our evidence is limited toward the shrines of later medieval saints. Wood, 'The Votive Scenario', 2011, p. 213.
5 Finucane, *Miracles and Pilgrims*, 1995, pp. 83–99.
6 On the etymology of the terms votive and ex voto, see Wood, 'Public and Private Dimensions', 2018, p. 70.
7 Bell and Dale, 'The Medieval Pilgrimage Business', 2011; Michele Bacci also analyses the connection between likeness and efficacy in the case of Italian votive giving. See Bacci 'Italian Ex-Votos and Pro-Anima Images in the Late Middle Ages', 2016, pp. 79–80. Verity Platt's claim that naturalism adds to the perceived effect of votive giving in ancient Greece rests on this concept of the lasting presence afforded by mimetic likeness. See Platt, 'Clever Devices and Cognitive Artefacts', 2018, p. 147.
8 The surviving wax ex-votos from Exeter cathedral still have fragments of string and, in some cases, wooded sticks attached. The strings poke out from the wax, indicating that these figures were made with the intention of being hung up near the shrine. See Radford, 'The Wax Images', 1949, p. 164; see also Blick, 'Votives, Images, Interaction', 2011, pp. 55–57.
9 Records of imported wax from the Hanseatic region make clear the high value ascribed to the substance. Most household wax used in Southern England was locally produced from tallow. In contrast, luxurious wax used in religious settings came from abroad. See Harwood, 'Trade and Consumption Patterns', 2008.
10 Hugo van der Velden offers a succinct differentiation of types of iconic portraits donated in the late Middle Ages: 'parts of the body were obviously donated in connection with specific maladies or injuries (with the probable exception of heads and portrait busts) whereas human figures and votive portraits had a wider application. In essence, however, there is no difference between these two types of images [...]'. Van der Velden, *The Donor's Image*, 2000, p. 219.
11 The phrase 'provisional subject' conforms to Emily Steiner's description of naming conventions in late medieval English literature. Steiner, 'Naming and Allegory', 2007, p. 257.
12 Schlosser, 'The History of Portraiture in Wax', 2008, p. 177.
13 On objects produced serially in late medieval and early modern Northern Europe, see Powell, 'A Point "Ceaselessly Pushed Back"', 2006.
14 Von Schlosser's essay was originally published in 1910 as 'Geschichte der Porträtbildnerei in Wachs', 1910–1911. Von Schlosser's publication gives significantly more attention to the use of wax as a portrait medium than another foundational essay connecting wax to early portraiture published earlier that same decade: Warburg's 1902 essay positing wax portraiture as central to the advent of portraits in early modern Italian religious spaces, published as *Bildniskunst und florentinisches Bürgertum*, 1902. This essay is now available as Aby Warburg, 'The Art of Portraiture', 1999. The roots of this discourse go back to the sixteenth century, when Giorgio Vasari first wrote of life-sized wax votive figures, see Vasari, *Le vite*, 1875–1885, vol. 3, pp. 373–375.
15 Freedberg, *The Power of Images*, 1989, p. 97.
16 Rawcliffe, *Medicine & Society*, 1997, pp. 21–23.
17 Finucane, *Miracles and Pilgrims*, 1995, pp. 130–152.
18 Webb, *Medieval European Pilgrimage*, 2002, pp. 52–56.
19 Wood, 'Public and Private', 2018, p. 75; Van der Velden, *The Donor's Image*, 2000, p. 193
20 Lightbown, 'Ex-Votos in Gold and Silver', 1979, p. 354.
21 Blick, 'Votives, Images, Interaction', 2011, p. 44; Wood, 'Public and Private', 2018, p. 69.
22 Radford, 'The Wax Images', 1949, pp. 164–168.

23 Finucane, *Miracles and Pilgrims*, 1995, p. 98.
24 Blick, 'Votives, Images, Interaction', 2011, p. 98; see also Webb, *Pilgrimage in Medieval England*, 2002, pp. 71–72.
25 Duffy, *The Stripping of the Altars*, 1992, p. 197.
26 Rawcliffe, *Medicine & Society*, 1997, pp. 21–23.
27 On the incorporation of material substances from shrines into souvenirs, see Webb, *Medieval European Pilgrimage*, 2002, pp. 164–166.
28 Horst Bredekamp further explains the connection between a body and its image: 'The notion that images can be fully valid bodies in another form and consistency led not only to the practice of iconoclasm but also to the diametrically opposed alternative: that absent individuals or institutions might be rendered present with the help of images. To this belongs the practice of the votive cult, in which persons, or parts of their bodies, were displayed in the effort to bring about their true healing or to ensure that a successful recovery from illness would endure'. Bredekamp, 'Substitutive Image Acts', 2018, p. 179.
29 Haviland and Parish, 'A Brief Account', 1970, p. 52.
30 Haviland and Parish, 'A Brief Account', 1970, p. 52.
31 Von Schlosser provides an example of the practical considerations that went into the decision to display an effigy instead of a preserved body. 'In his will dated 1415, the Duc de Berry directed that his funeral should be of the utmost simplicity, except – as he added with Gallic frankness – that if "my body cannot be kept without stinking too much, let there be made an effigy of it"'. Schlosser, 'The History of Portraiture', 2008, p. 198.
32 Lightbown, 'Gold and Silver', 1979, p. 354.
33 Blick, 'Votives, Images, Interaction', 2011, p. 37.
34 Freedberg, *The Power of Images*, 1989, p. 157.
35 Schlosser, 'The History of Portraiture', 2008, p. 177.
36 Schlosser, 'The History of Portraiture', 2008, 205.
37 Didi-Huberman, 'Ex Voto: Image, Organ, Time', 2007, pp. 7–16.
38 Aby Warburg, 'The Art of Portraiture', 1999, p. 190.
39 Park, 'Impressed Images', 1998, p. 258; Albertus Magnus, 'Commentary on Aristotle', 2002, p. 132.
40 Making wax into body parts required similar techniques of moulding and stamping, resulting in figurines that carried with them the identities of the votaries who bought and donated them. See Kumler, 'The Multiplication of the Species', 2011, p. 187.
41 Using different colours of wax and metal seal matrices enabled medieval people to leave a personal mark, and the seal was taken as a personal emblem for the person it represented. Brigitte Bedos-Rezak shows that seals could be functioned as a form of non-mimetic portraiture in the Middle Ages, giving specific, fixed, visual form to their subject despite the lack of mimetic likeness. See Bedos-Rezak, 'Medieval Identity', 2000. See also Bedos-Rezak, *When Ego Was Imago*, 2011, pp. 140–160.
42 Van der Velden, *The Donor's Image*, 2000, p. 248.
43 Van der Velden, *The Donor's Image*, 2000.
44 Blick, 'Votives, Images, Interaction', 2011, p. 34.
45 Marks, 'Wills and Windows', 2004, pp. 245–252.
46 Blick, 'Votives, Images, Interaction', 2011, p. 34.
47 Blick, 'Votives, Images, Interaction', 2011, p. 34; on an additional window at Canterbury cathedral that depicts a trindle, see Koopmans, 'Visions, Reliquaries', 2015, p. 50.
48 Van der Velden, *The Donor's Image*, 2000, p. 253.
49 Emanuele Lugli argues that the necessary acts of touch that come with measurement augment the efficacy of measured objects. See Lugli, *The Making of Measure*, 2019, p. 155.

50 Lugli, *The Making of Measure*, 2019, p. 229.
51 Blick, 'Votives, Images, Interaction', 2011, p. 34.
52 Bredekamp, 'Substitutive Image Acts', 2018, p. 137.
53 This, again, differs from the ways in which wax seals can produce an image of the individual they represent. See Bedos-Rezak, 'Ego, Ordo, Communitas', 2009.
54 Freedberg, *The Power of Images*, 1989, p. 97.
55 This need to represent an event through metonymy or metaphor is in keeping with Michele Bacci's discussion of individual and prototype in votive giving. See Bacci, 'L'individu et tant que Prototype', 2011, pp. 3–4.
56 Bacci, 'L'individu et tant que Prototype', 2011, p. 155.
57 Perkinson, *The Likeness of the King*, 2009; see also Freedberg, *The Power of Images*, 1989, pp. 192–245.
58 Perkinson, 'Rethinking the Origins of Portraiture', 2007.
59 Duffy, *The Stripping of the Altars*, 1992, p. 198; Pächt and Alexander, *Illuminated Manuscripts in the Bodleian Library*, 1973, no. 880, p. 77.
60 In many respects these depicted petitioners are more similar to the late medieval English 'wound man' than they are to typical scenes of votive giving. On the wound man, see Orlemanski, *Symptomatic Subjects*, 2019; see also Hartnell, 'Wording the Wound Man', 2017.
61 Duffy, *Stripping of the Altars*, 1992, p. 198
62 Freedberg, *The Power of Images*, 1989, p. 97.
63 Sapoznik, 'Bees in the medieval economy', 2019, p. 1153.
64 Blick, 'Votives, Images, Interaction', 2011, 32.
65 Wood, 'The Votive Scenario', 2011, p. 226.
66 Wood, 'The Votive Scenario', 2011, p. 223.

Source 2

Stefan Falimirz' *O ziołach* (1534): the first medical text published in Polish

Julia Czapla

In the 1480s, a new genre of medical texts called the *Gardens of Health* appeared.[1] These compendia described medicinal, culinary, and occasionally biological properties of plants and animals. Johannes Wonnecke von Cuba's first *Gart der Gesundheit* quoted numerous earlier texts, notably Pliny's *Historia naturalis* and Dioscorides's *De materia medica*. To make his text genuinely useful for medical practitioners – physicians, surgeons, barbers, midwives, apothecaries, and herbalists – he carefully separated fact from myth. Wonnecke also ensured that *Gart* featured new, accurate woodcuts created by local artists in Mainz, who based their images at least partly on observations of live plants and animals.

Gart turned out to be extremely popular. Until the 1530s new editions, translations and adaptations appeared regularly. In this case study I will present a Polish version of the *Gart* (Figure S2.1). Its full title is also a table of contents:

> *O ziołach y o moczy gich. O paleniu wodek z zioł. O oleykach przyprawianiu. O rzeczach zamorzkich. O zwierzętach, o ptaczech y o ribach. O kamieniu drogim. O urinie, o pulsie y o inych znamionach. O rodzeniu dziatek. O naucze gwiazdeczney. O stawianiu baniek. Y o puszczaniu krwie. O rządzeniu czasu powietrza morowego. O lekarzstwach doswiadczonych na wiele niemoczy. O naucze barwierzkiey.*[2]

Stefan Falimirz wrote it with the help of Andrzej Glaber (Jędrzej of Kobylin), Szymon of Łowicz, and Józef Zimmerman.[3] Florian Ungler, one of the most active Cracovian printers of the era, published it in 1534. Therefore, it is the oldest Polish medicinal text that precedes better known herbals by Marcin Siennik by thirty and thirty-four years respectively.[4]

Falimirz' compendium was quite popular as a simple and concise healthcare handbook. It was even adapted and reissued eight years later by Ungler's widow Helena, who inherited his printing shop.[5] This second

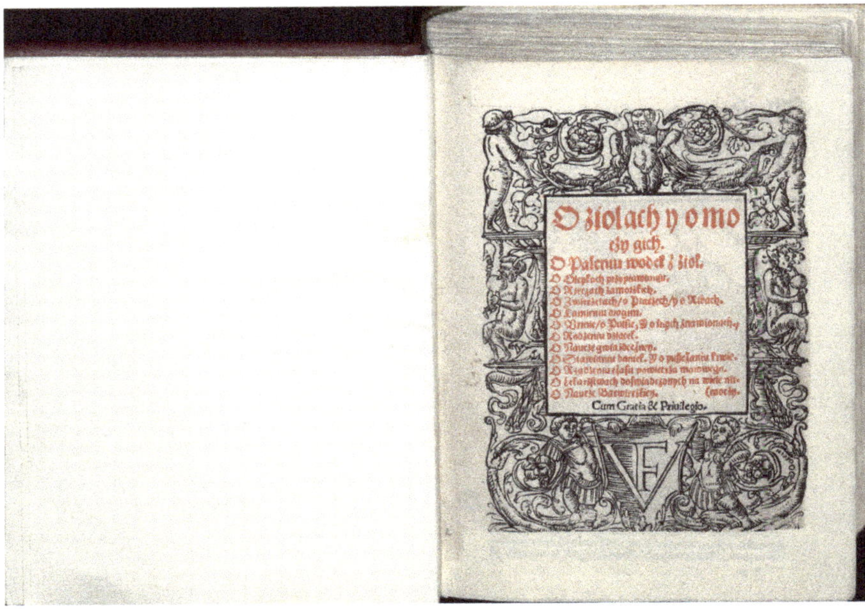

Figure S2.1 *O ziołach*, Kraków 1534, title page. Warszawa, Biblioteka Narodowa. Image credit: Warszawa, Biblioteka Narodowa

version was then reprinted in 1556.[6] In general, however, medical practitioners used it but not university-trained medical professionals. Marcin of Urzędów, a late sixteenth-century herbalist, deemed it outdated and full of unproven and fanciful stories. Historians of science rediscovered *O ziołach* only in the late nineteenth century.[7] Since then, it has proven valuable as primary source materials for historians of biology and medicine trying to identify Polish medieval and early modern names of plants and medical terminology.[8] There are also a few essays and articles on particular chapters of the compendium and its illustrations,[9] but no comprehensive study.

Unlike his successors in the field of Polish herbal and healthcare manuals, Falimirz most likely was not a medical professional. He lived as a courtier of the Polish magnate, and one of the richest men in the early sixteenth-century Poland, Jan Tęczyński, sword-bearer of Cracovian voivodeship and Podolian voivode (in 1534). Therefore, Falimirz spent a lot of time in Tenczyn (Tęczyński family estate) and the capital city, Cracow (situated twenty-four kilometres east of Tenczyn). He knew many nobles and intellectuals of Jagiellonian Poland. He decided to translate Latin *Hortus sanitatis* and adapt it for use in Cracow thanks to the encouragement of friends and acquaintances. Falimirz explicitly named his main motivation in the dedication for Tęczyński:

> Many cities in this famous Crown [of Poland], as well as elsewhere, have no physicians, no apothecaries. Probably many men who were virtuous and valuable to the republic would be cured. But since they have no medical advice, they have to leave this world before their time. (*Wiele miast w tey tho sławney Koronie iako y indzie Lekarzów y aptek mieć nie mogą. Snadzby się wiele zacznych ludzi a rzeczy pospolitey potrzebnych wyleczyło. Ale iże porady lekarzkiey nie maią: muszą przed czasem zchodzić z tego świata*).[10]

Falimirz produced an extensive compendium, filling its 435 folios with a wealth of pharmaceutical and medical knowledge. The chapters listed in the title discuss the following topics: properties of plants, methods of vodka distillation (here meaning production of essential oils), non-European plants and substances, mainly metals, salts, and balms, various animals and their properties, gems, diagnostic methods (analysing urine, measuring pulse, etc.), midwifery, astrology and weather, bloodletting and cupping, treatment of the plague (as well as early epidemic recommendations), drug preparation, and rudimentary surgery. Divided into two sections, the text focuses first on the properties of substances commonly found in apothecaries or sought for personal use, and then serves as a healthcare manual for barbers, midwives, and village healers without formal university training.

Almost six hundred woodcuts illustrate this all-encompassing compendium. Although some reproduce other illustrations, all blocks were made in Cracow. Ungler had one of the largest printing shops in early sixteenth-century Poland and he employed woodcutters.[11] Unfortunately, we know nothing about them – neither their names, their nationality, nor even how many there were. We can only guess it was an experienced local woodcutter with a few assistants. Although not a professional scientific illustrator on a par with some of his German contemporaries, he was a decent observer of nature and certainly had some experience creating scientific illustrations (in the early sixteenth-century sense of that term). He was probably the same person who made seventy woodcuts for Aemilius Macer's *De herbarium virtutibus* published by Ungler two years earlier.[12] Of course, he used various sources to illustrate *O ziołach*, most notably some edition of *Gart der Gesundheit* or its Latin adaptation, *Hortus sanitatis*. It is impossible to definitively claim which edition was used. Most Polish researchers suggested the first edition of *Hortus sanitatis* from 1491 as the primary source of inspiration.[13] However, Cracovian woodcuts show more similarities to later editions, mainly to German translations of *Hortus*. More specifically, it seems that at least some images were created specifically for Falimirz' compendium.

Full-page woodcuts accompany the compendium's title page and each chapter, summarising the chapter's content. The pharmaceutical section features images of various specimens and items set in landscapes or apothecary interiors, while the medicinal section includes depictions of procedures such as urine analysis, pulse measurement, and childbirth. Most chapters are richly illustrated, with the majority of the 260 woodcuts found in the chapter on plants (Figure S2.2). The illustrators used some blocks made for *De herbarium virtutibus* and copied over one hundred of them from the *Hortus*, making these conventional depictions. Plants are shown whole – from roots to leaves, often in bloom or bearing fruit. The decision to reproduce previously published images can be explained by Falimirz' wish to create a reliable source of information for people who would have no other source. Plants needed to be easily identified, or else the compendium would not have been helpful for a small-town herbalist or apothecary who needed to quickly recognise plants found in the wild or harvested in one's garden. That is why they were carefully copied. This chapter is accompanied by a short and unillustrated description of distillation methods.

Illustrators had more freedom in other pharmaceutical chapters. Non-European plants (seventy entries) and substances (twenty-two entries) that arrived in Cracow were already processed, and their images give the appearance as if they were observed there. These illustrations show plants from roots to leaves, but often in a wilted, dried, or damaged state. Falimirz knew little about substances from Asia and Africa, such as various minerals, so he depicted them generically as blobs in different shapes and sizes, or simply as containers like jars or barrels. He likely intended these images to be coloured to aid identification.

These two pharmaceutical chapters were more or less faithfully translated from the *Gart*. The fourth chapter, which covers animals – thirty-five

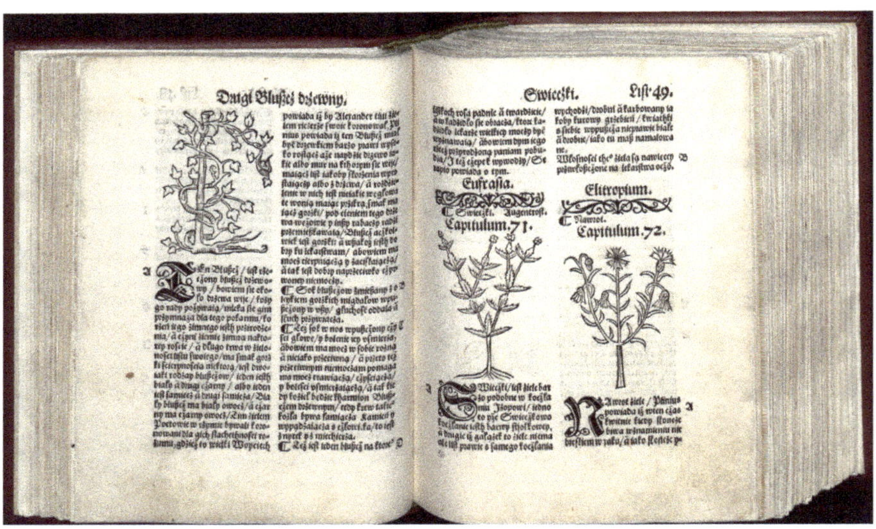

Figure S2.2 *O ziołach*, Kraków 1534., cap. 1, fols 48v–49r: Ivy, eyebright, goldenrod. Warszawa, Biblioteka Narodowa. Image credit: Warszawa, Biblioteka Narodowa

entries on quadrupeds, thirty-two on birds and other flying creatures, and forty-eight on fish and aquatic life – demanded greater attention from both Falimirz and his illustrators (Figure S2.3). These are primarily European animals, both domestic and wild. Unlike his German predecessors, Falimirz largely omitted Asian and African animals, as well as marine fauna.[14] Therefore, he excluded almost all legendary animals that crowded other treatises and compendia of the early sixteenth century, except for a 'sea dragon' that looks very much like a crocodile. Many animals unfamiliar in Cracow, such as whales and crocodiles, are depicted fantastically, while those kept in the royal menagerie in Zwierzyniec, like lions and camels, appear more realistic. However, Falimirz generally tended to describe animals he knew first hand and even included many freshwater fish typical of central Europe.[15]

The following chapter on precious stones describes forty-four gems. With no established conventions for depicting minerals – and no crystallographic knowledge to guide him – the Cracovian illustrator opted to show people assessing or using these substances, only occasionally depicting the minerals themselves. This approach was hardly original; at the time, rudimentary mineralogy formed part of pharmaceutical knowledge, and these entries and images may have been adapted from any edition of the *Hortus sanitatis*. These German illustrations also generally show people holding or procuring precious gems, stones, and metals, like a goldsmith showing the rings or a man mining the silver. However, they are far more

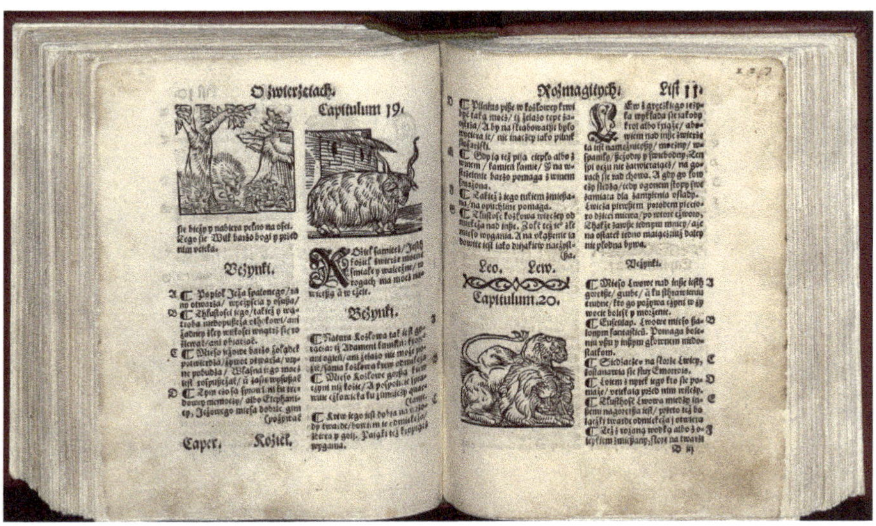

Figure S2.3 *O ziołach*, Kraków 1534, cap. 4, fols 10v–11r: hedgehog, goat, lion. Warszawa, Biblioteka Narodowa. Image credit: Warszawa, Biblioteka Narodowa

detailed than Cracovian images. This suggests that Ungler's illustrator may not have fully understood what he was meant to depict.

The medicinal part of the compendium begins with the chapter on rudimentary sixteenth-century diagnostics. The most common practices included visual and olfactory analysis of urine and blood. The colour of urine was the primary aspect. However, it was impossible to show it on black-and-white woodcuts. Falimirz gives thirty-one detailed descriptions based on *Hortus sanitatis*, but illustrates them with the images of glass bottles (Figure S2.4). Though the shadows are delicately marked, these illustrations were intended to be coloured as described in the text. Unlike urine analysis, pulse measurement and other diagnostic methods were relatively new at the time, so Falimirz devotes only a few pages to them. Full-page title woodcuts accompany this section, depicting physicians at work, along with illustrations showing an additional urine sample and a man defecating.

In the following chapter, Falimirz gives a description of the basics of midwifery (Figure S2.5). Like the botanical one, this chapter must have been essential, as for many readers it would have been the only source of information on pregnancy and childbirth. To ensure its reliability, Falimirz (or, more likely, Glaber) translated one of the most relevant works on the subject, namely Eucharius Rösslin's *Der Schwangeren Frauen und Hebammen Rosengarten*.[16] This treatise and its illustrations were considered a standard of the knowledge of obstetricians and 'paediatricians'. The verbatim translation contains nineteen carefully copied illustrations showing the child's position *in utero*, with the illustrators including an image of the birthing chair.

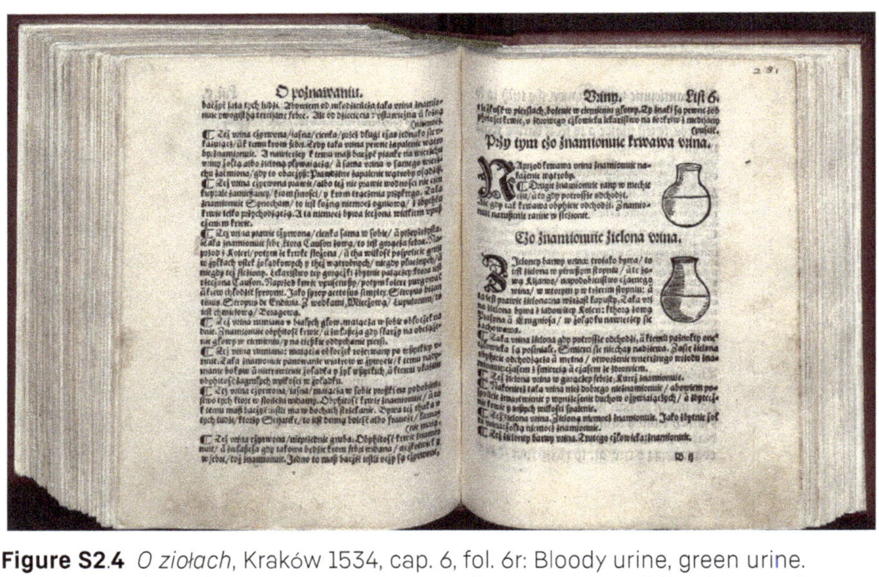

Figure S2.4 *O ziołach*, Kraków 1534, cap. 6, fol. 6r: Bloody urine, green urine. Warszawa, Biblioteka Narodowa. Image credit: Warszawa, Biblioteka Narodowa

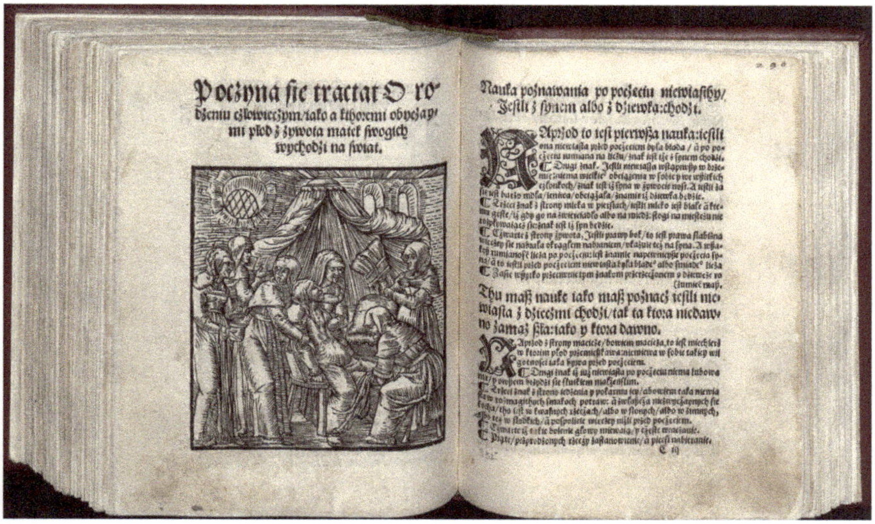

Figure S2.5 *O ziołach*, Kraków 1534, cap. 6, fol. 14v: Title page of the chapter on midwifery. Warszawa, Biblioteka Narodowa. Image credit: Warszawa, Biblioteka Narodowa

In sixteenth-century medicine, astrology and meteorology were considered parts of medical knowledge as they affected human health. The chapter on stars first discusses what happens each month. The depictions of these activities accompany these entries. The woodcuts are printed from the blocks made for the calendar published by Ungler in 1531.[17] The second part of this chapter presents a zodiac and planet table in which Falimirz describes the properties of all celestial bodies and their symbolic representations. He then briefly discusses the four seasons and adds another short table on the relationships between weather, seasons, and planets.

Unfortunately, it is unclear which text Falimirz actually translated, but in the following chapters, he shifts his focus to medical practices, beginning with descriptions of various bloodletting techniques illustrated by a woodcut of a naked man with an exposed chest and abdomen. The illustration gives a visual reference with the important bloodletting cuts marked (Figure S2.6). Falimirz next describes the practice of cupping, accompanied by an illustration demonstrating the proper positioning of cups. Much of this chapter details the medical recommendations and procedures relevant during times of plague, illustrated solely by an image depicting the bloodletting of an infected patient.[18] This chapter is inseparable from the two following it. The next one is a basic *pharmacopoeia* – a compendium of directions and recipes for drug-making. For easier use, Falimirz sorts them by affliction: salves for wounds and skin diseases, with basic surgical procedures described separately in the final chapter.

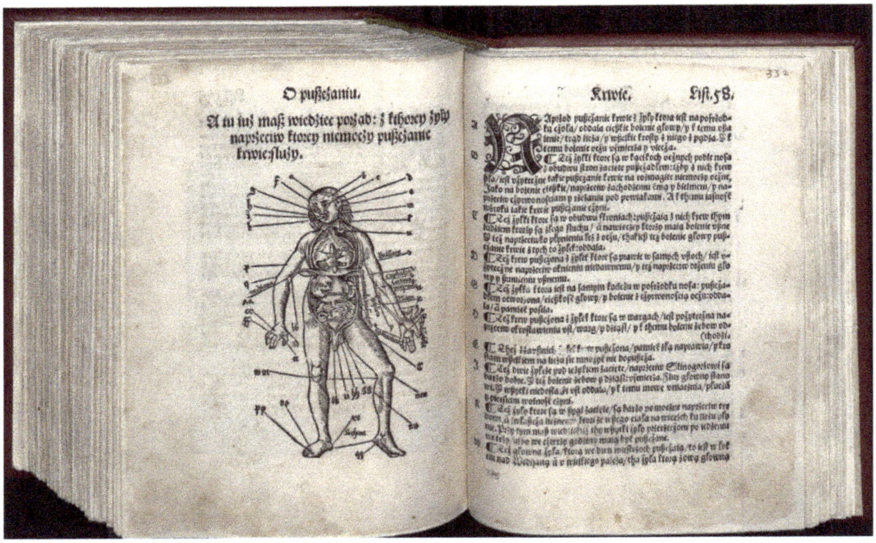

Figure S2.6 *O ziołach*, Kraków 1534, cap. 6, fol. 57v: Diagram of bloodletting. Warszawa, Biblioteka Narodowa. Image credit: Warszawa, Biblioteka Narodowa

Nobody can call *O ziołach* groundbreaking from a medicinal standpoint. However, it is undeniable that this compendium, as the first Polish text of the genre, was incredibly popular among Poles of the sixteenth century and should be considered one of the most important sources on the state of Polish medical knowledge of the era. *O ziołach* owes its popularity at least partially to its illustrations which must have been a great help for smalltown medical practitioners. To conclude, I wish to once more quote Falimirz who must have been extremely happy with his publication:

> my dear Florian not only did not skimp on great cost, but also – by his incessant care – looked after it, so that these Polish books were with utmost care, best and most beautifully adorned and beatified by new letters and wonderful figures. (*moy miły Florian swoiego wielkiego nakładu nie telko nie litował, Ale też ustawiczną robotą swą około tego tako pilnował, Jakoby nasnadniey, nalepiey, nachędożey nowemi Literami y czudnemi Figurami ty Polskie księgi ozdobił y ochędożył*).[19]

Notes

1 First German *Gart der Gesundheit* was published in Mainz in 1485 and its first Latin version, *Hortus sanitatis* in 1491. See Baumann and Baumann, *Die Mainzer Kräuterbuch-Inkunabeln*, 2010.

2 Falimirz, *O ziołach*, 1534. It was recently published as facsimile edition by Wiesław Wydra, see Falimirz, *O ziołach*, 2017. The full text is also available online in Polona (Polish National Library's digital library). The title can be translated as: 'On plants and their might. On distilling vodkas from herbs. On oils making. On things from beyond the seas. On animals, birds, and fish. On precious stones. On urine, pulse,

and other symptoms. On childbirth. On the science of stars. On cupping and blood-letting. On recommendations for the time of plague. On tried-and-true drugs for many ailments. On surgical knowledge.'

3 Hryniewiecki, 'Falimirz', 1948, pp. 354–355.

4 Siennik, *Lekarstwa doświadczone*, 1564, Siennik, *Herbarz*, 1568.

5 *O Ziolach tutecznych y zamorskich*, 1542. This edition – falsely attributed to Hieronim Spiczyński – was discussed primarily by Rostafiński, 'Nasza literatura', 1888, pp. 172–174, and most recently by Krzak-Weiss, 'Natura', 2020, pp. 207–211.

6 *O Ziolach tutecznych y zamorskich*, 1556.

7 It was first described by Rostafiński, 'Porównanie', 1888, pp. 117–125.

8 For example, Rostafiński, 'Porównanie', 1888, pp. 117–125; Rostafiński, *Nasza literatura*, 1888, pp. 166–171; Rostafiński, *Symbola*, vol. 2, 1900, pp. 66–72, 257–295; Jankowiak, 'Terminologia medyczna', 2000, pp. 37–50; Jankowiak, 'Szesnastowieczne słownictwo', 2005, pp. 151–158; Jankowiak, *Słownictwo medyczne*, 2005–2006; Jankowiak, 'Zapożyczenia', 2010, pp. 201–213.

9 For example, Kołodziejczyk, 'Das sogennante Herbarium', 1937, pp. 289–301; Szostak, 'Zielnik', 1977, pp. 7–50; Szostak, 'Zielnik', 1977, pp. 4–42; Roeske, 'Polskie drzeworyty', 1980, pp. 325–329; Krzysztofik, 'Elementy', 2015, pp. 89–112; Zemanek (et al.), 'Selected', 2009, pp. 179–183; Czapla, 'Niezwykłe zwierzęta', 2013, pp. 257–267; Szymański, 'Przyczynek', 2015, pp. 204–223; Krzak-Weiss, 'Natura', 2020, pp. 203–207; Czapla, 'Ikonografia owadów', 2021, pp. 24–29.

10 Falimirz, *O ziołach*, fol. 2r.

11 *O ziołach* is not his only illustrated work, although by far the largest one. On Ungler's printing activity and publications, see Bułhak, 'Ungler', 1983, pp. 307–311.

12 Macer, *De herbarium virtutibus*, 1532. It was the first herbal published in Poland. See Krzak-Weiss, 'Natura', 2020, pp. 201–203.

13 Kołodziejczyk, 'Das sogennante Herbarium', 1937, p. 300.

14 There are only twenty-four non-European animals, as listed and discussed in Czapla, 'Niezwykłe zwierzęta', 2013, pp. 357–367.

15 Falimirz, *O ziołach*, 1534, fols 41r–46r.

16 He most likely used the Augsburg edition published in 1528 (Krzak-Weiss, 'Natura', 2020, p. 205). Cf. Górnicki, 'Zarys piśmiennictwa', 1939–1947, pp. 75–75, who suggested 1532 Latin translation, *De partu hominis*.

17 Cf. Chojecka, 'Krakowska grafika', 1963, pp. 356–357.

18 While *morowe powietrze* is generally translated as plague (a disease caused by *Yersinia pestis*), the recommendations seem to be more relevant to malaria.

19 Falimirz, *O ziołach*, 1534, fol. 2r.

3

The anatomy of whiteness in late medieval Italy

Robert Brennan

Skin colour was a significant issue in medieval medicine. In one respect it signified disease: yellow skin, for example, could be a sign of cholera.[1] In another respect it indicated the 'complexion' (*complexio*) of an individual patient: the overall balance in a given body between the elemental qualities of hot, cold, wet, and dry.[2] Paler skin was generally identified with colder, wetter complexions, whereas darker skin was identified with hotter, drier complexions. By extension, medical writers often attributed the white skin of Northern Europeans to the coldness and wetness of their environment, while attributing the black skin of sub-Saharan Africans to the heat and dryness of equatorial regions. On this basis, they drew sweeping conclusions about the physical, behavioural, and mental proclivities of the world's peoples.[3]

Recent scholarship in the history of science has identified this complexional framework, which was passed down from the tradition of Greco-Roman medicine, as a significant factor in the development of racialised thinking in Europe.[4] Meanwhile, another important body of scholarship has traced the invention of whiteness as a category of European identity back to thirteenth-century France, drawing largely on artistic and literary sources.[5] Questions have been raised as to whether these two traditions – one artistic and literary, the other medical and scientific – bear any direct relation to one another.[6] This essay will argue for the plausibility of such a connection at one canonically important juncture in European art history: Florentine painting in the era of Cimabue (c. 1240–1302) and Giotto (c. 1267–1337).

To set up this connection, the essay proceeds through three parts. The first section draws upon visual evidence to establish anatomy – and in particular, soft-tissue anatomy – as an area of active exchange between painters and physicians in the period. The second section then turns to the writings of Florentine physicians, in order to link medical understandings of white skin with concurrent developments in painting. The third section concludes by considering several wider social implications of these developments, focusing in particular on the relationship between whiteness and gender.[7]

At the outset it is important to acknowledge the difficulties of such an argument. In an important essay, Daniela Bohde has highlighted the absence of any phrase that could be translated as 'skin colour' in Italian art writing from the fifteenth to seventeenth centuries, showing that the sources focus overwhelmingly on 'flesh' (*carne*), and hardly ever on 'skin' (*pelle*).[8] Subsequently these findings have been invoked to dismiss considerations of race from scholarship on flesh tones in late medieval art.[9] This essay does not dispute Bohde's analysis of the artistic literature, but instead draws attention to a different body of sources: a tradition of Florentine medical writing, contemporary with Cimabue and Giotto, in which distinctions between 'skin' and 'flesh' (*cutis* and *caro*), as well as discussions of 'skin colour' (*color cutis*), coincide directly with references to visual art.

Painted crosses

The transition from Cimabue to Giotto has long been regarded as a pivotal moment in the history of Italian painting. The earliest known writer to comment upon it was Dante Alighieri, a contemporary of both artists, who observed that 'in painting, Cimabue thought he held the field, and now it is Giotto they acclaim'.[10] Later on in the 1380s and 1390s, Filippo Villani wrote the earliest surviving history of Florentine painting, in which the passage from Cimabue to Giotto looms large as a central development.[11] In the centuries that followed, subsequent histories of Florentine painting largely followed suit.[12] For example, the 1550 edition of Giorgio Vasari's *Lives of the Artists* begins with a biography of Cimabue, but characterises Giotto as a primary instigator of 'modern art'.[13]

All of these writers were familiar with Cimabue and Giotto's works in Florence. Among them, one particularly prominent juxtaposition was a pair of monumental crucifixes made for two of Florence's most important churches: one by Cimabue for the Franciscan Church of Santa Croce, the other by Giotto for the Dominican Church of Santa Maria Novella (Figures 3.1 and 3.2). The relationship between these two crosses is exceedingly complex and multifaceted. Evaluating it is complicated by the extensive damaged suffered by Cimabue's work during the flood of the Arno river in 1966, as well as continuing debates over chronology: some scholars divide the two works by more than a decade, while others date them within a span of as little as a few years.[14] In what follows, I wish to discuss just one narrowly selective aspect of the comparison, which concerns the two artists' treatment of anatomy.

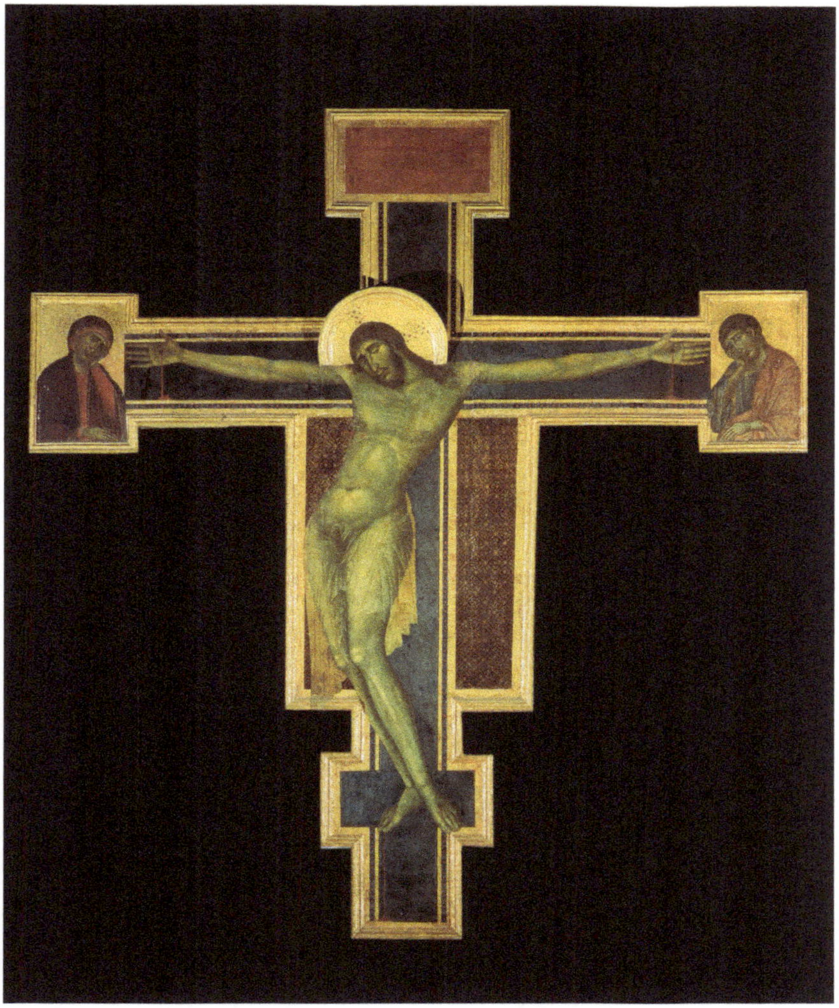

Figure 3.1 Cimabue, Crucifix, before 1288. Florence, Santa Croce (photograph before 1966). Image credit: Wikipedia Commons

Giotto was clearly thinking differently about the body as a skeletal structure, weighing it down and bending it strictly at the joints, in contrast to the gracefully meandering curve of the body in Cimabue's painting. Cimabue derives this curvature from a tradition of Byzantine imagery that artists like Giunta Pisano had introduced into Italy around the 1230s.[15] From the carpentry of the two crosses, it appears that Giotto began his work with a similar sort of Byzantinising curve in mind, only to change directions midway through, in favour of the more rigorously analytic interplay of gravitational force and anatomical structure that we see today.[16]

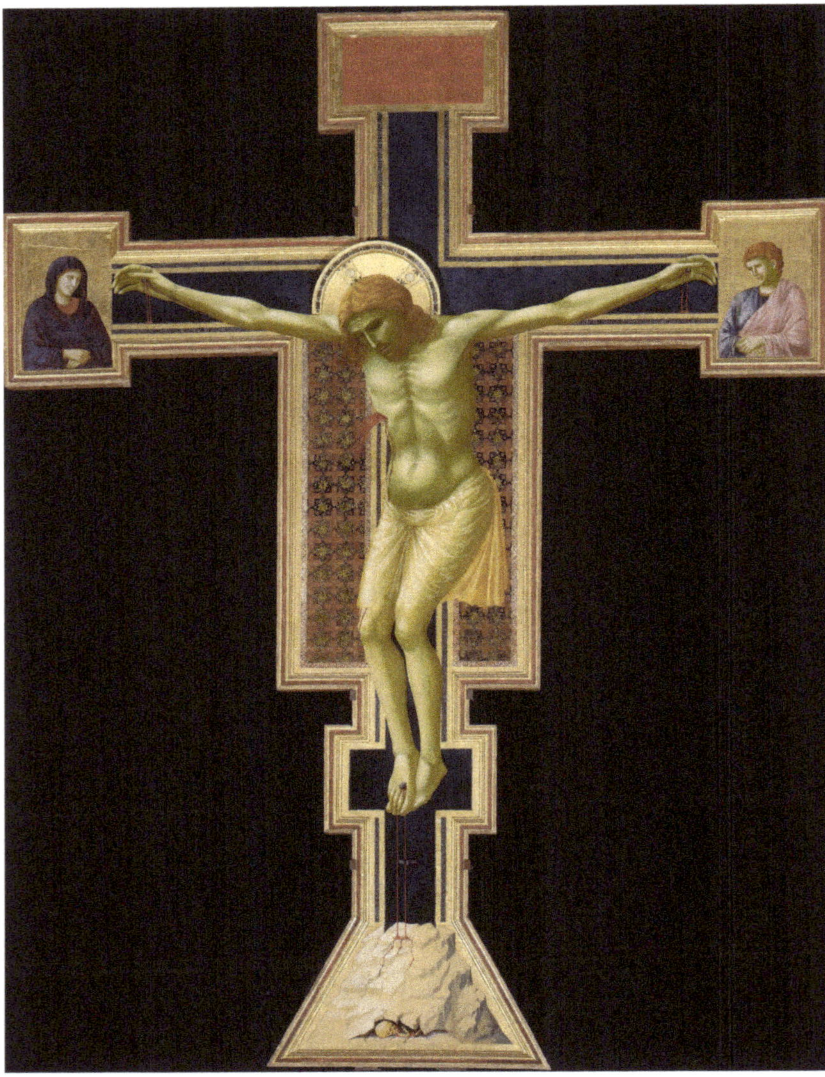

Figure 3.2 Giotto, Crucifix, after 1288, Florence, Santa Maria Novella. Image credit: Wikipedia Commons

Art historians have often linked this parting of ways to a famous passage in Cennino Cennini's *Libro dell'arte* (c. 1400), which states that Giotto 'changed the art from Greek into Latin, and made it modern'.[17]

As is well known, however, this difference is far from absolute, for Cimabue's cross already manifests a pronounced interest in anatomical details.[18] This becomes particularly evident on comparison with an earlier cross Cimabue had painted for the Dominicans of Arezzo, datable between about 1260 and 1272 (Figure 3.3).[19] Whereas at Arezzo, the muscles tend

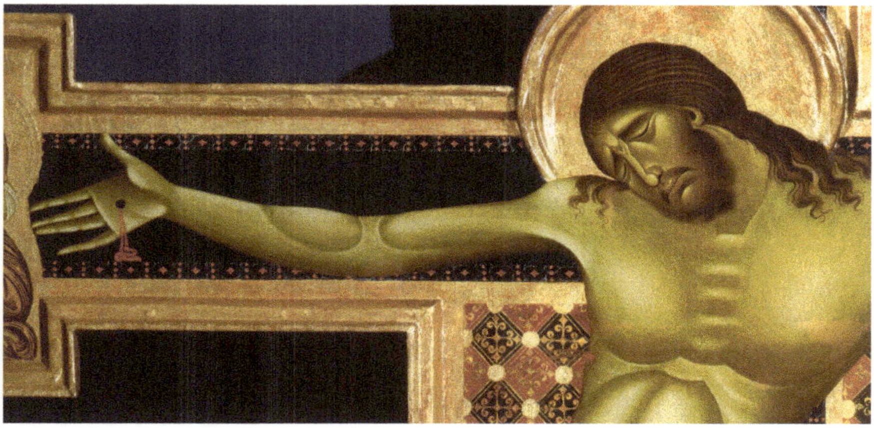

Figure 3.3.a Detail, Cimabue, Crucifix, c. 1260–1272. Arezzo, San Domenico. Image credit: Photo Scala, Florence [artwork in public domain]

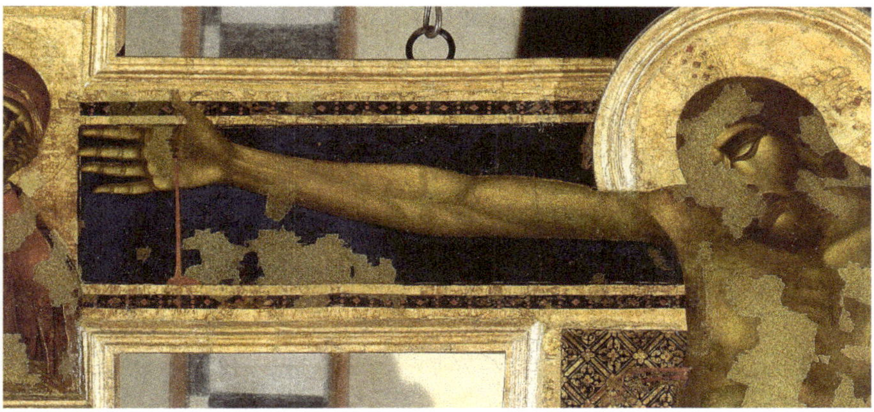

Figure 3.3.b Detail, Cimabue, Crucifix, before 1288. Florence, Santa Croce (current state). Image credit: Photo Scala, Florence [artwork in public domain]

to swell into abstract, crisply delineated volumes, at Santa Croce they consist almost entirely of smoothly blended tonal transitions that express distinctive anatomical functions. In Arezzo, for example, the lower contour of the arm bends like a chord hung between the nail and the shoulder socket, indifferent not only to the body's weight, but also to the semicircular bulges of muscle that sprout symmetrically around the elbow above. At Santa Croce, by contrast, the arm straightens out, tugged tight against the nail by a tension that passes visibly from the pectoral to the bicep through the 'Y'-shaped transition at the elbow and on to the tendons at the wrist. This is the same basic shift toward a functional conception of anatomy that would lead Giotto to rethink the structure of the torso and lower body at Santa Maria Novella.

In the decades after Giotto's early work for the Dominicans, he and his followers continued to develop and refine these principles in several more monumental crucifixes for Florentine churches (e.g., Figure 3.4). The Franciscans of Santa Croce in turn responded with a new monumental cross that pushed such anatomical investigations even further (Figure 3.5). Datable to the later 1320s, and generally attributed to a painter known as the Figline Master,[20] the work follows the precedent laid down by Giotto in some respects, such as the twisting musculature of the arms. But the Figline Master delves much deeper into such details as the veins and arteries of the arm, or the topography of the hand, where every last crease of skin is precisely tailored to the cusping of the palm and fingers around the

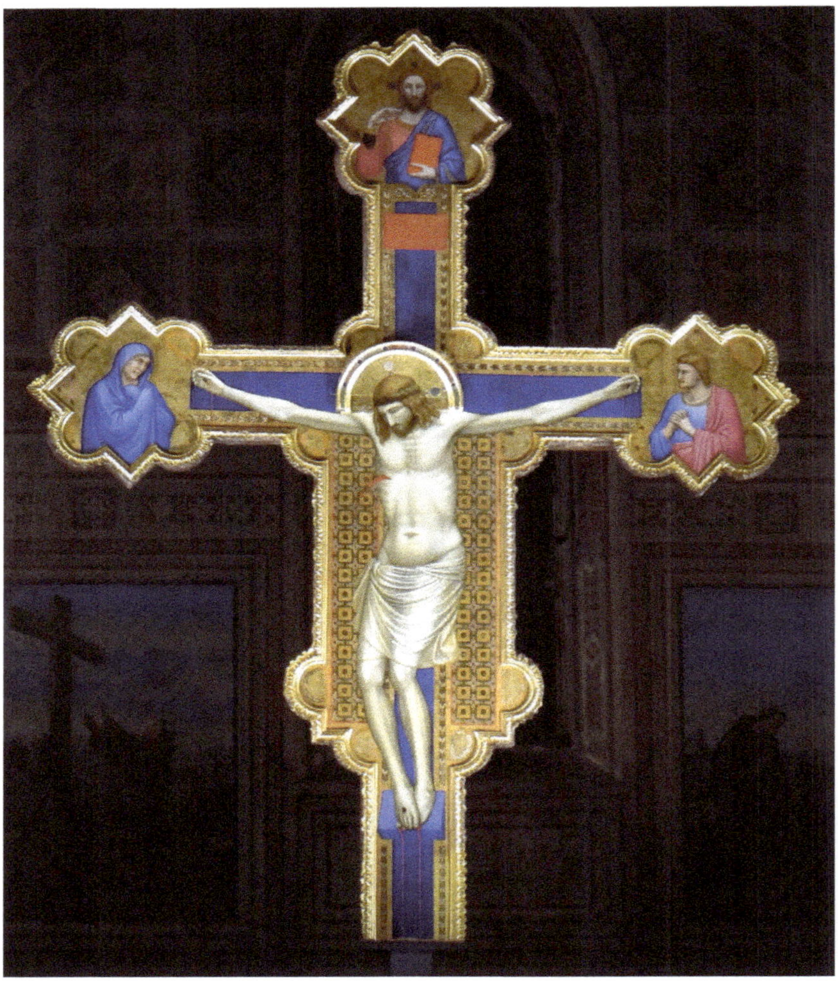

Figure 3.4 Detail, Giotto, Crucifix, c. 1315–1320. Florence, Ognissanti. Image credit: Wikipedia Commons

nail (Figure 3.6).[21] At the same time, he entirely rethinks the skeletal structure of the torso. The articulation of the rib cage is now so precise that an exact anatomical match can be found for each and every one of the true and false ribs (Figure 3.5).[22]

In light of these developments, it is easy to imagine how the history of Florentine painting in this period could be narrated as a series of ever deeper convergences with anatomical science. Such a story is in fact already hinted at by the earliest extant history of painting in Florence – the aforementioned text by Filippo Villani, written in the 1380s and 1390s. Villani's narrative begins with the transition from Cimabue to Giotto, but it is the later transition from Giotto to his followers that leads him to invoke

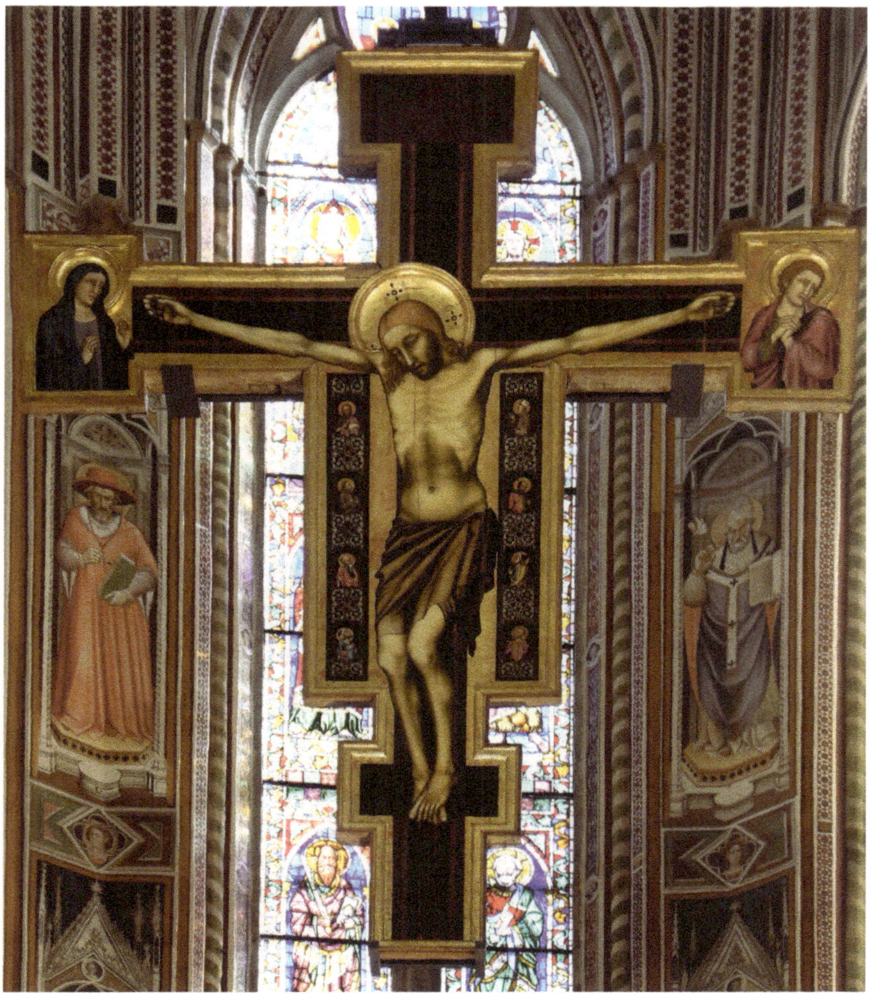

Figure 3.5 Figline Master, Crucifix, c. 1325–1330. Florence, Santa Croce. Image credit: Wikipedia Commons

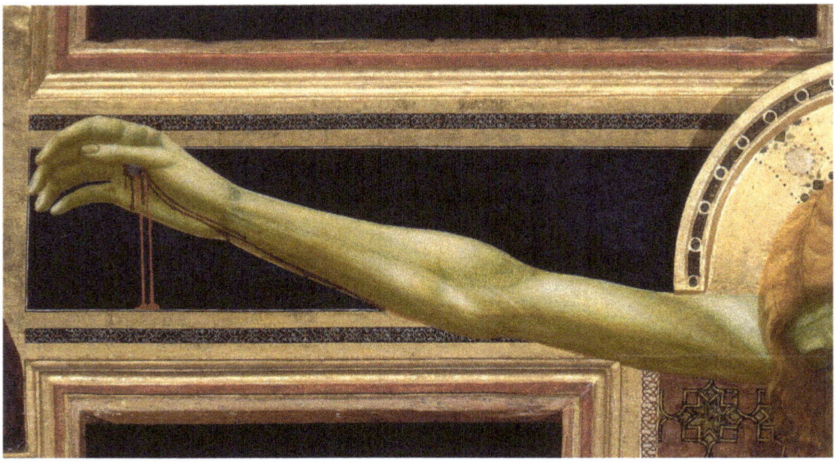

Figure 3.6.a Detail, Giotto, Crucifix, after 1288. Florence, Santa Maria Novella. Image credit: Photo Scala, Florence/Fondo Edifici di Culto – Min. dell'Interno [artwork in public domain]

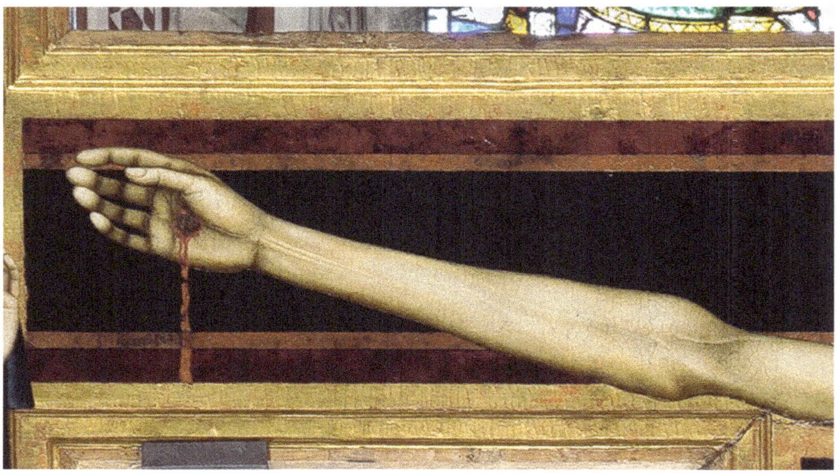

Figure 3.6.b Detail, Figline Master, Crucifix, c. 1325–1330. Florence, Santa Croce. Image credit: Photo Scala, Florence/Fondo Edifici di Culto – Min. dell'Interno [artwork in public domain]

anatomy. The passage concerns an artist named Stefano Fiorentino, a student of Giotto whose work is largely lost today.[23] What Villani says about Stefano is nevertheless relevant to the work of other anatomically inclined painters of this generation, such as the Figline Master:

> Stefano, the ape of nature, excelled in so great an imitation of [nature] that in the human bodies figured by him, the arteries, veins, nerves, and every last minute lineament are accurately gathered by physicians.[24]

Scholars have long understood this passage to mean that Stefano's figures were so lifelike that doctors used them to study anatomy.[25] Not long after Villani, however, the writings of Florentine artists suggest something more like a reciprocal exchange. In his aforementioned *Libro dell'arte* (c. 1400), Cennini has a chapter on 'the measures that a perfectly made body of man must have', in which he attempts to quantify the total number of bones in the body.[26] A few decades later, in his *Commentaries* on art, Lorenzo Ghiberti quotes extensively from the skeletal anatomy of two of the most authoritative medical writers of the period, Averroes and Avicenna.[27]

The crosses discussed thus far leave little doubt that skeletal anatomy had been an intense preoccupation among Tuscan painters for over a century by Ghiberti's time.[28] And yet when Villani describes the interest that physicians took in painting, he points to a strikingly different subcategory of human anatomy: 'arteries, veins, nerves, and every last minute lineament'. On first glance, one might dismiss this comment as a mere rhetorical flourish, as if to say, 'every last conceivable detail'. However, the crosses surveyed above demonstrate the persistence of an equally intensive interest in this same sphere of soft tissue anatomy, sustained across several generations of leading Tuscan painters, from Cimabue to Giotto and the Figline Master. From Villani's account, it would be easy to chalk this interest up to a straightforward pursuit of naturalism. If we turn to the works of Florentine medical writers during this same period, however, a more complicated range of interests comes into view.

For a relevant corpus of medical writings, we need look no further than Villani himself, who outlines a history of Florentine medicine in the same treatise as his history of painting. Villani's chapter on medicine begins with Taddeo Alderotti (d. 1295), then moves on to Alderotti's pupils, Pietro Torrigiano (d. c. 1320) and Dino del Garbo (d. 1327), before concluding with the latter's son and pupil, Tommaso del Garbo (d. 1370).[29] While all of these physicians taught at universities outside of Florence, they maintained close ties with their hometown, and in some cases, their biographies overlap rather closely with the paintings observed thus far. Dino del Garbo, for example, was well connected with the Franciscans of Santa Croce, and was living in Florence when the Figline Master was painting his cross for the church.[30] A testament of these connections is a portrait of Dino from a lost fresco in the nave of Santa Croce, where he appeared among the saved in a *Last Judgment* by Andrea di Orcagna.[31] It thus seems likely that Dino's portrait stood in direct view of at least one, if not both, of the monumental crosses by Cimabue and the Figline Master, whose locations in the church are undocumented, but are usually thought to have been installed around the rood screen or high altar.[32]

Medical perspectives

Much of what Florentine physicians have to say about visual art was prompted by references in earlier medical authorities, such as Hippocrates,

Galen, and Avicenna. A prominent example can be found in Galen's many discussions of 'balanced complexion' (*complexio aequalis*). To say that a given patient had a hot or cold complexion was to presuppose a normative, perfectly equilibrated complexion, against which variations could be named and judged. Galen understood this 'balanced complexion' as a purely theoretical construct: an ideal, a matter of logical necessity – not a complexion that one would ever actually expect to see in practice. For this reason, he repeatedly compares it to the ideal, normative status of Polykleitos's *Canon* in the art of sculpture.[33] As a result, virtually every medical theorist of this period found it necessary to comment on the artistic achievements of Polykleitos (see Source 3). And as they worked through the complications of Galen's concept, the discussion also increasingly came to converge with contemporary developments in painting.

In a treatise datable between 1277 and 1283, Taddeo Alderotti highlighted a basic difficulty posed by Galen's concept of balanced complexion: a contradiction regarding the skin colour that Galen attributes to it.[34] As Alderotti observes, Galen sometimes describes the skin of a perfectly balanced complexion as 'midway between white and dark' (*medius inter album et brunum*), whereas elsewhere, he writes of it as 'mixed of white and red' (*ex rubeo et albo commixtus*).[35] Alderotti resolves the contradiction by deciding in favour of white and red, but struggles to establish a definitive theoretical justification.[36] Along the way, however, he introduces a range of natural-philosophical principles relating to colour, as well as a reference to painting.

This reference occurs at a point in the argument where Alderotti seeks to distinguish between three different causes of colour in the body. First, there are colours caused by the humours. Second, there are colours that arise out of mixtures between different humours or elements. Third, in contrast to mixture, there is also the possibility of superimposition: 'certain colors are generated through overlaying (*supernatationem*), as when painters place one color on top of another and there results a third color'.[37] Alderotti adapts this threefold distinction directly from a passage in Aristotle's treatise, *De sensu et sensato*, including the point about painting.[38] In doing so, however, he significantly alters its meaning. Aristotle's discussion of painterly superimposition was typically understood in terms of motifs involving an overlay of discrete natural phenomena, such as the depiction of fish underwater.[39] Taddeo instead brings it to bear on the rendering of human skin. As such, he aligns it squarely with the standard method of blending flesh tones in a tempera or fresco painting among leading Italian painters of these same decades. To create a smooth transition from light to shade, the common practice was to lay down a darker base layer and superimpose it with a lighter tone that dissipated into the shadows.[40]

Alderotti articulates this principle of superimposition amidst a series of rather scattered, disparate reflections on colour. Subsequently, however, Florentine physicians went on to adapt it into a standard argument in favour of whiteness as a sign of perfectly balanced complexion. The crucial step seems to have been taken by Pietro Torrigiano in his widely influential *Plus quam commentum* (completed around 1320).[41] Torrigiano's argument begins by classifying skin among the parts of the body that Galen calls *radicalia*:

> [Galen] calls those members *radicalia*, which are hard and white, similar in color to semen, and called *radicalia* as if to say generated out of the 'root' (*ex radice*) – that is, the bones, cartilage, fat, nerves, and things of this kind.[42]

Having established this classification, he proceeds to the following conclusion:

> skin is by nature white, like the other members that Galen calls *radicalia* [...] but the blood and the flesh of the muscles, which are covered by the skin [...] are red; on the surface, the result will be a color mixed from both, because the skin itself, being thin, admits the color of whatever it touches.[43]

To make this case, Torrigiano adopts standard Galenic principles.[44] And yet the underlying idea of colour superimposition is one that his teacher, Alderotti, had introduced to this same discussion through an analogy with painterly technique. In fact, Torrigiano's reasoning comes remarkably close to the way that painters were thinking about skin colour at this time. In the *Ognissanti Madonna*, for example, datable to around 1310, Giotto goes out of his way to reveal bare flesh at the corner of the Virgin's eyes, as if to explain the presence of that same rosy-pink colour at the creases of the eyelids, or submerged beneath the semi-transparent white surface of the cheeks.[45]

This conception of perfectly complexioned skin was shared by Dino del Garbo and his son, Tommaso. Although much of Dino's work on the subject remains unpublished or lost, his views are summarised in Tommaso's *Summa medicinalis*, a work left incomplete at the time of his death in 1370. As Tommaso explains, Dino laid particular emphasis on the Galenic principle that 'among all parts of the body, skin is closest to the absolutely balanced state (*temperamento ad pondus*)', and should thus be used as a standard against which the complexion of all other parts can be judged.[46] The basis of this argument was precisely the same as Torrigiano's:

> the complexion of skin is such [...] not according to its own innate complexion, seeing as it is cold and dry, because it is nervous [tissue], but according to the complexion which results in it through the proximity of its own complexion to the blood, flesh, and spirit contained in the veins and arteries that are dispersed through it.[47]

For Dino and Tommaso, in other words, the superimposition of skin and flesh not only accounted for the white and red colour of perfectly complexioned skin; it also made skin into the primary indicator – the touchstone or 'canon', as it were – for all internal distinctions between the complexion of a body's parts.

From the thirteenth into the fourteenth century, then, Florentine physicians sought to explain the natural perfection of white skin by analogising it not only with Polykleitos' *Canon*, but also with painterly techniques for the layering of flesh tones. Meanwhile, over the course of this same period, painters increasingly turned to white and red as standard hues for the modelling of flesh. At the outset of this broad development lies the emphatically yellow skin of Cimabue's Arezzo cross (Figure 3.3a) – a hue that had dominated the flesh tones of many successive generations of Byzantinising

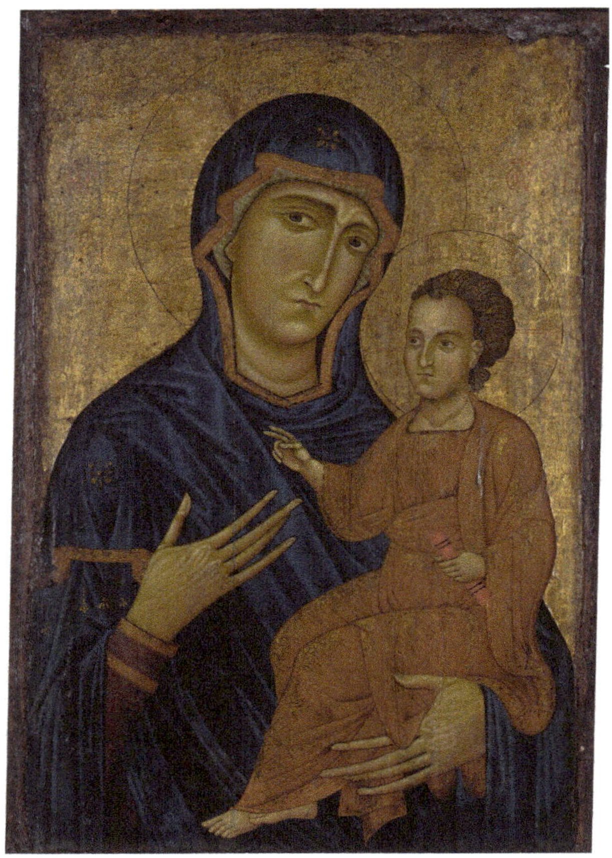

Figure 3.7 Berlinghiero, Madonna and Child, c. 1230. New York, Metropolitan Museum of Art. Image credit: The Metropolitan Museum of Art

painters in Italy, such as Berlinghiero (d. 1236), Giunta Pisano (d. c. 1260), and Guido of Siena (d. 1290) (Figure 3.7). The transition from yellow to white unfolded unevenly over the second half of the thirteenth century but came to be standardised by the early decades of the fourteenth, in works like the *Ognissanti Madonna*. This association of yellow skin with Greek painting is confirmed by contemporary written sources. In one thirteenth-century handbook on manuscript illumination, for example, the primary characteristic of 'Greek' painting is the predominance of ochre in the flesh tones.[48] When Cennini describes Giotto's technique for modelling the face of the Virgin Mary, by contrast, the flesh tones consist exclusively of white and red.[49]

The interplay of medical theory and painterly technique initiated by Alderotti may go some way to explaining this broader convergence. However, it is important to recognise that medical theories of complexion could have played into painting through the mediation of many other adjacent fields of knowledge, such as theology.[50] Leading Franciscan and Dominican theologians, such as Bonaventure and Thomas Aquinas, had argued that Christ, in Aquinas' words, 'had the optimal complexion, because his body was fashioned miraculously by the operation of the Holy Spirit'.[51] Such arguments were particularly prominent in mendicant interpretations of the Passion. Christ was said to have experienced the greatest possible suffering not because of the uniqueness of the tortures he endured, but rather, in Bonaventure's words, 'on account of the maximal balance of his complexion', which made his perceptive faculties maximally sensitive to pain. The concentration of pain in 'his hands and feet' likewise guaranteed that 'the affliction was maximal, on account of the nerves and muscles that congregate there, where sensation is especially strong'.[52]

It is easy to see how this theological principle could have guided the ever subtler, more sensitive attention that Cimabue, Giotto, and the Figline Master paid to the soft tissue of Christ's hands and feet. If so, the same must be said of the lightening of Christ's skin throughout this same period, a development that comes to fruition in works by artists like Giotto and the Figline Master in the early decades of the fourteenth century (Figures 3.4 and 3.5). Admittedly, there remains a marked contrast in these crosses between the rosy white flesh of John and Mary in the side panels, and the comparatively white, yet morbidly 'livid', at times yellow-green skin of the crucified Christ.[53] The contrast is particularly strong in Giotto's cross at Santa Maria Novella, where a sheen of white skin hovers over a maelstrom of red, green, and yellow underlayers, as if to signal the depletion and involution of the body's vital energies.[54] And yet even here, a conscious nod to complexional theory can be discerned in Christ's bright orange-red hair – a characteristic that has long been recognised as marking an 'extraordinary break' within the broader iconographic tradition.[55] Indeed, the colour is all the more puzzling given the sinister, anti-Semitic associations that red hair often bore in this period.[56] However, in the same passage that Galen describes white and red skin as a sign of balanced complexion, he immediately adds 'red and moderately curly hair' (*capilli vero rubei et mediocriter mixti crispi*) – a feature that was repeated and widely affirmed by Florentine physicians in these decades.[57]

In at least one instance, a mendicant preacher is said to have outlined a complexional argument of precisely this type in the nave of Santa Croce itself.[58] The sermon is recounted in a *novella* by the Florentine writer, Franco Sacchetti, where it is attributed to an 'excellent master in theology' named Niccola di Cicilia, who passed through Florence in the 1370s.[59] Despite the likely proximity of Cimabue and the Figline Master's crosses, the focus of Niccola's sermon lay entirely on another crucifix that hung in a private chapel on the south side of the nave: a copy of the miracle-working *Volto Santo*, whose model in Lucca was traditionally attributed to the hand of Nicodemus.[60] And yet the sermon was all about the illegitimacy of this putatively ancient, highly venerated image. For as Sacchetti explains, Niccola and his associates argued 'that our Lord was the most beautiful body there ever was, in both his face and every member, and that this *Volto Santo*, which looked like a big mask, was the opposite'.[61] Niccola's dismissal of the authoritative cult image thus rested squarely on the superlative beauty of Christ: a beauty manifest not only in the anatomically differentiated muscles and bones that artists like Cimabue, Giotto, and the Figline Master had been striving after for nearly a century by this time, but also in Christ's increasingly white skin, whose 'perfection' now stood as a veritable axiom of medical science.

Gender, economics, cosmetics

Medical discourse constitutes just one of many frames of reference that Italian painters and their audiences would have brought to bear on flesh tones during this period – the present study certainly makes no claims to comprehensiveness.[62] In the future, much work remains to be done on the question of how this particular, medical conception of whiteness related to painterly representations of people of the global majority, for example, or to contemporary practices of slavery in Italy.[63] By isolating the relation of painting and medicine, the essay has nevertheless revealed a striking correspondence between medieval and modern ideas of whiteness. For what emerges out of these sources is not only an aesthetic preference for white skin, but also its elevation to the status of a biological norm – a standard against which the particularities of any given body were to be perceived, ordered, and ranked. In this, a clear analogy emerges with modern notions of whiteness as 'the universalist measure against which all other identities become particular'.[64]

Whether there is any connection between these historically distant regimes of whiteness is a question that lies far beyond the scope of the present essay.[65] However, to propose such a correspondence is also, inevitably, to draw attention toward a glaring disjunction: the starkly different social, political, and economic *functions* that whiteness must have performed before and after the rise of modern European imperialism, and in particular, Atlantic slavery. How then did medieval ideas of whiteness interact with broader socio-economic conditions? To conclude, I will consider just one small facet of this vast question, in order to suggest how the particular connections between painting and medicine analysed throughout this essay might help to shed some light upon it.

The broad shift of colour palette outlined earlier in this essay, from yellow to white, had different implications for men than it did for women, even though the stylistic trajectory was virtually the same for both genders. The Virgin Mary represented a normative standard among women, comparable to that of Christ among men, for as many theologians had argued, she too had been graced with a perfectly balanced complexion.[66] Unlike Christ, however, as the Virgin's skin changed from yellow to white, she also began to put on the costume of contemporary Italian women, and subsequently, to assume the hairstyles, physiognomy, and fashionable accoutrements of young Italian ladies (e.g., Figure 3.8). In

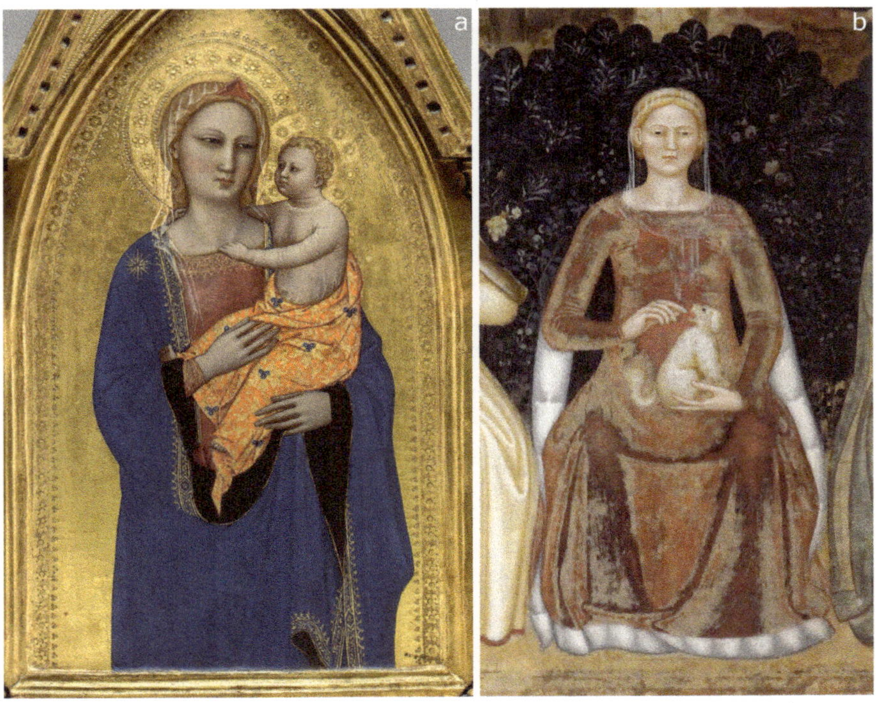

Figure 3.8.a Detail, Nardo di Cione, Madonna and Child, c. 1360, Washington, National Gallery of Art. Image credit: The National Gallery of Art
Figure 3.8.b Detail, Andrea di Bonaiuto, Noblewoman and Dog, from The Militant and Triumphant Church, 1366–1367. Florence, Santa Maria Novella, Spanish Chapel. Image credit: Wikipedia Commons

other words, the Virgin was brought down to earth – made to appear more like a real-life, fourteenth-century woman – in precisely the same pictures that lent her an explicitly artificial, unattainable, scientifically engineered complexion.

I have argued that the manufacture of this ideal involved an active exchange between painting and medical knowledge. It is significant, then, that both painters and physicians had a direct, professional interest in female beauty practices. Florentine doctors, from Taddeo Alderotti forward, often included recipes for skin-whitening cosmetics in their *consilia* – the closest surviving approximation of their prescriptions for individual patients.[67] Painters could present themselves as purveyors of cosmetics as well, as in the following passage from Cennini's *Libro dell'arte*: 'You would have occasion, in the service of young ladies, especially those of Tuscany, to demonstrate a certain colour to which they take a fancy, and which they often use to beautify themselves, with certain waters [...]'.[68]

It is difficult to know how much painters and physicians actually profited off of these interactions. Cennini's phrasing ('in the service [...]') suggests an informal mode of exchange, in which cosmetic advice served to cement relationships with elite patrons rather than generate immediate monetary returns.[69] A similar type of relationship may well stand behind the cosmetic writings of doctors like Alderotti, who was notorious for his cultivation of noble patronage, despite his humble upbringing.[70] In his *Consilia*, for example, when describing a 'cure for blemishes of the face', Alderotti notes that the recipe was concocted 'for a certain high-ranking German woman' (*pro quadam domina theotonica*).[71]

An account of such relationships can be gleaned in at least one medical treatise of the period, written by the French surgeon Henri de Mondeville between 1306 and 1320. Mondeville spent most of his life working at French universities and courts, but his outlook is not irrelevant to the Italian physicians under consideration here, for he was intimately familiar with the work of Italian doctors from Alderotti's circle.[72] The passage occurs in the introduction to a long chapter on cosmetics, which is mostly concerned with face-whitening, or as Mondeville calls it, 'cures for the dark colour of a face':[73]

> this decoration is against God and against justice, nor does it have much to do with curing disease, but is done for deception and fraud, so I will skip through it quickly, for I do not like it. And nevertheless if a surgeon should dwell in some provinces or cities, where there is an abundance of wealth and courtly women, and [if] he is famous for knowing how to do these things sufficiently, he can gather from this the greatest profit and favour among the ruling women, because it is no small thing these days. Without it nothing is done, and without it no one is in the grace of rulers, and for this one is favoured more than the grace of the Pope or divine grace itself.[74]

In Mondeville's view, then, cosmetics are morally wrong, yet economically necessary for the practice of medicine.[75] This position is clearly aimed to shift blame away from the doctor and onto the patient. But what makes it extraordinary is Mondeville's description of the psychological factors involved. For as he explains, skin whitening is part of [...]

> [...] the common adornment, which is generally and indifferently used by all women, whether they need it or not, even though they are not disfigured by any notable blemish, because there is no woman who is so beautiful that she is content with her own beauty.[76]

For the purposes of this essay, it matters little whether Mondeville is exaggerating, or whether we are truly to believe that no woman – not a single one – saw herself as living up to the beauty standards of the time. More important is the underlying principle that the passage lays bare: the idea that cosmetics can be a source of infinite profit as a result of an infinite, inexhaustible demand, a demand that is in turn driven by the establishment of a patently unattainable ideal.

In my opinion it can be no coincidence that this principle, which resonates so deeply with the beauty industry of our own time, is articulated in the fourteenth century by a doctor, who, like the painters of the era, openly stood to benefit from the exploitation of beauty standards. Surely there must have been women, and perhaps also male doctors and painters, who sought to resist this kind of exploitation, but this would be a story for another essay.[77] The aim of the present analysis has simply been to suggest that the establishment of whiteness as an authoritative, anatomically rationalised standard of beauty was a matter of active exchange between painters and physicians in this period.

Notes

1 See generally Hickley, 'Medical Diagnosis and the Colour Yellow', 2015, pp. 1–17.
2 On the theory of complexion in late medieval Italian medicine, see Siraisi, *Taddeo Alderotti and His Pupils*, 1981, 255–61; Chandelier and Robert, 'Nature humaine et complexion du corps', 2013, pp. 474–510. On the concept more generally, see Groebner, '*Complexio*/Complexion', 2004.
3 For example, Galen, *De complexionibus*, 1976, pp. 86–87 (II.6); *On Temperaments*, trans. Ian Johnston, 2020, pp. 182–185; Bartholomeus Anglicus (d. 1272), *De rerum proprietatibus*, 1601, p. 648; for these and other examples, see van der Lugt, 'La peau noire dans la science medievale', 2005, pp. 439–475.
4 Eliav-Feldon, Isaac, and Ziegler, eds, *The Origins of Racism in the West*, 2009; Kennedy and Lewis-Jones, eds, *The Routledge Handbook of Identity*, 2016.
5 Heng, *The Invention of Race in the European Middle Ages*, 2018, pp. 181–256, building on Caviness, 'From the Self-Invention of the Whiteman in the Thirteenth Century', 2008, pp. 1–33.
6 Weeda, 'Geographical determinism, ethnicity and religion, c. 1100–1300 CE', 2016, p. 96.

7 For literary aspects of this relationship in fourteenth-century Italy, see Clines, 'Dido and Laura in Carthage', 2023, with previous bibliography.
8 Bohde, 'Le tinte delle carni', 2007, pp. 41–63, with the note on 'skin color' at p. 42. Cf. Gadebusch Bondio, 'La carne di fuori', 2005.
9 For example, Fend, *Fleshing out Surfaces*, 2016, p. 22.
10 Dante, *Purgatorio*, XI.94–96; see Pfisterer, *Donatello und die Entdeckung der Stile*, 2002, pp. 54–55, for differences between Dante and later sources.
11 Villani, *De origine civitatis Florentie*, 1997, pp. 153–154, 411–412. See Baxandall, *Giotto and the Orators*, 1971, pp. 77–78; Schwarz and Theis, *Giottus Pictor*, 2004, vol. 1, pp. 287–290.
12 For example, Ghiberti, *I commentarii*, 1998, pp. 83–84.
13 Vasari, *Le vite*, 1966–87, vol. 2, pp. 35–44, 97.
14 For an overview of debates on chronology, see Gaeta, *Giotto und die* croci dipinte, 2013, pp. 54, 84–85. On the conservation of Cimabue's work, see Jakobs, 'Restaurierung und Zeitgeschmack', 1988, pp. 53–67.
15 Gaeta, *Giotto und die* croci dipinte, 2013, pp. 47, 56. For the broader impact of Byzantine crucifixion imagery in Italy during this period, see Belting, *The Image and Its Public in the Middle Ages*, 1990; Derbes, *Picturing the Passion in Late Medieval Italy*, 1996.
16 Ciatti, 'The Restoration and the Study of the Crucifix', 2002, pp. 32–34; however, Gaeta, *Giotto und die* croci dipinte, 2013, pp. 70–73, 77, questions aspects of this interpretation.
17 Cennini, *Il libro dell'arte*, 2003, p. 63. For the connection with these crucifixes, see e.g., Cannon, *Religious Poverty*, 2013, pp. 64–65.
18 See Flora, *Cimabue and the Franciscans*, 2018, pp. 171–184, with previous bibliography.
19 For the date, see Cannon, *Religious Poverty*, 2013, p. 59; for its state of preservation, see Maetzke, *Cimabue ad Arezzo*, 2001.
20 On the date of the Figline Master's cross, see Tartuferi in Tartuferi and D'Arelli (eds), *L'arte di Francesco*, 2015, pp. 214–215; Tartuferi, 'Il crocifisso di Santa Croce nel percorso del Maestro di Figline', 2016, p. 204; Polzer, 'The Figline Master Revisited', 2018, p. 48. Extensive restoration work on the cross was completed by the Opificio delle Pietre Dure in 2012.
21 These details anticipate the hands of Christ painted several decades later by Giovanni da Milano on the keystone of the Rinuccini Chapel in the sacristy of the same church.
22 That is, the true and vertebrochondral ribs, omitting only the floating ribs.
23 On Stefano Fiorentino, see Volpe, 'Il lungo percorso del "dipingere dolcissimo e tanto unito"', 1983, esp. pp. 244–252; Bellosi, 'Giottino e la pittura di filiazione giottesca', 2006, pp. 347–368.
24 Villani, *De origine civitatis Florentie*, 1997, p. 412: 'Stephanus, nature symia, tanta eius ymitatione valuit, ut etiam a physicis in figuratis per eum corporibus humanis arterie, vene, nervi et queque minutissima lineamenta proprie colligantur, et ita ut ymaginibus suis, Giotto teste, sola aeris attractio atque respiratio deficere videantur'.
25 For example, Panofsky, 'Artist, Scientist, Genius', 1962, p. 142; Seiler, 'Giotto – das unerreichte Vorbild?', 2012, p. 66.
26 Cennini, *Il libro dell'arte*, 2003, p. 118; for his sources, see Baroni, Rinaldi, and Travaglio, 'Formation, Transmission and Genres in the Recipe Books', 2018, p. 22, note 28.
27 Bergdolt (ed.), *Der dritte Kommentar Lorenzo Ghibertis*, 1988, pp. 532–547. On skeletal anatomy, see Lugli, 'Measuring the Bones', 2015, pp. 346–363.
28 Cf. Vasari, *Le vite*, 1966–1987, vol. 2, p. 118, on a work by Giotto's student, Puccio Capanna, at San Domenico in Pistoia, featuring 'un Crucifisso, una Madonna et un San Giovanni [...] et a' piedi un'ossatura di morto intera nella quale, che fu

cosa inusitata in que' tempi, mostrò Puccio aver tentato di vedere i fondamenti dell'arte'.

29 Villani, *De origine civitatis Florentie*, 1997, pp. 388–396.

30 Augusto De Ferrari's article on Dino in *Dizionario Biografico degli Italiani*, vol. 36, Rome 1988, notes that he was raised in the neighbourhood of Santa Croce, and buried in the church; see also Siraisi, *Taddeo Alderotti and His Pupils*, 1981, pp. 31–33, for Taddeo Alderotti's connections with Santa Croce.

31 Vasari, *Le vite*, 1966–1987, vol. 2, p. 221: '[...] fra i medesimi è maestro Dino del Garbo, medico allora eccellentissimo, vestito come allora usavano i dottori e con una berretta rossa in capo foderata di vai, e tenuto per mano da un Angelo, con altri assai ritratti che non si riconoscono'. On the work, only fragments of which survive, see Kreytenberg, *Orcagna*, 2000, pp. 39–62, with a discussion of Dino's portrait at 46.

32 See generally Donal Cooper, '"In medio ecclesiae"', 2000. On the location of Giotto's cross at Santa Maria Novella, see Gaeta, *Giotto und die* croci dipinte, 2013, pp. 97–112; Cannon, *Religious Poverty*, 2013, pp. 48–51; and for the Figline Master's cross, see Offner, 'The Master of the Fogg Pietà', 1927, p. 57 note 2.

33 For a list of relevant passages in Galen, see Brennan, *Painting as a Modern Art*, 2019, p. 195 note 70.

34 For the date, see Siraisi, *Taddeo Alderotti and His Pupils*, 1981, p. 40.

35 For the Latin see the following note. The references are to *Microtechne* II.14 (ἡ χροιὰ μὲν ἐξ ἐρυθροῦ καὶ λευκοῦ συμμιγής) and *De complexionibus* II.1 (καὶ μέλανος τὴν χρόαν καὶ λευκοῦ), in Galen, *Opera omnia*, 1821–1833, vol. 1, pp. 342, 577.

36 Alderotti, *In Galeni micratechnen comentarij*, 1522, fols 98v–99v. See also Alderotti, *Expositiones in arduum aphorismorum Ipocratis*, 1527, fols 369r–v, where the argument remains similarly unresolved.

37 Alderotti, *Expositiones in arduum aphorismorum Ipocratis*, 1527, fol. 369v: 'quidam vero generantur per supernatationem sicut quando pictores ponunt unum colorem super alium et resultat ibi tertius color [...] haec verba leguntur in libro de sensu et sensato'.

38 Aristotle, *De sensu et sensato*, 440a7.

39 For example, Thomas Aquinas, *In Aristotelis* [...] *commentaria*, 1866, vol. 3, p. 164.

40 For example, Cennini, *Il libro dell'arte*, 2003, p. 115.

41 For the date, see Jacquart, 'Cœur ou cerveau?', 2003, p. 84.

42 Torrigiano, *Plus quam commentum*, 1557, fol. 73r: '[Galenus] vocat autem radicalia illa membra, quae sunt dura et alba, similata spermati in colore, et dicta quidem radicalia quasi genita ex radice, sicut ossa, chartilagines, panniculi, nervi et huiusmodi'.

43 Torrigiano, *Plus quam commentum*, 1557, fol. 76r: 'signa complexionis aequalis [...] sunt haec, scilicet color commistus ex albo et rubeo: temperantia enim musculorum efficit hunc colorem in cute, quia, cum cutis sit natura alba ad modum membrorum, quae Galenus vocat radicalia, propter calorem, cum exiccaverit humidum sanguineum, ex quo fiunt, dealbare ipsum per ulteriorem decoctionem in ipso: sanguis autem et caro musculorum, quae a cute teguntur, cum sortita fuerint temperamentum conueniens [sic], sint rubea, resultabit in superficie color commistus ex utroque, cum cutis quidem tenuis existens admittat colorem eorum, quae tangit'. Cf. Torrigiano, *Plus quam commentum*, 1557, fol. 29r: 'Sed bonus color est, qui est ex albo et rufo mistus: nam, cum membra, quae Galenus vocat radicalia, sint alba, frigiditati et siccitati attenentia, caro vero et sanguis sint rubea, accidit ex eorum mistione color apparens in exterioribus ex utroque colore commistus'.

44 See e.g., Galen, *De complexionibus*, 1976, pp. 47, 86 (I.9, II.6); trans. Johnston, pp. 98–99, 183. Dino del Garbo similarly cites Galen's *Tegni* and *De ingenio sanitatis* in arguing 'quod cutis est membrum spermaticum': *Expositio super tertia et quarta fen IV libri canonis Avicennae*, 1496, fol. 70r, cf. 96r. For further discussion of the transparency of skin, and other related principles, among doctors of this period,

see Jacquart, 'A la recherche de la peau dans le discours médical de la fin du Moyen Âge', 2005, esp. pp. 495–496.

45 On the state of conservation in the Virgin's face, see Peroni, 'La "Maesta" di Ognissanti', 1984, p. 30; Seracini, 'Diagnostica', 1984, pp. 99–101, where the area around the eyes appears to have suffered less damage than elsewhere. The colors as presently restored can also be confirmed through comparison with the much better-preserved face of the child (on this point, see also Del Serra, 'Il restauro', 1984, p. 88).

46 Tommaso del Garbo, *Summa medicinalis*, 1529, fol. 9v: 'Et dicit Dinus quod sicut homo magis appropinquat: sic inter omnia membra corporis cutis est propinquior temperamento ad pondus et temperata cutis plus omni alia cute'. Tommaso del Garbo, *Summa medicinalis*, 1529, fol. 67v: 'Et dicit ad hoc Dynus [...] quod duplex est regula determinandi complexiones membrorum: una inquantum ipsa sunt principium operationum: et talis regula determinandi de complexionibus est corpus temperatum [...]. Alia est regula determinandi complexiones in relatione ad equale ab temperamento et illa est cutis'. Cf. Galen, *De complexionibus*, 1976, pp. 42–43, 46 (I.9); trans. Johnston, pp. 90–93, 97–99.

47 Tommaso del Garbo, *Summa medicinalis*, 1529, fol. 9v: 'et talis est complexio cutis secundum quam ipsa iudicatur temperatior aliis membris non secundum sui propriam et innatam complexionem: cum illa sit frigida et sicca: cum sit nervosa. Sed secundum complexionem que in ea resultat ex sua propria complexione ex vicinitate sanguinis carnis et spiritus contenti in venis et arteriis dispersis per ipsam'.

48 Travaglio, 'Il "Liber colorum secundum magistrum Bernardum [...]"', 2008, p. 34, with an Italian translation at p. 41. In the first of two sets of instructions for painting faces, described as a method 'for making a good, Greek flesh tone' ('ad faciendum bonam incarnaturam graecam'), one begins with an undercoat of green, then models the facial features in an ocher-based brown, and finishes with a flesh tone of ocher mixed with red and white. By contrast, the second method, free of geographic designation ('ad faciendum aliam bonam incarnaturam'), begins by laying green into the shadows and then simply overlays it with flesh tones of red and white.

49 Cennini, *Il libro dell'arte*, 2003, pp. 118–119; see Brennan, *Painting as a Modern Art*, 2019, pp. 74–85, for comparison with a Byzantine treatise known in Europe during the period.

50 Equally relevant is vernacular poetry, with which many of these doctors, such as Dino and Torrigiano, were involved: see Siraisi, *Taddeo Alderotti and His Pupils*, 1981, pp. 75, 82–86.

51 Thomas Aquinas, *Summa theologica*, in *Opera omnia*, 1903, p. 443 (III, q. 46, a. 6): 'nam et secundum corpus erat optime complexionatus, cum corpus eius fuerit formatum miraculose operatione spiritus sancti'. Cf. Dante, *Paradiso*, XIII.43–48.

52 Bonaventura, *Commentaria in quatuor libros sententiarum*, 1887, vol. 3, p. 349: '[...] manus eius et pedes [...] in quibus maxima erat afflictio propter nervos et musculos ibidem concurrentes, in quibus praecipue viget sensus. [...] maxima erat afflictio propter maximam complexionis aequalitatem et propter sensus vivacitatem'. The passage surrounding the quotation from Aquinas in the previous note covers all of these same points. For previous discussion in relation to these crosses, see Gaeta, *Giotto und die* croci dipinte, 2013, pp. 58–59, 116–121. On the theological tradition more broadly, see Resnick, 'Ps.-Albert the Great on the Physiognomy of Jesus and Mary', 2002, pp. 217–240; van der Lugt, *Le ver, le demon et la vierge*, Paris 2004, pp. 456, 460, 468–469; Cohen, *The Modulated Scream*, 2010, pp. 202–208, 211. The maximal perceptual sensitivity of the balanced complexion is explicitly noted by Galen, *De complexionibus*, 1976, p. 52 (II.1); trans. Johnston, pp. 110–111.

53 On the 'livid' state of Christ's perfectly complexioned, yet crucified body, see e.g., Bridget of Sweden (d. 1373), *Revelationes caelestes seraphicae*, 1680, p. 17: 'Itaque cum filius meus sic laceratus et liuidus staret, solum cor recens erat, quia optime

et fortissime nature erat. De mea enim carne corpus mundissimum et optime complexionatum sumpsit'.

54 The lightest layers of Christ's flesh tones consist of 99% lead white, mixing with yellow ochre toward the shadows, whereas those of Mary and John consist of lead white and vermilion: see Moioli and Seccaroni, 'X-ray fluorescence (XRF) for analysis of pigments', 2002, pp. 376, 378, table 1; Matteini, Moles, Lanterna, Nepoti, Rizzi, and Tosini, 'Characteristics of the materials and techniques', 2002, pp. 388, 390; Gaeta, *Giotto und die* croci dipinte, 2013, pp. 76–77, 82. The flesh tones of the Ognissanti cross do likewise contain ocher in areas of shading, but the resulting hue is far less yellow than in Byzantinising works of the previous century: see Bracco, Ciappi, and Hilling, 'La pittura della *Croce* di Ognissanti', 2010, pp. 122–123.

55 Gaeta, *Giotto und die* croci dipinte, 2013, p. 76. On the pigments, see Matteini (et al.), 'Characteristics of the materials and techniques', 2002, p. 393 ('orange-red ochre layers on a yellow base'), and Bracco (et al.), 'La pittura della *Croce* di Ognissanti', 2010, p. 124, with the same pigments for Christ's hair in the Ognissanti cross.

56 Mellinkoff, 'Judas's Red Hair and the Jews', 1982, pp. 31–46; Mellinkoff, *Outcasts*, 1993, pp. 145–160.

57 Galen, *Microtechne*, in *Opera omnia* 1821–1833, vol. 1, p. 342 (II.14); Alderotti, *In Galeni micratechnen commentarij*, 1522, fol. 94v; Torrigiano, *Plus quam commentum*, 1557, fol. 76r. For contrary opinions in earlier scholastic literature, see Resnick, 'Ps.-Albert the Great on the Physiognomy of Jesus and Mary', 2002, pp. 237–238.

58 *Pace* Cohen, p. 211. For other sermons relevant to these crosses, see Cannon, *Religious Poverty*, 2013, pp. 51–53, 63–64; cf. Iannella, 'Malatia e salute nella predicazione', 1995, pp. 177–216.

59 Sacchetti describes the circumstances of the sermon as follows: 'Capitò questo maestro Niccola nella nostra città per una questione che aveva mosso contro a lui uno Inquisitore de' frati predicatori in Cicilia; e andavasi a diffinire in Corte dinanzi al Sommo Pontefice, nel tempo ch'e' Fiorentini ebbono Guerra co' pastori della Chiesa' (Sacchetti, *Trecentonovelle*, 2000, p. 187 (Novella LXXIII)). For context, see Burr, *Spiritual Franciscans*, 2003, pp. 163, 179–181.

60 On the chapel, see Giura, 'Notizie su due cappelle perdute', 2011, pp. 38–39. The patron, Dino di Geri Cigliamochi, was apparently a wider target of derision: see e.g., Davidsohn, *Geschichte von Florenz*, 1896–1927, vol. 4, p. 218. For copies of the *Volto Santo*, which took a diverse range of painted and sculptural forms by this period, see e.g., Lazzarini, *Il Volto Santo di Lucca*, 1982, pp. 97–118, 173–181; Martinelli, *L'immagine del Volto Santo di Luca*, 2016.

61 Sacchetti, *Trecentonovelle*, 2000, p. 188 (Novella LXXIII): 'che il nostro Signore e di viso e d'ogni membro fu il piú bel corpo che fusse mai e che questo Volto santo che parea uno mascherone era il contrario'.

62 Even within this narrow frame of reference, many important issues remain to be explored. Given Heng and Caviness' work on thirteenth-century France, for example, it is significant that Giotto's cross has long been associated with French artistic influence: see Gaeta, *Giotto und die* croci dipinte, 2013, pp. 86–97.

63 On slavery in late medieval Italy and its relation to skin colour, see e.g., Epstein, *Speaking of Slavery*, 2001, pp. 79–80, 183–191; cf. Patton, 'What did Medieval Slavery Look Like?', 2022. On the politics of the Black body in thirteenth-century Italian art, see e.g., Kaplan, 'Black Africans in Hohenstaufen Iconography', 1987.

64 Bowles, 'Blinded by the White', 2001, p. 39.

65 See generally Whitaker, *Black Metaphors*, 2019, esp. pp. 1–22; Heng, *The Invention of Race in the European Middle Ages*, 2018; Kim, 'The Politics of the Medieval Preracial', 2021; Lopez-Jantzen, 'Historiography, Periodization, and Race', 2021; Clines, 'Dido and Laura in Carthage', 2023.

66 For example, Resnick, 'Ps.-Albert the Great on the Physiognomy of Jesus and Mary', 2002, pp. 228–240, esp. 237.

67 Alderotti, *Libello per conservare la sanità del corpo*, 1852, pp. 6–7 ('le mani e la facia laverai coll'acqua fredda, però che ti farà buono colore e chiaro [...]. Lo tuo corpo adornerai di belli vestimenti, però che l'animo tuo si ne rallegrarà molto'), and note 72 below. On the genre, see Siraisi, *Taddeo Alderotti and His Pupils*, 1981, pp. 271–274.

68 Cennini, *Il libro dell'arte*, 2003, p. 204: 'Egli acchaderebbe in servigio delle giovani donne, spezialmente di quelle di Toschana, di dimostrare alchuno colore del quale ànno vagheza, e usano di farsi belle d'alchune aque [...]'. For a recent discussion of the passage, see Sammern, 'Treating Bodily Impurities', 2023, pp. 121–122.

69 Cennini worked as a court artist for the Carrara in Padua (Frezzato in Cennini, *Il libro dell'arte*, 2003, pp. 11–17).

70 Villani, *De origine civitatis Florentie*, 1997, pp. 388–391; Siraisi, *Taddeo Alderotti and His Pupils*, 1981, p. 38.

71 Alderotti, *I 'Consilia'*, 1937, p. 195 (CXLVI).

72 Siraisi, *Taddeo Alderotti and His Pupils*, 1981, pp. 51–52.

73 Henri de Mondeville, *Die Chirurgie*, 1892, p. 405: 'De primo, scilicet de ornatu communi faciei, recurrendum est ad capitulum de ornatu virorum, ubi fit sermo de cura coloris obscuri faciei [...]'.

74 Henri de Mondeville, *Die Chirurgie*, 1892, pp. 398–399: 'ista decoratio est contra Deum et justitiam nec est ut plurimum cura morbi sed fit propter deceptionem et fraudem, ideo breviter pertransibo, et quoniam mihi non placet; et tamen si cyrurgicus moraretur in provinciis aliquibus aut civitatibus, ubi esset copia divitum et curialium mulierum et haberet famam, quod sciret sufficienter de talibus operari, ipse posset reportare inde maximum commodum et gratiam dominarum, quod non est modicum his diebus, quoniam sine ipsa factum est nihil et sine ipsa nemo potest esse dominis gratiosus et ideo eligibilior est in casu quam sit gratia summi pontificis aut divina'.

75 Henri de Mondeville's argument parallels Galen, *Miamir* I.3, but since the latter does not yet seem to have been translated, the connection has been doubted: see McVaugh, *The Rational Surgery of the Middle Ages*, 2006, p. 220; Demaitre, 'Skin and the City', 2011, pp. 100–102. For the wider aesthetic implications of this line of thought, see Lichtenstein, 'Making Up Representation', 1987.

76 Henri de Mondeville, *Die Chirurgie*, 1892, p. 405: 'Primum sit ornatus communis, qui comuniter et indifferenter fit ab omnibus, sive indigent sive non, quamvis nullo vitio notabili deturpentur, quoniam non est aliqua, quae ita pulchra, quod propria pulchritudine sit contenta'.

77 For example, Brennan, *Painting as a Modern Art*, 2019, p. 166.

4

'I advocate the frequent viewing of [...] green': Ficino, green walls and early modern 'chromotherapy'

Katharine Stahlbuhk

Introduction

Ut pictura medicina, 'as in painting so in medicine'. This chapter builds on the introduction of this volume, exploring how, in the early modern period, the act of observing and being surrounded by green walls – often embellished with figurative decorations – was regarded as a therapeutic practice for the eyes. Before delving into this form of 'chromotherapy' through a close examination of pivotal medical and philosophical texts from antiquity to the Renaissance, in conjunction with the common use of green walls in the fourteenth and fifteenth centuries, it is worth noting that the concept of 'colour' itself is anything but straightforward.[1] As Leonardo da Vinci warns in his *Libro di pittura*, 'colour will never be seen with ease', concisely indicating what has always driven and simultaneously complicated the study of colour:[2] namely, that colour as an optically conveyed sensory impression is always determined by subjective factors. Simultaneously, colour and its impression are dependent on a multitude of external physical conditions; in particular its perception is decisively shaped by social and cultural preconditions alongside linguistic meanings and ascriptions. Seeing and speaking about colour thus always proves a complex process that not only touches on perceptivity, but is also closely connected to aesthetic, epistemic, ethical, and political questions and problems.[3]

Speaking generically of 'green walls', the possible range of green tones – which spans from intense to rich to brownish-dirty hues and presumably impacts (and impacted) the beholder differently – must similarly be taken into account. Focusing on the Italian peninsula and on green wall surfaces in fresco or any other lime-painting technique, it is possible to nuance a 'spectrum' based on the employed pigments – mainly green earth and other mineral pigment mixtures – to determine the colour appearance in a relatively light green, ranging from sage to olive tones, possibly with a slight blue or even brownish tinge or hue.[4]

It is also worth noting that people in the fifteenth century were doubtless conscious of the influence a colour could have on their mindset or mental condition. In 1496 Girolamo Savonarola preached a sermon in which he speaks allegorically of eyeglasses. He treats the risks and benefits of such a 'filter', which if good (*buoni*) will always let 'your intellect see well'.[5] Interestingly, Savonarola refers not to transparent but to coloured lenses underlining that through red eyeglasses the whole book would appear red while reading, and through green lenses everything would appear to be green. While he does not further elaborate on green, Savonarola identifies red and yellow as dangerous colours: the former being the eyeglasses of wrath, and the latter of envy or avarice.[6]

But what of green? A line in Pliny suggests that Savonarola (and, presumably, his contemporaries) might have seen green as a 'good' colour for the lenses of eyeglasses. One that would enhance a reader's comprehension and the 'just' judgment of the text. Indeed, Pliny, after apparently referring to green-lensed eyeglasses ('"Smaragdi" are generally concave in shape'), specifies that 'Nero used to watch fights between gladiators in a reflecting "smaragdus"'.[7] Did this tint thus offer more enjoyment and better apprehension of the combat? Certainly, the belief in the direct impact of specific colours, attested to by similar sources, is reflected in the profusion of green spaces in the late medieval and early modern period, and allow us to understand a conscious employment of colour akin to a form of chromotherapy.

A significant number of 'green spaces' feature the so-called *verdeterra* murals (Figure 4.1), a technique I have dealt with extensively as an important phenomenon of Quattrocento painting.[8] At the centre of my previous study are nearly monochrome mural paintings representing (mainly) sacred scenes, whose colour reduction cannot be explained with the evocation of other materials like marble or similar stones. The reduction of the employed palette to (mostly) green and greenish pigment mixtures can be related to monastic ideals of poverty and simplicity. A subsequent inclusion in observant church politics from the 1430s onwards enhanced the widespread diffusion of this type of decoration in cloisters and chapels.[9] Beside the monastic ideals, the chromatic appearance of those murals is likewise 'rooted' in the sources to be analysed in the following pages.

But, in order to foreground the medical aspect of colour vision, the focus of the present chapter is not on green figurative painting, but rather on (simple) green-washed walls. That the exposure to a particular colour has a direct effect on the viewer is, in the case of rooms with walls decorated with either greenery, with green figurative cycles or with just a green encompassing tint, taken to extremes, as the beholder literally enters a 'colour space' that enfolds him or her almost entirely. Such an experience

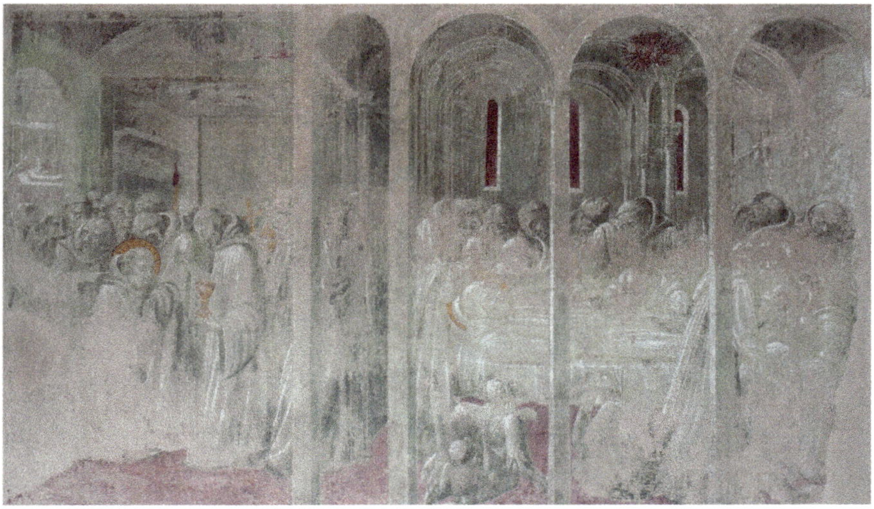

Figure 4.1 Pietro di Giovanni d'Ambrosio, Last Communion and Death of Hieronymus, c. 1442–1443, fresco. San Salvatore, Lecceto (Siena). Image credit: Damien Cerutti

is of great importance in understanding the holistic approach to health or well-being, which treated body and mind.

Green spaces and their ancient sources

In the following paragraph, I will provide a brief overview of the categories of similar green spaces to underline their peculiarity, while also highlighting their diffusion. In parallel, ancient sources as well as contemporary testimonies will be mentioned, in order to explain the use of this specific colour.

One such green-coloured space that had an important follow-up in the fifteenth century is the convent library of San Marco in Florence.[10] Around 1440 Michelozzo created a new form of humanist library for the observant convent of the Florentine Dominicans, making the inheritance of the erudite Niccolò Niccoli available to readers as, rhetorically speaking, one of the first de-facto 'public' libraries since antiquity.[11] The new building served not only as an architectural container for storing the codices, but also allowed for their consultation and study in an appropriate, stimulating ambience. As such, Michelozzo created a structure similar to a three-aisled basilica; moreover, thanks to restorations carried out shortly before the year 2000, restorers discovered that Michelozzo's library originally had completely green-washed walls. The whitewash, mixed with *terra verde* (green earth), tinted the walls in a light shade of sage.[12] This library – in its architectural and chromatic design – became a model for numerous other convent libraries over the course of the Quattrocento including Santa

Maria delle Grazie in Milan and San Domenico in Bologna, as well as the Biblioteca Malatestiana in Cesena, just to name a few.[13] The last example of the Malatestiana is particularly noteworthy due to its state of preservation (Figure 4.2), and hence offers the possibility to comprehend and appreciate the original effect of similar colour spaces.[14]

Not only do the well-preserved remnants of such green wash attest to the spread of this practice, but a significant number of paintings also bear witness to it. A notable example is Melozzo da Forlì's *Sixtus IV Appointing Platina as Prefect of the Vatican Library* (1477), which was originally located on the northern wall of the Sala Latina in the newly established *Biblioteca Sistina* (1475). It was detached at the end of the nineteenth century and is now housed in the Pinacoteca Vaticana. Behind the group of portrayed figures framed by a sumptuous portico, it is possible to identify the proper reading room with round-arched windows and a tinted green wall.[15] As Sergio Bettini specifies, the archival documents testify that the walls of the Sala Latina were originally painted in just such an 'emerald green'.[16]

At first glance this chromatic choice may appear to be merely a matter of taste. However, as Magnolia Scudieri, Michele Ciliberto, and later Bettini have demonstrated,[17] the use of green in convent libraries (and in the Vatican Library) is driven not only by aesthetic pleasure or beauty but, more importantly, by the aesthesis of green. This explains why the design of the library of San Marco and of all its successors is closely associated with the calming meditation-enhancing effects of green, often regarded

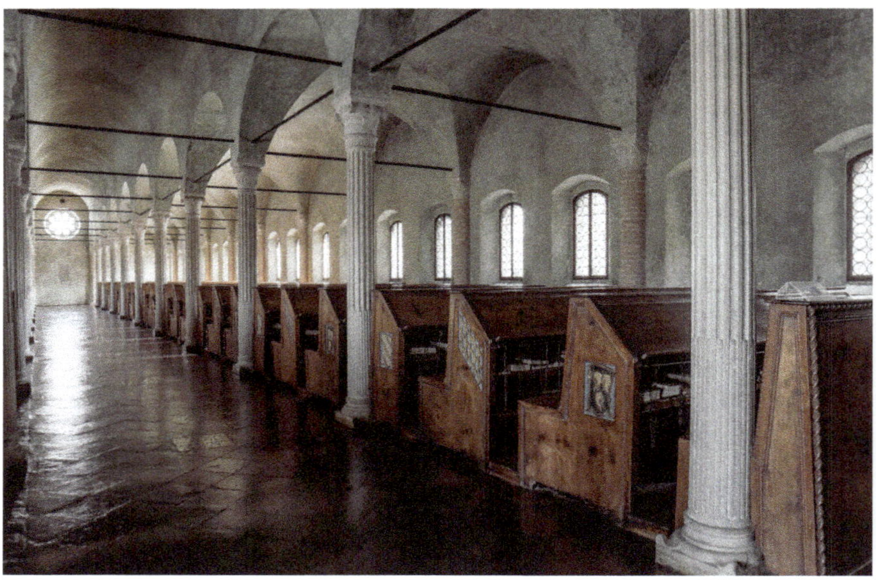

Figure 4.2 Biblioteca Maltestiana: Reading Room, c. 1452. San Francesco, Cesena. Image credit: Wikipedia Commons

as a middle or mediating colour. A contemporary comment on the colour choice brings us closer to the therapeutic implications of this way of acting: a note by the Bishop of Gaeta, Francesco Patrizi, in his *De Institutione rei publicae*, published in 1471 and dedicated to Sixtus IV, the Pope portrayed in Melozzo's mural, states that: 'the walls [of the libraries] are decorated with [...] green paint, since all gradations of green are pleasing to the eyes and conducive to concentration'.[18] This apparently well-known and accepted quality mentioned by Patrizi draws on a basic text of medieval wisdom. An entry in the *Encyclopaedia of Isidore of Seville* suggests that green marble was specifically used for library floors to enhance vision: '[T]he more experienced of architects would not think of putting gilt ceiling panels in libraries, or any paving stones other of Carystean marble, because the glitter of gold wearies the eyes, and the green of the Carystean marble refreshes them' (VI, 11, 2).[19]

Due to its 'eye-refreshing' effect, green became associated with concentration and intellectuality, which likely contributed to the widespread use of green walls in libraries and *studioli*. Alongside surviving evidence, archival sources, and restoration reports, this diffusion has been attested to also in numerous miniatures and paintings, especially those depicting Church Fathers or monks in their studies, where the surrounding architecture evokes the green walls used in libraries. This is the case, for instance, in Sandro Botticelli's representation of *Saint Augustine* in the Church of Ognissanti in Florence or in Vittore Carpaccio's rendition of the same saint in the Scuola di San Giorgio degli Schiavoni in Venice.

The practice of enhancing the study space with green colour led to the creation of particularly notable green-monochrome rooms, such as the little *studiolo* that once completed the Camera d'Oro in Torrechiara Castle near Parma. Through some monochrome paintings on the green plaster surrounding a window of the huge and richly decorated chamber, and through movable (now lost) wood panels likewise tinted in green and decorated with monochrome figures, the owner Pier Maria Rossi could enclose himself in an intimate green setting surrounded by a cycle of *Illustrious Men* from Aristotle to Dante.[20] According to this, not only green plaster, but also wood and, as one might easily suppose, green curtains or drapes accompanied or better facilitated thinking and writing processes. A beautiful illumination of *Vincent of Beauvais in His Study* (Figure 4.3) illustrates, through the hangings in front of the book shelves and the cloth on the table in front of him, such a versatility (and geographic diffusion) of 'green items' in similar ambiences. Especially for these kinds of representations regarding the religious sphere, besides Isidore, an important source, written in the thirteenth century is William Durand's *Rationale*, where he declares that green is the colour of contemplation (*uiridis contemplationem*).[21] From this point of view it is worth considering pictorial works like Fra Angelico's *Mocking of Christ* (Figure 4.4), where in the foreground Mary and Saint

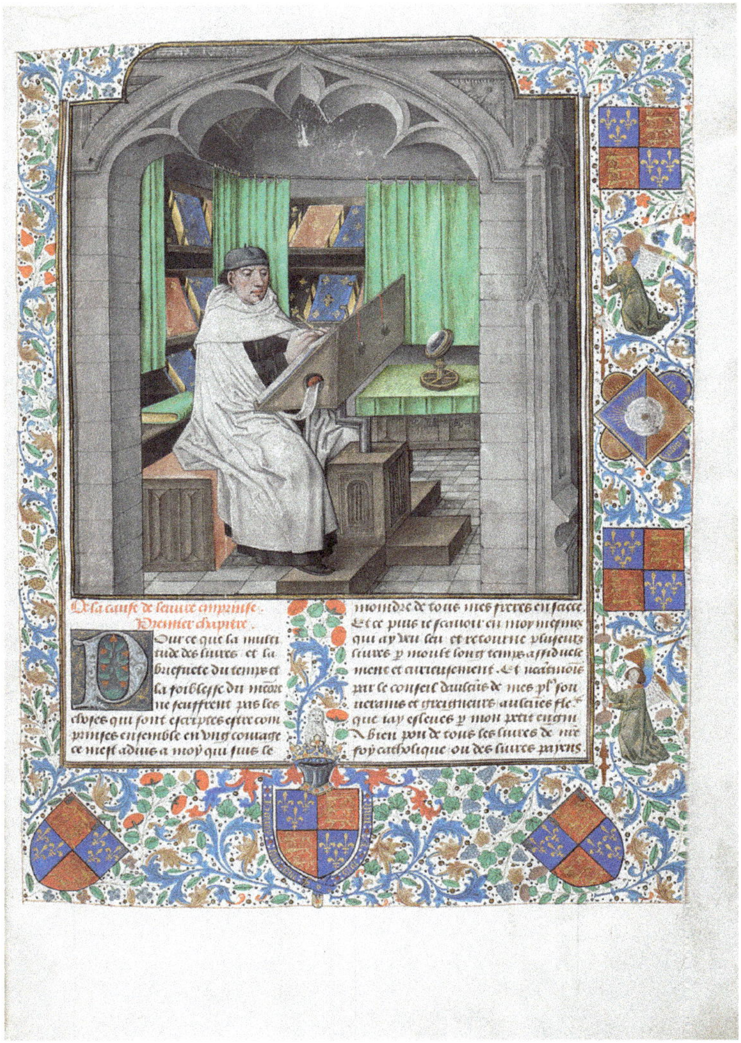

Figure 4.3 Vincent of Beauvais in His Study, in: Vincent of Beauvais, *Speculum historiale*, translated into French by Jean de Vignay, Bruges, c. 1478–1480. British Library, Royal 14 E. i, vol. 1, f. 3. Image credit: Wikipedia Commons

Dominic contemplate the torment of Jesus depicted as a 'vision' in front of a green cloth.[22]

The above-mentioned examples leave no doubt regarding the intentionality of green in similar spaces. Nonetheless, one must take note that the greenwashing of walls was not confined to libraries or studies: a second typology of green spaces includes the papal bedchamber. Here, the concentration-enhancing effects of the colour have a lesser importance, rather

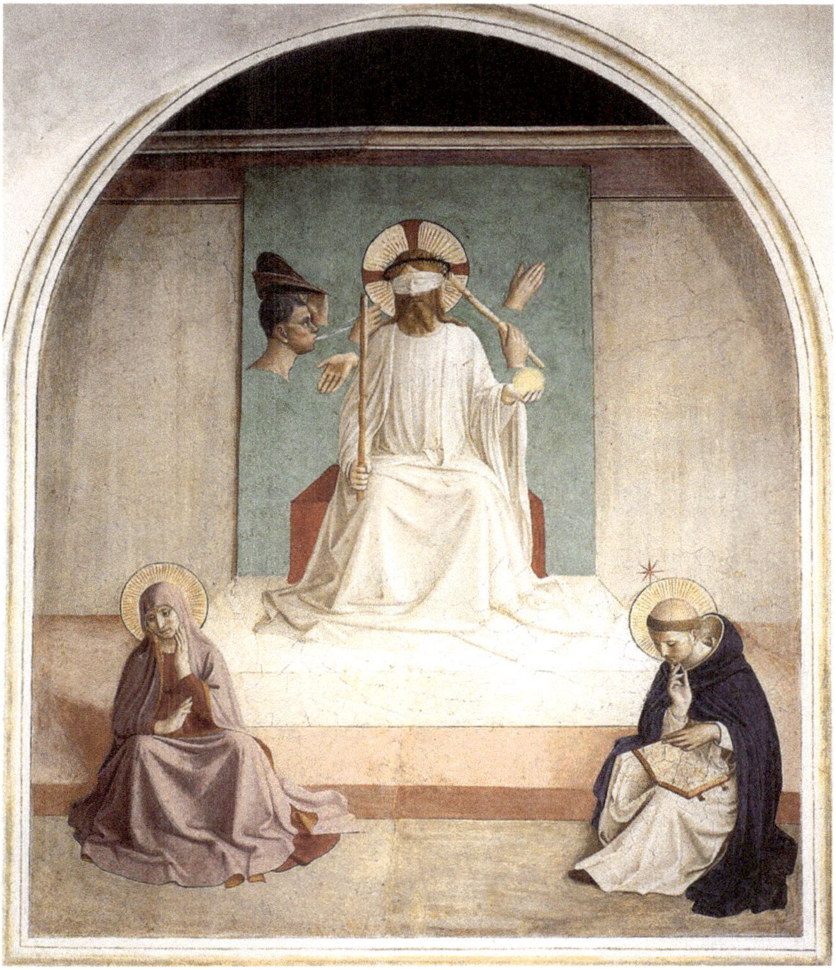

Figure 4.4 Beato Angelico, Mocking of Christ, c. 1440–1441, fresco. San Marco, Florence. Image credit: Wikipedia Commons

the calming and contemplative features of the middle colour green keep their validity also in the wall tint of a bedroom. For example, the *cubiculum* (bedchamber) of Martin V in Santa Maria Novella was painted in this way as documents attest, which tell of a certain Giovanni di Guccio and his assistants, who were paid in 1419 to cover the walls of the papal bedroom with green earth (*etiam pinserunt muros dicte camere ubi dormit Papa de verde terra*).[23] A vague idea of how this might have looked is offered in one *formella* of the Armadio di Santa Croce by Taddeo Gaddi (c. 1335–1340) which shows the *Dream of Innocent III*. The back wall of the room, where the sleeping Pope lies in his bed, is green, which, as specified also in the above-mentioned documents, is adorned with the papal coat of arms. This type of wall design thus dates back at least to the fourteenth century and might, to a certain extent, be related to the *foliage* decorations of the *cubiculum* of Benedict XII in Avignon, where the documents also attest work at the green paintings in the papal chamber (*picturae viridis camera pape*) for the years 1337 and 1339.[24] After Avignon and Florence, finally the Roman papal palace under Eugene IV also had a green-decorated bedchamber as numerous documents refer to a *viridarium*, which can possibly be identified with the *cubiculum*.[25]

Conceptually, the series of green rooms can be extended to include the practice of fictional tendril decoration, where the colour green, as a symbol of nature and vegetation, becomes predominant. In a broader discourse, similar connotations of wall designs also resonate in late medieval and later examples, such as Leonardo da Vinci's *Sala delle Asse* in the Castello Sforzesco (1498), and even in the now lost side wall decoration of the *Camera Verde* in Palazzo Vecchio, Florence, from the 1540s.[26] Referring to an allusion to nature through the colour green, and anticipating that, in this third typology of green spaces (often semi-open ones and loggias), the calming and invigorating effects were major motivations for such decoration, a look into the fifth book of Vitruvius' *De Architectura* offers an intriguing comment. In the description of porticoes, though from a slightly different perspective, this antique source confirms, or better, anticipates the aforementioned quotes of Isidore and Durandus:

> In fact the areas between the porticoes which will be open to the sky should, it seems, be enlivened with greenery; open-air walks are very healthy, particularly for the eyes, since the refined and rarefied air emanating from plants flows into the body because it is in motion, and *sharpens our vision; and by removing the heavy discharge from the eyes, leaves our sight acute and images sharp*. (V, 9, 5)[27]

Aristotle, Marsilio Ficino, and the therapeutic effects of green

The clear abundance of green walls in the fifteenth century – libraries, studies, bedrooms, loggias, cloisters, and chapels – allows us to assume that the positive, therapeutic effect of similarly coloured walls was widely known and practised. Indeed, not only ancient and medieval sources like Vitruvius or Isidore refer to the benefits of green, but, as has been emphasised through the example of Savonarola's eyeglasses or the recommendation of Patrizi to Sixtus IV, also contemporary voices highlight the ophthalmological aspect. The question emerges: why in this epoque, broadly calculating from the Trecento to the Cinquecento, did green rooms encounter such favour? Indeed, the root of all subsequent interpretations and associations acknowledged to the colour green goes back to antiquity, more precisely to Aristotle, who formulates his thoughts on colours and spectra mainly in *On Sense and Sensible Objects* (442a)[28] and in *Meteorologica*, whereby the first text speaks of a seven-coloured spectrum between brightness and darkness and the second of a three-coloured one, where green is placed in the centre:

> Nor do more than two rainbows occur at the same time. Of two such simultaneous rainbows each is three-coloured, [...] these colours are almost the only ones that painters cannot manufacture; for they produce some colours by a mixture of others, but *red, green and [purple/purpure]* cannot be produced in this way, and these are the colours of the rainbow – though between the red and green band there often appears a yellow one. (371b–372a)[29]

Aristotle insists on the intermediate colour green, positioned between black and white, in his *On Plants*, where he writes with respect to the colour of trees:

> The green colour must be the most common characteristic in trees. For we see that, as whiteness is their most common characteristic within, so is greenness without. This is because they use material which is nearer and more ripe. Greenness must be present in all plants, because their material draws and thins the wood of the tree, and the heat causes a rapid ripening, and some moisture survives there, which appears on the outside; this is the greenness which appears in plants, unless the ripening becomes greater. But it is midway in power between the leaves and the wood. Greenness is not destroyed, if there is moisture in it, which arises from the nature of the earth. From both these causes the green develops. A proof of this is that the bark of the tree, when it gets dry, turns black, but within it is white. In trees *between these two colours is a green colour* on the surface. (II, VIII)[30]

Green being classified as the colour in the centre of the spectrum, as the middle tone,[31] might have easily influenced the ascriptions of calming and balancing effects in the centuries to come. That is why, before analysing another Aristotelian citation on green, I want to focus on one fifteenth-century text which bares the necessary requisites to function as authoritative, contemporary source, while even baring an explicit therapeutic intention: Marsilio Ficino, in the second book *On the Long Life* (*De vita longa*) of his *De vita libri tres* finished in 1489 and dedicated to Lorenzo de' Medici, describes the potential power of green things, which have a refreshing and rejuvenating effect on the observer.[32] It is important to emphasise that, on the one hand, Ficino's *De Vita* is part of a long standing tradition, embedded in medieval culture and especially the second book under consideration here relies heavily on the *De retardanda senectute* by Arnaldus de Villa Nova and, through him, on the eponymous work by Roger Bacon.[33] On the other hand Ficino's treatise became extremely popular and was soon (partially) translated into Italian and other European languages.[34] That is why, even though Ficino's approach to green introduces no fundamental novelty, he serves as an important exponent for illustrating the general understanding of this colour's beneficial properties. Thus, his text contributes to a better understanding of the popularity and diffusion of green spaces during the fifteenth century. When considering early modern chromotherapy within the many green spaces of the period, it is important to note that Ficino was well acquainted with green monochrome painting and green-washed walls. Most of the known figurative cycles were executed in Florence and the surrounding area – including his deanery of San Cristoforo in Novoli which bears several green monochrome murals.[35] Ficino also likely used the green-tinted study room of the Biblioteca di San Marco mentioned previously.

While Ficino does not comment directly on such works of art or green rooms, in a broader discourse on colour perception, it is remarkable that an entire chapter is devoted to green. No other colour receives comparable attention from the Tuscan Neoplatonist. Although Ficino refers to the colour of nature – the title includes a clear reference to 'green fields' – he is not concerned with the health-promoting factors such as the cleanliness of the air or the tranquillity of the rural setting mentioned several times in his treatise *On Life*, but explicitly with the colour green (*colour viridis*).[36]

Before properly delving into Ficino's thoughts on green, it is necessary to emphasise the significance of the sense of sight – which includes colour vision – within his *De vita*. He calls it 'the principal part of the animal spirit',[37] hence, of fundamental importance in Ficino's holistic approach to medicine. The study of medicine, and consequently pharmaceutical knowledge, form the basis of Ficino's treatise on healthcare, the *Three Books on Life*. The *Books* have been aptly described as 'a key text of early modern esotericism'.[38] Originally conceived as independent works, the second book, dedicated to Ficino's long-time friend and patron Filippo Valori,[39] deals with life-prolonging measures. In twenty chapters, Ficino primarily discusses nutritional topics, points out the importance of regular digestion, mentions remedies of various kinds, and reminds his addressees to 'avoid both continual thinking and sexual intercourse' due to their old age.[40]

Like the first and third books, the second *On Long Life* is based on the works of Galen of Pergamon and thus on the Hippocratic humoral doctrine. According to this theory, human health is guaranteed when there is a balance of the four humours.[41] The preservation of health – or balance – is, of course, the cardinal priority in Ficino's treatise on life-prolonging actions. According to Ficino, a balanced lifestyle includes 'natural remedies' such as fresh air and walking, but he also includes exposure to a certain colour and its corrective effects. In particular, Ficino recommends that the erudite strive to maintain a clear mind even in advanced age. For this, it is necessary to 'nourish' oneself with things such as fragrances, light wine, light, and colours.[42]

In this context, it is particularly noteworthy that Ficino's 'therapy of the intellectual' does not refer to colour effects in general, but explicitly emphasises the power of green. This is not only evident in the fourteenth chapter of the *liber secundus*, but in several points in *De vita triplici*. For example, in the first book, Ficino describes various factors that contribute to the increase of 'black bile', which he associates with the danger of melancholy. This, according to the tenth chapter, also includes 'whatever offends the sight',[43] thus once again hinting at the intimate connection between sight and mental condition. Ficino then lists possible measures to counteract melancholy. Among other things, there is the hint 'to calm and to cheer the dissonant and the sorrowful mind with constant and harmonious lyre and song', as well as 'horseback riding, [...], and the constant company of agreeable people'.[44] But also: 'I advocate the frequent viewing of shining water and of green or red colour'.[45]

The fourteenth chapter of the second book – *Confabulatio senum sub Venere per virentia prata* ('Conversation of the Old People Traversing the Green Fields under the Leadership of Venus') – is introduced by Ficino with old men in the company of Venus taking a walk. The goddess of love first addresses her companions with mockery and salaciously ambivalent oracles, only to strike a more serious note giving her interlocutors 'this to meditate on: the nature of green things'.[46] The introductory tale of the joking characters out in nature provides Ficino with the necessary framework to abstract from the objects – the green plants with their youthful, life-giving character – and deal specifically with the colour itself. Hence, he has Venus say: 'While we are walking among the green things, let us figure out why the colour green more than others foments the sight and healthfully delights it'.[47] This assertion alone is central given the abundance of 'green spaces' in Ficino's place of residence, fifteenth-century Florence. Indeed, the intention of the chapter seeks 'scientifically' to explain the reason for this. '[L]et us ask why' (*nobis cogitandum*)[48] is immediately followed by an explanation of the function of visual rays in contact with light or darkness. If neither complete light nor absolute darkness is favourable to the rays of vision, the middle colour of the spectrum is green according to Aristotle. In that tradition, Ficino concludes: '[T]he colour green tempering most of all black with white, furnishes the one effect and the other, equally delighting and conserving the sight'.[49] The positioning of green in the harmonious middle position between white/light and black/darkness is followed by a similar derivation of the special position of green things in relation to their (surface) structure. The green colour has 'soft and withal tender quality, just like water'.[50] Thus, when looking at green things, the rays of the eye would neither be injured nor dissolved in the distance, as is the case with hard and rough objects/colours. 'Finally, things [...], like water and green things, with their softness soothe the liquid rays of the eyes. [...] And so it rejoices in water; it is delighted by mirrors similar to water and green things'.[51] Ficino states: 'Why I have gone into all this?' and continues,

> That you may understand that the frequent use of green, since it recreates the spirit of sight, which is in a way the principal part of the animal spirit, refreshes also the animal spirit itself. And we will also remember that if the colour green, which among the colors is the middle grade and the most tempered, is so good for the animal spirit, much more will those things which through their qualities are the most temperate help the natural and vital spirits to conduce greatly towards our life. [...]. Through tempered things, therefore, the life which resides in the spirit is recreated; through tempered things the spirit is conformed to celestial things.[52]

The 'frequent use of green' (*frequentum viridium usum*) thought in relation of being surrounded by green walls very aptly sums up the holistic sensory experience of green-decorated spaces, enforced by Ficino's comment that the sight of green things is of benefit not only to the eyes, but also for the life spirit itself. In conclusion, it can be said that green was attributed a dual value: calmness and power. The calming effect due to the colour's position in the middle of the spectrum, and the power-generating effect can be explained 'etymologically' with *viribus* meaning power and *viridibus* or *viriditas* meaning green power.

As noted earlier, Ficino's statements are not new, nor do they represent an isolated case in the early modern period and are well embedded in the Aristotelian tradition. Indeed, the main ancient source from which all the following apparently draw their knowledge are (Pseudo-) Aristotle's *Problemata physica*. The thirty-first book deals with problems with the eyes, and in section 19, we find the question: 'Why does our vision deteriorate if we stare at other things, but improve if we look at green and grassy things such as vegetables, and the like?'[53] The answer shows how close Ficino's interpretation remains to this source:

> Is it because we can stare least at white and black (for both harm the sight), but such colours are intermediate between these; so that, our vision being now intermediate, we are not rendered impotent by it, but rather improved? Perhaps, as is the case with bodies, we suffer because of too violent exercise, but the mean puts us in the best position, and similarly with sight. For when we stare at solid objects we strain the sight, but when we look at liquid objects we do not strain it, because there is nothing to interrupt the vision. Now green objects are only moderately solid and there is sufficient moisture in them. So they do no harm and they encourage the sight to rest on them, because the mixture of colour is well adjusted to the vision. (XXXI, 19)[54]

The evidence for the medical employment of green 'things' becomes even clearer in Aristotle's *On Marvellous Things Heard*, where he explicitly recalls that malachite 'fetches a price comparable with gold; for it is a *drug* used for the eyes' (58).[55] In the *Naturalis historia* Pliny follows Aristotle, where in his thirty-seventh book he explains the beneficial effect of looking at emeralds:

> Certainly, no colour has a more pleasing appearance. For although we gaze eagerly at young plants and at leaves, we look at 'smaragdi' with all the more pleasure because, compared with them, there is nothing whatsoever that is more intensely green. Moreover, they alone of gems, when we look at them intently, satisfy the eye without cloying it. Indeed, even after straining our sight by looking at another object, we can restore it to its normal state by looking at a 'smaragdus'; and engravers of gemstones find that this is the most agreeable means of refreshing their eyes: so soothing to their feeling of fatigue is the mellow green colour of the stone. (XXXVII, 16, 64)[56]

As for the *Problems*, almost verbatim quotations can be traced in Ficino for Pliny; especially with regard to the comparison of colour with water and mirrors.[57] In order to highlight the continuity and diffusion of such ideas, beside Ficino, it is worthwhile to take a few more early modern sources into account. The Bolognese physician and astrologer Girolamo Manfredi, even in a much more synthetic way than Ficino, referrs similarly to the beneficial effect of the green colour on the human eye.[58] In his medical history, written in the vernacular in 1474 and commonly known as *Il Perché*, he poses the question: 'Why is our vision better in green colours than in white or black?' His answer is less literary or humanistically charged than in *De vita triplici*, but in essence gives the same Aristotelian reasoning:

> Each extreme weakens the feelings, and the tempered medium strengthens, because the extremes desperately move the sense organ, as too much white dissolves and the strong black has too much of a unifying and flattening effect. But the middle colour, like the green, moves moderately, neither too dissolving nor too unifying, but greatly strengthening the sense of sight.[59]

This strand of reasoning runs through the medical-encyclopaedic treatises of the following decades and centuries. An example from the sixteenth century is the *De rerum varitetate* by the erudite Girolamo Cardano from 1557: 'green improves the vitality and invigorates the eyesight'.[60] And in the following century the poet Alessandro Tassoni writes in his *De' pensieri diversi* in explicit reference to Aristotle and Cardano:

> [T]hat green, as the colour of the middle and of moderation, refreshes the eye, and that white and black, as the outermost, produce the opposite effect. But this opinion of Aristotle includes not only the green, but also all the other colours of the middle; and yet the other colours do not delight so much as the green does. (V, 13)[61]

The *longue durée* of these attributions to the colour green (which remain to this day in esoteric guides) is ultimately shown by *Die Augenheilkunde der Alten* (The Ophthalmology of the Ancients) by the Silesian ophthalmologist, and expert in colour sense and colour blindness, Hugo Magnus from 1901, who refers to Aristotle:

> Let us look at [Aristotle] a little more closely, because we are finally uncovering the source of an assumption that is still generally held to be true today. [...], it would also – he continues – be very healthy for the eyes if one were to look at greenery more often. [...] This Aristotelian view of the ophthalmo-hygienic benefit of green colour, which, as we have just seen, really did arise from the quaintest presuppositions, *has now become a dogma* not only for antiquity but also for modern times.[62]

Green: colour of nature, colour of vitality and eternity

In conclusion, at least a brief comment on the semantics of the colour green in a religious context should be remarked upon in order to highlight the interconnection and overlap of the religious and medical spheres. In the Christian context, the so-called gemstone allegory, for example, traces a broad reception of Pliny's *Natural History*. One of the most extensive sources in this regard are the writings of Hildegard of Bingen, who, thanks to her widely read treatise, certainly has a direct connection to the abovementioned encyclopaedias. Hildegard, foreshadowing Ficino, writes:

> If the blood and water in a person's eyes are too distressed, whether through old age or through illness, the person should go out to a green meadow and look at it until his eyes become wet as if from weeping: For the green of that meadow removes the dimness from the eyes, and makes them clean and clear again.[63]

Hence, her interpretation of the colour green mostly stems from the analogy or similarity with the plant world. It stands for freshness and vitality in contrast to the dry and dead. Hildegard's concept of *viriditas* or 'green power' develops exactly from this idea.[64] In the same way, the meaning of the colour green appears in general in Christian gemstone allegory; specifically in relation to the green jasper[65] and the emerald. Their chromatic similarity to the colourfulness of vegetation implies the positive connotation of something withered. Thus, they usually stand for faith, contemplation, eternal life, and hope. Attributions of this kind can be found in numerous stone books and commentaries on the *Apocalypse* and, insofar as the therapeutic effects of the colours of those stones are alluded to, even in this case have ancient roots. In addition to Pliny, Theophrastus should be remembered, who insisted on the healing effect of the emerald 'good for the eyes, and for this reason people carry seals made of it, so as to see better'.[66] And Christian exegetics follow this opinion.[67]

The green jasper, on the other hand, stands for faith, since, according to John's *Revelation*, the foundation of the Heavenly Jerusalem consists of it.[68] This equation – jasper equals faith – is made explicit in Richard of St Victor, who comments on that passage: 'for first the jasper is put, here it signifies faith' (*primus etenim ponitur jaspis, qui significat fidem*).[69] The author's insistence on the jasper in the description of the Holy City of Heaven goes further specifying that also the walls of the city are built of this stone:

> [T]he holy city Jerusalem coming down out of heaven from God, [...] its radiance like a most rare jewel, like a jasper, clear as crystal. It had a great, high wall, with twelve gates, [...]. The wall was built of jasper, while the city was pure gold, like clear glass. (Apoc. 21, 10–18)

Richard of St Victor's commentary reads as follows: 'The wall is identical with Christ, identical with the union of the Word and the Incarnate, and it is built with jasper, that is, not with an ordinary stone, but with this green stone, since Christ promised man green, eternal immortality'.[70]

The symbolism of green walls is, after all, deeply anchored in Christian exegesis and finds one of the most significant 'applications' of its complexity in the green monochrome painting of the Quattrocento (Figure 4.5), where it embodies an ascetic-contemplative ideal. But even in a room embellished by simple, green-coloured walls (Figure 4.2), the pervasiveness of

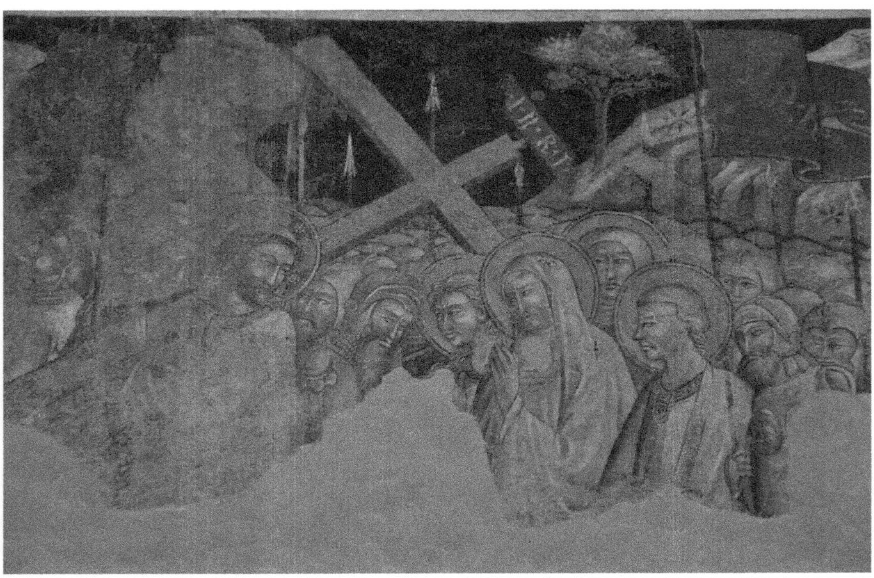

Figure 4.5 Pietro and Antonio Miniato, Carrying of the Cross, c. 1440, fresco, once Compagnia di San Girolamo. San Francesco, Prato. Image credit: Katharine Stahlbuhk

such a colour-presence makes the beholder physically experience the colour. The positive effects on body and mind ascribed to green in the above cited texts substantiates this claim that a form of chromotherapy was being practised throughout the Quattrocento.

Notes

1 In the vast literature on colour cf. esp. Gage, *Colour and Culture*, 1993; and the studies on various colours by Michel Pastoureau like that on *Green* (2014).
2 Leonardo da Vinci, *Trattato*, ed. 1890, §433, p. 144: 'Il colore non si vedrà mai semplice' (English translation is mine).
3 This paragraph is a free citation from the *Editorial* I wrote together with Hana Gründler and Franziska Lampe for the first issue 2022 of the *kritische berichte*.
4 Cf. Lalli, Innocenti, 'La Terra Verde', 2021; Vittorini Orgeas, 'La tecnica in terraverde', 2021; Eastaugh (et al.), *Pigment Compendium*, 2008, p. 641.
5 Savonarola, 'Predica XXVIII', in: *Prediche*, ed. 1962, vol. 2, pp. 362–397, here pp. 378–379: 'Colui che legge con li occhiali, ha dinanzi el libro aperto e li occhiali tra li occhi e il libro, [...]. Così dunque, come se tu avessi li occhiali rossi, tutto el libro ti pareria rosso, e se fussino verdi, pareria el libro verde, e così d'altri colori. [...]. Se tu hai dunque buoni occhiali, lo intelletto tuo vedrà sempre bene, e coì e contra se tu li arai cattivi. Piglia uno paio di occhiali gialli, e tu vedrai ogni cosa gialla, se tu hai li occhiali rossi, tu vedrai ogni cosa rossa. Li occhiali gialli sono li fantasmati della invidia, o vuoi della avarizia; li rossi, della ira, perché dalle passioni dell'anima dentro si formano li fantasmati conformi a quelle passioni, [...]'.
6 Savonarola, 'Predica XXVIII', in: *Prediche*, ed. 1962, vol. 2, pp. 362–397, here pp. 378–379.
7 Pliny, *Natural History*, ed. 1962, pp. 213–215. Scholars still discuss whether Pliny refers to glasses, to a mirror, or if it just a misunderstanding, cf. Woods, 'Pliny, Nero', 2006.
8 Cf. Stahlbuhk, *Oltre il colore*, 2021.
9 Stahlbuhk, *Oltre il colore*, 2021, pp. 123–188; Stahlbuhk, 'The Mode of Painting', 2021.
10 On the library cf. e.g., Canali, 'Brunelleschi, Michelozzo, Alberti', 1998; Scudieri, 'La Biblioteca', 2000.
11 Cf. Ullman and Stadter, *The Public Library*, 1972. Obviously, the definition of such a space as 'public' is at odds with our contemporary understanding of the term. On the complexity of the diverse notions of a public using and dwelling in pre- and early modern libraries see Molino, *L'impero di carta*, 2017, pp. 9–36.
12 Scudieri, 'La Biblioteca', 2000, p. 24, who mentions also the remains of a slight reddish lines, probably to evoke a sense of fictive stone/marble (Scudieri, 'La Biblioteca', 2000, p. 26).
13 For San Domenico in Bologna cf. Alce, D'Amato, *La Biblioteca*, 1961, pp. 42–43 with the document which attests the purchase of 350 *libbre* of green earth. For the Malatestiana cf. Baldacchini, *La biblioteca*, 1992. Furthermore, there have been e.g. that in San Giovanni in Canale in Piacenza and of Sant'Andrea in Faenza. This last one, in the sixteenth century, has been described as with *le pareti tinti di verde* (Razzi, 'Diario di viaggio', 1971, p. 90).
14 Concerning the green convent libraries, it is important to point out that there have been also such green spaces decorated with figurative monochrome murals as is best preserved in San Barnaba in Brescia. Cf. Panazza, *Il convento*, 1990; Seveso, 'La biblioteca', 2005.
15 This detail was first noted by Bettini, 'In Biblioteca', 2010, p. 59.

16 Bettini, 'In Biblioteca', 2010. Document published in Redig de Campos, *I palazzi Vaticani*, 1967, p. 60.
17 Scudieri, Ciliberto, 'Un'ipotesi per il verde', 2000; Bettini, 'In Biblioteca', 2010.
18 Bettini, 'In Biblioteca', 2010, pp. 60, 65 n. 18; English translation is mine.
19 Isidore, *Etymologies*, ed. 2006, p. 141. Cf. Scudieri, Ciliberto, 'Un'ipotesi per il verde', 2000.
20 On Torrechiara cf. Holthaus, 'La camera d'oro', 1991; Campbell, 'Pier Maria Rossi's Treasure', 2005; Zanichelli, 'La committenza dei Rossi', 2007.
21 Durand, *Rationale*, ed. 1995, p. 48 (I, iii, 39).
22 Especially on green textiles – in private households as well as in confraternities and the like – there would be a lot to say. Rebekah Compton mentions e.g. green verdure textiles in the Palazzo Medici (Compton, 'Green Gardens', 2021, pp. 136–137); for green cloths in religious settings cf. Stahlbuhk, *Oltre il colore*, 2021, pp. 55–59, 303–304.
23 AOSMF, II, 1 75, fol. 46v, available online via http://duomo.mpiwg-berlin.mpg.de (accessed 5 August 2025).
24 Cf. Castelnuovo, *Un pittore*, 1991, p. 35.
25 Cf. Weddigen, *Raffaels Papageienzimmer*, 2006, pp. 65–66.
26 Connections between the Sala delle Asse and the papal chamber in Avignon notes also Iacobone, 'La Sala delle Asse', 2019. Cf. also Alberti, 'Dai Giardini dipinti', 2019; Pedersen, 'The Sala delle Asse', 2019. For the Camera Verde cf. Edelstein, 'The camera verde', 2003.
27 Vitruvius, *On Architecture*, ed. 2009, p. 151 (emphasis is mine). A relation between the green walls of the libraries and this ancient source supposed already Bettini, 'In Biblioteca', 2010, p. 61.
28 Aristotle, 'On Sense', ed. 1975, p. 245.
29 Aristotle, *Meteorologica*, ed. 1978, p. 243 (emphasis is mine). The edition by Lee translates 'ἁλουργὸν' as 'blue'. Instead, it should be intended as purpure or reddish purple.
30 Aristotle, 'On Plants', ed. 1980, p. 219 (emphasis is mine).
31 See also the contributions by Jonietz and Brennan in the present volume, considering the colour spectrum or the middle tones in relation to medical analysis and healthy (skin) colour.
32 Ficino, *Three Books*, 1989. On Ficino's chapter with a special focus on Venus see also Compton, 'Green Gardens', 2021.
33 Cf. Clark, 'Roger Bacon', 1986.
34 Cf. Akopyan, Malkova, 'Medicine, Astology', 2022.
35 Stahlbuhk, *Oltre il colore*, 2021, pp. 271–273; Schäffner, *Terra Verde*, 2009, p. 319.
36 Ficino, *Three Books*, 1989, p. 204.
37 Ficino, *Three Books*, 1989, p. 207. Obviously, Ficino relies here, e.g., on Augustine, who asserted: 'Let us, therefore, rely principally on the testimony of the eyes, for this sense of the body far excels the rest, and comes closer to spiritual vision, though it differs from it in kind' (*De trinitate* XI, 1); cf. Saint Augustine, *The Trinity*, ed. 2010, p. 316.
38 Boenke, 'Einleitung', 2012, p. 8. For the interest or awareness on the part of the physicians regarding colour vision, and specifically on the colour of nature, see also Federici's comments in the present volume.
39 On their friendship, cf. Jurdjevic, 'Prophets and Politicians', 2004.
40 Ficino, *Three Books*, 1989, p. 215.
41 Cf. the first Part in Klibansky, Panofsky, Saxl, *Saturn and Melancholy*, 1964. See also Brennan's contribution in the present volume regarding skin colour in relation to the four humours.
42 Cf. Boenke, 'Einleitung', p. 13.
43 Ficino, *Three Books*, 1989, p. 133.
44 Ficino, *Three Books*, 1989, p. 135–137.

45 Ficino, *Three Books*, 1989, p. 135. For the additional mention of green's complementary colour red cf. Stahlbuhk, *Oltre il colore*, 2021, p. 116.
46 Ficino, *Three Books*, 1989, p. 205.
47 Ficino, *Three Books*, 1989.
48 Ficino, *Three Books*, 1989, p. 204.
49 Ficino, *Three Books*, 1989, p. 205.
50 Ficino, *Three Books*, 1989.
51 Ficino, *Three Books*, 1989, p. 205–207.
52 Ficino, *Three Books*, 1989, p. 207.
53 Aristotle, *Problems*, ed. 1965, p. 193.
54 Aristotle, *Problems*, ed. 1965, pp. 193–195.
55 Aristotle, 'On Marvelous Things Heard', ed. 1980, p. 261 (emphasis is mine).
56 Pliny, *Natural History*, ed. 1962, p. 213. The translation justly prefers to leave the term 'smaragdus', as our modern understanding of 'emerald' does not entirely correspond to what the ancients listed under the term 'smaragdus', where a variety of green coloured stones could be named like this. The same Pliny lists twelve different 'types' of emerald (XXXVII, 65). Cf. Comment n. 23 in: Theophrastus, *On Stones*, ed. 1956, pp. 97–98.
57 Cf. Pliny, *Natural History*, ed. 1962, pp. 213–215.
58 On Manfredi cf. Trombetti, 'Manfredi', 2007; Durato, *Mai sotto Saturno*, 2008.
59 Manfredi, IL PERCHÉ, ed. 1678, p. 289; English translation is mine.
60 Cardano, *De rerum varietate*, 1557, p. 113; English translation is mine. On Cardano cf. McLean, *Girolamo Cardano*, 2004; Baldi (ed.), *Girolamo Cardano*, 1999.
61 Tassoni, *De' Pensieri diversi*, 1665, p. 132.
62 Magnus, *Die Augenheilkunde*, 2015 (1901), pp. 116–117; English translation and emphasis are mine.
63 Hildegard, *Heilkunde*, ed. 1957, pp. 252; English translation is mine.
64 On Hildegard and colour, cf. Meier, 'Die Bedeutung der Farben', 1972, pp. 280–290; Meier, *Gemma spiritualis*, Munich 1977.
65 As stated for the emerald, the identification of the stones mentioned in the ancient sources rarely fits with our modern classification system and corresponding nomenclature. The 'iaspis', when mentioned in the sources, refers to a green translucent stone, not to an opaque silica of different possible colours, as we classify it today. Cf. Comment n. 27 in: Theophrastus, *On Stones*, ed. 1956, pp. 107–108.
66 Theophrastus, *On Stones*, ed. 1956, p. 50.
67 Cf. the cited sources in Schleusener-Eichholz, *Das Auge*, 1985, pp. 485–462, 474–475.
68 Apoc. 21, 19: 'The foundations of the wall of the city were adorned with every kind of jewel. The first was jasper, [...]'.
69 Richard of St Victor, *In apocalypsim Joannis* [col. 0871B], cited in Šedinová, 'The Symbolism', 1999, p. 83.
70 Šedinová, 'The Symbolism', 1999, the English translation is mine.

Source 3

The *Canon* of Polykleitos in Galen, ʿAlī ibn Raḍwān, and their Florentine readers

Robert Brennan

The vast majority of medical writings that survive from Roman antiquity were written in Greek by Galen of Pergamon (129–c. 216 CE). Within this extensive corpus, Galen repeatedly discusses the work of Polykleitos, a Greek sculptor active in the fifth century BCE. The most comprehensive – and today, best known – of these passages occurs in Galen's treatise, *On the Doctrines of Hippocrates and Plato* (c. 162–66 CE). Here, the sculptor comes up amidst a discussion of the Stoic philosopher, Chrysippus of Soli (c. 279–c. 206 BCE):

> [Chrysippus] says that health of body is proportion in things that are hot, cold, dry, and wet, which are obviously elements of bodies; but he believes that beauty does not lie in the proportion of the elements but of the members: of finger, obviously, to finger, of all the fingers to palm and wrist, of these to forearm, of forearm to upper arm, and of all to all, as is written in Polykleitos' *Canon*. Polykleitos first gave us full information in that book about all the proportions of the body, then he confirmed his account in action by fashioning a statue in accordance with the demands of the theory; and he gave to the statue, as he did to the treatise, the name *Canon*.[1]

On the Doctrines of Hippocrates and Plato was well-known in the medieval Islamic world, having been translated into Arabic by Ḥunayn ibn Isḥāq in the ninth century.[2] The above-cited account of Polykleitos is in fact thought to stand behind the title of Ibn Sīnā's widely influential medical treatise of 1027, *The Canon of Medicine* (*al-Qānūn fī al-Ṭibb*).[3] However, *On the Doctrines* was not translated into Latin until the sixteenth century, and Greek manuscripts of the work did not circulate widely in Latin Christendom before that time.[4] Nevertheless, Latin readers could read about Polykleitos and his *Canon* in a range of other works by Galen and his Arabic commentators, some of which became standard texts in university medical curricula across Europe during the thirteenth and fourteenth centuries.[5]

Knowledge of ancient art – and in particular, individual artists like Polykleitos – was scarce in Europe at this time. The present-day identification of Polykleitos' *Canon* with the *Doryphoros* (*Spear-Bearer*), a lost bronze statue known through marble copies, was not made until the nineteenth century.[6] It was not until the second half of the fourteenth century that key sources on ancient art, such as the relevant sections of Pliny's *Natural History*, started to be studied intensively.[7] Well into the fifteenth century, the name 'Polykleitos' still typically served as a vague token of artistic achievement, interchangeable with other quasi-legendary figures like Pheidias or Apelles.[8] Medical discourse represents a significant exception to this broader state of affairs.

Galen repeatedly discusses Polykleitos in relation to the medical concept of 'balanced complexion': a theoretical standard of health against which the particular condition of any given patient was to be judged. The works in which he invokes Polykleitos are too numerous to be discussed comprehensively here.[9] Instead, I will focus on one particularly prominent passage in Galen's *Art of Medicine*, a treatise known by many names in this period, including *Ars medica*, *Ars parva*, *Tegni*, and *Microtechne*. Galen presents this work as a comprehensive introduction to the medical profession, and it served as a centrepiece of medical curricula at many universities throughout the period.[10] In what follows, I will provide transcriptions and translations of the two principle Latin translations of the passage on Polykleitos, followed by a widely read commentary by ʿAlī ibn Raḍwān (c. 988–c. 1061, known in Latin as 'Haly'),[11] as well as two commentaries by Florentine professors of medicine, Taddeo Alderotti (d. 1295) and Pietro Torrigiano (d. c. 1320).

From the outset it should be noted that none of these texts exist in modern critical editions. My transcriptions derive from editions printed in the Renaissance, and must be considered provisional, subject to correction upon more detailed philological analysis of a wider range of editions and manuscripts. For ease of reading, I have resolved all abbreviations, modernised punctuation, and unified most spellings across the Latin texts.

Reference to Polykleitos is made in the fifth chapter of *The Art of Medicine*, where Galen describes the signs that indicate 'balanced complexion' throughout the body as a whole, as opposed to the preceding sections, which had addressed individual parts.[12] Two Latin translations of this passage were available to medieval readers. The first, known as the *translatio antiqua*, was completed in the twelfth century by an unknown translator working from the Greek text; the second, known as the *translatio arabica*, was completed by Gerard of Cremona (c. 1114–1187) from the Arabic translation of Ḥunayn ibn Isḥāq (809–873, known in Latin as 'Johannitus').[13] The *translatio antiqua* reads as follows:

> Signa competentis craseos secundum totam habitudinem animalis: Color quidem ex rubeo et albo commixtus, capilli vero et rubei et mediocriter crispi ut in pluribus, mediocritas vero carnositatis in quantitate et qualitate. Medium enim perfecte est huiusmodi corpus omnium superfluitatum ut dicantur et intelligantur. Adhuc enim spissum dicitur et tenue, similiter adhuc et multam carnem hominis et paucam, et crassum[14] et durum et molle et pilosum et nudum. Nihil igitur horum est mediocre, sed quale Policleti regula ad summum venit mediocritatis universe, ut tangentibus quidem neque molle appareat neque durum, neque calidum neque frigidum; videntibus vero neque pilosum neque nudum, neque crassum neque gracile, aut aliquam aliam habens intemperantiam.[15]

> The signs of an agreeable balance in the whole condition of the animal [are as follows]: a colour mixed out of red and white, hair that is red and midway curly as in many [cases], a middle state of fleshiness, both in quantity and in quality. Indeed, a body of this sort is the mean of all superfluities, such that the latter may be described and understood. Furthermore it is said to be both thick and thin, to have much flesh and little, and to be hard and soft, hairy and hairless. It is therefore characteristic of these [latter categories] that they are not at all moderate; rather, only something like the rule of Polykleitos reaches the height of moderation universally. To those touching it, it feels neither soft nor hard nor hot nor cold; to those viewing it, neither hairy nor hairless, neither fat nor skinny, nor having any other intemperateness.

Gerard of Cremona's *translatio arabica* differs in a number of respects, such as its characterisation of Polykleitos and his work:

> Ego quidem dico quod signa complexionis in corpore toto sunt quod color est compositus ex albedine et rubedine, capilli sunt flavi ad rubedinem et crispitudinem temperati secundum plurimum, et quod caro est temperata in qualitate sua et quantitate sua, quoniam hoc corpus est medium inter omnes species superfluitatum, propterea, quia omnis superfluitas non dicitur nec intelligitur nisi comparatione ad ipsum; quod est, quia corpus spissum non dicitur quia spissum est nisi per comparationem ad hoc corpus, et similiter extenuatum non dicitur quia est extenuatum nisi per comparationem ad ipsum. Et secundum hoc exemplum comparatur ad ipsum multam carnem habens et paucam carnem, et crassum et macrum, et molle et durum, et pilosum et nudum pilis. Et non est aliquod horum corporum aequale, sed aequale est quod est secundum exemplum quod praeparavit Polycletus, et nominavit ipsum Canonem, qui consecutus est ultimum aequalitatis totius, donec fit, quando tangitur, ut non appareat quia est molle, neque quia est durum, neque quia est calidum, neque quia est frigidum; et quando aspicitur ad ipsum, non invenitur pilosum neque nudum pilis, neque grossum neque gracile, neque vincit super eum aliquid superfluitatis.[16]

> Certainly I tell you that the signs of [balanced] complexion in the whole body are that the colour is composed of white and red; the hair is blond, tempered

> toward red and curliness, as is often [the case]; and the flesh is tempered in both its quality and in its quantity, since this body is the medium among all types of superfluities, in the sense that any superfluity is not described or understood [as such] without comparison to it. That is, a thick body is not said to be thick except through comparison to this body, and similarly, a thin body is not said to be thin except through comparison to it. And accordingly, it is as compared to this model (*exemplum*) that [a body] has much flesh or little flesh, is fat or skinny, soft or hard, hairy or hairless. None of these [latter] bodies are balanced – rather, the balanced one is that which is in accordance with the model that Polykleitos prepared and nominated as the *Canon*, which reaches the limit of all balance, such that when it is touched, it feels neither soft nor hard, neither hot nor cold, and when it is looked at, it is found to be neither hairy nor hairless, neither fat nor thin, and not the slightest bit of superfluity gets the better of it.

In both translations, the passage provides little direct information about Polykleitos: it does not specifically clarify that he was a sculptor, for example. Latin readers could have acquired such knowledge elsewhere in Galen or other ancient authors, but explanations were readily available in standard Arabic commentaries on the text. One such commentary by ʿAlī ibn Raḍwān (c. 988–c. 1061), which was also translated into Latin by Gerard of Cremona in the twelfth century,[17] reads as follows:

> Ista sunt signa corporis quod est in meliori formarum. Et hoc corpus, quamvis non sit inventum secundum veritatem, est tamen canon, ad quem comparatur totum, quod est in medicina, sicut fecit Polycletus. Iste enim fecit statuam in ultimo quod possibile est ab aequalitate, et posuit eam canonem, per quem perveniatur in operatione statuarum. Cum ergo dicit medicus, in cibo aut medicina aut in signo aut in causa, quod est aequale aut calidum aut frigidum aut humidum aut siccum, et quanta sit summa gradus eius in caliditate sua aut in frigiditate aut in alio ab illo, tunc illud non est nisi secundum comparationem eius cum meliori formarum, quia melior formarum est canon medicorum secundum intentionem logicorum.[18]

> These are the signs of the body in the best of forms. And this body, although it is not found in reality, is nevertheless the measure (*canon*) to which everything in medicine is compared, like the one Polykleitos made. For the latter made a statue at the limit of what is possible in terms of balance, and set it as the measure of what is to be reached in the working of statues. Therefore, when a doctor says about a food or a medicine or a symptom or a cause that it is balanced or hot or cold or wet or dry, and what degree of hotness or coldness it is, and so on, then this is not so except according to how it compares with the best of forms, since the best of forms is the measure of physicians, understood in the sense of the logicians.

ʿAlī ibn Raḍwān not only supplies further information about Polykleitos, but also neatly summarises the broader significance of the *Canon* as a work that grounds the scope and potential of sculpture as an art. In his view, moreover, what makes the 'balanced complexion' akin to Polykleitos' *Canon* is that it is an ideal – 'not found in reality' – whose authority derives from an inner conceptual necessity, rooted ultimately in the science of logic.

Florentine interpretations of the passage reflect commentaries like that of ʿAlī ibn Raḍwān, while also expressing their own, historically specific attitudes toward visual art. Taddeo Alderotti, a founding figure of Florentine medical tradition, who taught at the University of Bologna from the 1260s into the 1290s, began writing a commentary on Galen's *Art of Medicine* sometime before 1283.[19] In his account of the passage on Polykleitos, he begins with a literal interpretation that consists largely of quotations and paraphrases from the *translatio antiqua*.[20] He then works through a series of doubts and difficulties that the passage raises. It is here that he discusses the question of why the colour of perfectly complexioned skin is white and red (discussed in Chapter 3 of this book). Later on in this same section, he also addresses Polykleitos:

> [...] sed tale quale est Polycleti regula. Polycletus fuit quidam carpentarius qui fecit unam statuam adeo moderatam quod ad ipsam comparabantur omnes alie statue. Similiter ad illud corpus comparantur omnia alia corpora. Non solum hominum, sed ciborum potuum et medicinarum et ponuntur in gradu per maiorem et minorem recessum ab eo.[21]

> [...] but such a body is like the rule of Polykleitos. Polykleitos was a certain carpenter who made a statue so moderated that all other statues were compared to it. Likewise, to this body all other bodies are compared, not only of men but also of foods and drinks and medicines, and they are ranked as greater or lesser in relation to it.

Much could be said about Taddeo's use of terminology (e.g., *carpentarius*), as well as the relationship between this principle and broader notions of art (*ars*) that pervaded both university education and the guild system in this period. Given the correspondence with ʿAlī ibn Raḍwān, whom Alderotti cites frequently elsewhere throughout the text, the passage also suggests how Arabic medical texts could serve as authoritative sources about the history and theory of art in this period – a significant connection in light of the contemporaneous proliferation of pseudo-Arabic script in Italian art.[22]

The most authoritative commentary on the *Art of Medicine* by a Florentine physician in this period was undoubtedly the monumental *Plus quam commentum*, completed by Pietro Torrigiano before his death around 1320. As indicated by the title (literally, 'more than a commentary'), Torrigiano brought an unprecedented range of philosophical and scientific reflection to the task of commentating Galen's text.[23] He also approaches the passage in a fundamentally different way than Alderotti. Explicitly citing ʿAlī ibn Raḍwān, he insists on reading the passage as a continuation of the immediately preceding section in Galen's text, which concerns the complexion of muscles.[24] This continuity is significant for many reasons, including the topic of skin colour addressed in Chapter 3 of this book. For in the preceding passage on muscles, Galen had explicitly addressed the relationship between climate and ethnicity, prompting both ʿAlī ibn Raḍwān and Torrigiano to compare and contrast the white skin of Slavic peoples with the black skin of Africans.[25] This same continuity also guides Torrigiano into his extended reflection on the anatomy of white skin in the section on Polykleitos:[26]

> SIGNA COMPETENTIS etc infra. Signa complexionis aequalis secundum habitudinem totius corporis denotatae in musculis sunt haec, scilicet color commistus ex albo et rubeo: temperantia enim musculorum efficit hunc colorem in cute, quia, cum cutis sit natura alba ad modum membrorum, quae Galenus vocat radicalia, propter calorem, cum ex[s]iccaverit humidum sanguineum, ex quo fiunt, dealbare ipsum per ulteriorem decoctionem in ipso: sanguis autem et caro musculorum, quae a cute teguntur, cum sortita fuerint temperamentum conveniens, sint rubea, resultabit in superficie color commistus ex utroque, cum cutis quidem tenuis existens admittat colorem eorum, quae tangit. Deinde dicit, CAPILLI VERO etc infra. Et ex signis eius sunt capilli rubei et mediocriter crispi in pluribus. Et causa huius in promptu est ex praedictis,[27] apud recolentem, quod color rubeus medius est inter album et nigrum, quorum unus frigiditatem, alter caliditatem annunciat: recolentem quoque, quod crispitudo siccitatem significat, simplicitas vero humiditatem. Dicit autem in pluribus, propter quandoque fieri tortuositatem pororum causam in talibus superfluae crispitudinis, nequaquam augmentata siccitate. Est autem et hic sciendum, quod tales capilli non sunt necessarium signum temperantiae omnium musculorum corporis, sed principalius eorum, qui in capite. Deinde dixit, MEDIOCRITAS VERO etc infra. Et ex signis est mediocritas carnositatis in qualitate et quantitate. Deinde dixit huius causam unam communem, et dixit, MEDIUM ENIM etc infra. Et ideo est habens mediocritatem carnositatis quia hoc corpus est perfecte medium inter omnes tales superfluitates, adeo ut oporteat omnem superfluitatem dici et intelligi tanquam ad ipsum relatum; omnis enim superfluitas ad medium comparatur, ut non dicatur superfluum, nisi quod super medium excellit. Deinde exemplificat, et dicit, ETENIM etc infra, quia spissum et tenue, multae carnis et paucae, crassum et macrum, durum et molle, pilosum et nudum, et huiusmodi non dicuntur nisi per comparationem ad ipsum secundum quantitatem separationis ab ipso. Deinde volens declarare mediocre, ostendit illud per quoddam simile, et dicit, NIHIL IGITUR horum etc infra, nihil igitur nunc dictorum, scilicet spissum et tenue etc, est mediocre, cum ipsa sint extrema abextrinsecus existentia, et dicta per comparationem ad illud, talia, sed mediocre est illud, quod venit ad summum universae mediocritatis, discernibile ad tactum vel visum, vel aliquem sensum, ut ad tactum neque sit molle, neque durum, temperantiam habens inter passivas: neque calidum, neque frigidum, temperantiam habens inter activas. Ad visum vero neque sit pilosum neque nudum, neque grossum neque gracile, neque alicuius alterius superfluitatis habens denominationem, sed temperantiam in utrisque, et sit, qualis regula Polycleti statuifici. Hic enim (sicut dicitur) in memoriam Helenae fecit statuam tantae pulchritudinis, ut nulla posset ei attribui deformitas, et posuit eam regulam statuarum, ut diceretur pulchrior per maiorem appropinquationem ad ipsam.[28]

'The signs of an agreeable, etc.'. The signs of a balanced complexion according to the condition of the whole body as denoted in the muscles are these: namely, a colour mixed of white and red. For the balance of the muscles creates this colour in the skin, because skin is by nature white, like the other members that Galen calls *radicalia*, on account of the heat, so since when the wet bloody [substance] from which they [i.e. *radicalia*] are made has dried out, it [comes] to whiten as it boils down within itself, but the blood and the flesh of the muscles, which are covered by the skin, insofar as they have an agreeable temperament, are red; on the surface, the result will be a colour mixed from both, because the skin itself, being thin, admits the colour of whatever it touches. Then he says 'the hair, etc.'. Among its signs are red and moderately curly hair, as in many [cases]. And the cause of this is readily apparent from what was said above,[29] recalling that the colour red is midway between black and white, of which one indicates coldness, the other hotness, and recalling also that curliness signifies dryness, and straightness wetness. And he says 'in many [cases]' because at times the tortuosity of the pores becomes the cause of superfluous curliness in such men, even if the dryness is increased. Here however it must be known that such hair is not a necessary sign of balance for all muscles of the body, but more specifically those which are in the head. Then he says 'a middle state etc.': also among the signs is the balance of fleshiness in quality and quantity. Then he says that the cause of this is one and the same, and says 'the mean, etc.': that is, it has a balance of flesh since this body is perfectly in the middle of all such superfluities, such that it is necessary for all superfluity to be named and understood as if in relation to this; for all superfluity is compared to a medium, in order that it not be called superfluous unless it exceeds the mean. Then he exemplifies, and says 'Furthermore etc.': that thick and thin, much and little flesh, fat and skinny, hard and soft, hairy and hairless, and things of this kind are not denominated except through comparison to this [balanced body], according to their quantity of separation from it. Then wishing to explain the medium, he demonstrates it through a certain similitude, and says, 'none therefore of these etc.': none therefore of what has now been said – that is, fat and thin etc. – is the mean, since these are extremes that exist extrinsically, and are only called as such through comparison to it, whereas the mean is that which comes to the height of universal balance, discernable to touch or sight, or any sense, as [for example] to touch, it neither becomes soft nor hard, having a balance between passive [qualities], and similarly neither hot nor cold, having a balance between active [qualities]; to vision indeed neither is it hairy nor hairless, nor wide nor slender, nor does it possess the name of any other superfluity, but balance in both, and it is like the rule of Polykleitos the statue-maker. For this man, as is said, made a statue in memory of Helen that was of such beauty that no deformity could be attributed to it, and he established it as a rule for statues, in order that [a statue] would be called more beautiful insofar as it drew nearer to it.

Torrigiano's account of Polykleitos introduces the concept of 'beauty' (*pulchritudo*), while preserving the rigorous, neither–nor logic of Galen and 'Alī ibn Raḍwān. In this way, it offers a surprisingly analytic precedent for notions of ineffable beauty that would become prominent in later phases of European art theory.[30] The emphasis on beauty arises in tandem with assumptions about gender that are relevant to the art of Torrigiano's own, early fourteenth-century moment.[31] The effort to link Polykleitos with a statue of Helen – however fanciful – likewise recalls emergent practices of antiquarianism, for already by the second half of the fourteenth century, a Venus Pudica statue was on display 'in a private house in Florence' that contemporaries attributed to Polykleitos.[32] By embedding the discussion in an overtly racialised conceptual framework, Torrigiano also anticipates the medical and scientific literature of eighteenth- and nineteenth-century Europe, in which classical sculptures were often placed at the apex of illustrated racial hierarchies.[33]

Notes

1 Galen, *On the Doctrines*, 1981, p. 309; for the date, see Galen, *On the Doctrines*, 1981, p. 46. On the passage, see Pollitt, *The Art of Ancient Greece*, 1990, 76. Here and throughout I modify the spelling of Polykleitos' name and italicise the alleged name of his work ('Canon') for consistency.
2 De Lacy in Galen, *On the Doctrines*, 1981, pp. 42–46.
3 Strohmaier, 'Avicenna between Galen and Aristotle', 2019, pp. 217–218.
4 Nutton, '*De placitis Hippocratis et Platonis* in the Renaissance', 1988, pp. 281–309.
5 See recently McVaugh, 'Galen in the Medieval Universities, 1200–1400', 2019, pp. 381–392.
6 Moon, *Polykleitos, the Doryphoros, and Tradition*, 1995.
7 McHam, *Pliny and the Artistic Culture*, 2013, pp. 63–64, with bibliography.
8 Pfisterer, 'Phidias und Polyklet von Dante bis Vasari', 1996, pp. 69–97; Pfisterer, *Donatello und die Entdeckung der Stile*, 2002, pp. 184–201, 216, 226–232, 254–259.
9 For an overview of texts available to Latin readers in the late Middle Ages, see Kaye, *A History of Balance*, 2014, pp. 160–161, 175–176.
10 See Ottosson, *Scholastic Medicine and Philosophy*, 1984.
11 ʿAlī ibn Raḍwān is to be distinguished from the famous Persian medical writer, ʿAlī ibn Abbās al-Majūsī (d. c. 982–994), who was known in Latin as 'Haly Abbas'.
12 For the Greek text and corresponding English translation of the passage, see Galen, *On the Constitution*, 2016, p. 211.
13 Kaye, *A History of Balance*, 2014, pp. 139–140.
14 This stray category is omitted in the translation below.
15 Galen, *Opera*, 1490, vol. 1, fol. 26ra.
16 Torrigiano, *Plus quam commentum*, 1557, fol. 189r (D).
17 Ottosson, *Scholastic Medicine and Philosophy*, 1984, 26, pp. 102–103; Hasse, *Success and Suppression*, 2016, pp. 373–374.
18 Torrigiano, *Plus quam commentum*, 1557, fol. 189v (E).
19 Siraisi, *Taddeo Alderotti and His Pupils*, 1981, pp. 35, 40.
20 Alderotti, *In Galeni micratechnen*, 1522, fol. 98ra.
21 Alderotti, *In Galeni micratechnen*, 1522, fol. 100rb.
22 For examples, with previous bibliography, see recently Schulz, 'Schriftgestöber und geritztes Gold', 2018, pp. 215–243; Moore, 'Kufesque between Pilgrimage and Polemic', 2021, pp. 152–215; Napolitano, 'Dall'ottone alla tempera', 2022, pp. 31–60.
23 On the intellectual scope of Torrigiano's commentary, see recently Utamura, 'Revisiting the Exegetical Tradition of Galen's Prologue', 2020, pp. 352–375, with previous bibliography.

24 Torrigiano, *Plus quam commentum*, 1557, fol. 75v: 'Propter quod (sicut dicit Hali) cum dicimus totius corporis habitudinem, tunc plurimum, quod significamus, est musculus [...]'.

25 Torrigiano, *Plus quam commentum*, 1557, fol. 189r ('Alī ibn Raḍwān) and fol. 76r (Torrigiano): 'Manifestum enim est quod in regione Sclavorum cutis et pilus albescunt, quantumcumque musculi ab ea contecti sint calidi: in regione vero Aethiopum nigrescunt, quantumcumque sint frigidi'. This racial dimension is consistent with other passages in Torrigiano's treatise, on which see Biller, 'Proto-Racial Thought in Medieval Science', 2009, p. 166.

26 This is the same passage discussed above in Chapter 3 of this book. It should be noted that these principles concerning skin colour had already been outlined at an earlier point in the treatise: Torrigiano, *Plus quam commentum*, 1557, fol. 29r.

27 See the prior discussion of hair colour at Torrigiano, *Plus quam commentum*, 1557, fols 47r–54r, esp. 48r.

28 Torrigiano, *Plus quam commentum*, 1557, fols 76r–v.

29 See note 27 above.

30 For example, Sammern and Saviello, 'Einleitung: Der schöne Körper als Kunstprodukt', 2019, pp. 9–11.

31 See e.g., Brennan, *Painting as a Modern Art*, 2019, pp. 130–150, with further medically oriented discussions of Polykleitos at pp. 184, 194–198.

32 Significantly, however, Benvenuto da Imola, who describes the statue and its setting, opposes this attribution on the basis of what he had read in Pliny: 'Ego autem vidi Florentiae in domo privata statuam Veneris de marmore mirabilem in eo habitu in quo olim pingebatur Venus. Erat enim mulier speciosissima nuda, tenens manum sinistram ad pudenda, dexteram vero ad mammillas, et dicebatur esse opus Polycleti, quod non credo, quia ut dictum est Polycletus sculpsit in aere, non in marmore [...]' (*Comentum super Dantis Aldigherij comoediam*, 1887, vol. 3, p. 280). Instead, he attributes it to Praxiteles.

33 See e.g., Bindman, *Ape to Apollo*, 2002.

5

The uroscopic colour palette: Dominicus de Ragusa, Gentile da Fabriano, and painterly knowledge of urine

Fabian Jonietz

In the fifteenth century, if one asked which art most fully epitomised the principle of dissimulation, the answer might not necessarily have been painting. In 1469, the physician Giovanni d'Arezzo described how patients were misled by 'so-called doctors' (*illudunt namque huius dicti medici vulgus cum medicinis*), who might, for instance, claim to detect from a urinalysis that the patient had eaten figs or donkey flesh. In reality, they reached such conclusions simply by observing remnants of the fruit or freshly butchered animal skin.[1] Conversely, in another medical treatise written around 1495, Gabriele Zerbi recommended that doctors should exaggerate the complexity of diagnosis in front of laymen, and secretly delay the process for a whole day by ordering a morning sample of urine, even if this was not actually necessary.[2]

The methods of urinalysis, which rested on ancient Roman-Greek and modern Arabic theories, had likewise been invoked repeatedly among patients – and in fact, far earlier – as a way of dissimulating doubts about the competence of doctors. The treatise *De cautelis medicorum*, composed around 1300, already contains a warning that some patients might present doctors with other people's urine, or even that of animals, in order to test their methods.[3] Numerous incompetent charlatans undermined furthermore the status of the profession as Giovanni d'Arezzo's criticism makes clear. He contrasts dubious physicians with the esteemed arts of painting and sculpture: in these fields, skill is evident, as the works are displayed for all to judge, while physicians – famously – bury their mistakes.[4]

Such relationships and comparisons perhaps furnish the foundation of a novella by Boccaccio (*Decameron* VIII.9), in which the painters Buffalmacco and Bruno di Giovanni fool the physician Simone, whose shop sign with an image of a urine glass or *matula* announces his profession. Over the course of the story, the painters' cosmetically applied wounds ensure that this expert of urinalysis ends up falling into a cesspool, or, as an early fifteenth-century illustrator imagined it, a toilet (Figure 5.1).[5]

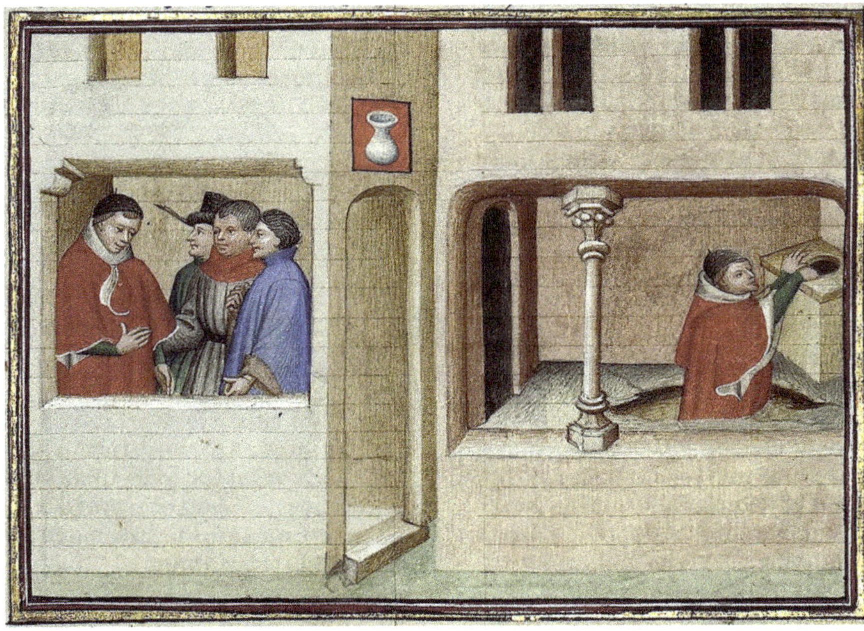

Figure 5.1 Giovanni Boccaccio, *Decameron* (illustration to Novella VIII.9), 1414/18. Vatican, Biblioteca Apostolica Vaticana, Pal. lat. 1989, fol. 253v. Image credit: Wikipedia Commons

Together, these examples indicate several levels of affinity between controversies surrounding the methods of urinalysis and classic motifs within the artistic tradition. This chapter investigates the relationship between the medical practice of urinalysis and painters' specialised knowledge of materials and colours, focusing the analysis on four areas. The methods of urinalysis are based not only on smell and taste, but perhaps even more importantly on vision – viscosity, sediment, and not least the colour of the urine as observed in a glass *matula*.[6] Beginning in the early fifteenth century with a previously unknown collaboration between a doctor and a famous painter, Gentile da Fabriano, I examine various sources and contexts that demonstrate the expertise of visual artists in the field of excrement products – a genuine knowledge thoroughly bound up with the practices of the early modern workshop. For physicians and intellectuals, however, it was equally important that such painterly expertise was confirmed by a pseudo-antique, seemingly authoritative statement attributed to a founding figure of ancient medicine. Connections between the written characterisation of colours and the actual colouring of uroscopic treatises likewise demonstrate the important role that medical experts played in the systemisation and codification of nuanced colour gradients, as well as the diffusion of this specialised knowledge beyond the readership of fellow physicians.

On a more general level, this chapter also aims to counter the stark focus of art historical research on the anatomical studies of early modern artists. The anatomical paradigm, as this reductive view can be characterised, occludes the fact that painters and sculptors were concerned with much more than the correct representation of human proportions:[7] already in Lorenzo Ghiberti's *Commentarii*, the author lists the sciences that painters need to know and distinguishes knowledge of correct anatomical representation *(Notomia)* from the equally necessary knowledge of a general theory of the human body (*Medicina*).[8]

Since the 1400s, as I will argue, it was in the interest of artists to understand and truthfully represent a wide range of bodily phenomena, including mental conditions and states of excitement that could manifest themselves through the emission of sweat, the colouring of the skin, the tightening of the muscles, or the protrusion of the eyes.[9] For example, certain artists made a name for themselves by representing bodies that seemed lifelike not primarily due to anatomically correct representation, but rather because the figures salivated or spit, or defecated under the visible strain of the whole body.[10] Pliny mentions the ability to represent sweat as a special sign of lifelikeness in the work of Parrhasios (*ut sudare videatur*).[11] In the fifteenth century, this praise was taken up directly by Bartolomeo Facio in his celebration of works by Jan van Eyck (*in balneo... anus quae sudare uideatur*) and Rogier van der Weyden (*mulier in balneo sudans*), and was also raised to the status of a norm by Leon Battista Alberti in his treatise on painting.[12]

Later it was said of Renaissance artists like Raphael and Titian that physicians who observed their paintings could correctly draw conclusions about the acute illnesses of the people depicted:[13] again only a variation of Pliny's praise of Apelles, who portrayed his subjects so lifelike that physiognomists were able to predict their remaining years of life.[14] The depiction of such precarious states of health, contrary to canonical ideas of beauty, indicates an ideal mode of representation that goes beyond mimesis, embracing a different model – that of 'lifelikeness'. The representation of the body in a medical state as close as possible to the living person also made the figure's appearance congruous with its future developments and actions. Precisely for this reason, the method of urinalysis was directly linked with the theory of astrological prognostication – whose practitioners were traditionally deemed children of Mercury along with physicians and painters, who in many images are shown practicing their arts together as a group (Figure 5.2).

Twenty shades of urine

That early modern painters had an understanding of medicine that far exceeded anatomy can also be gathered from representations of

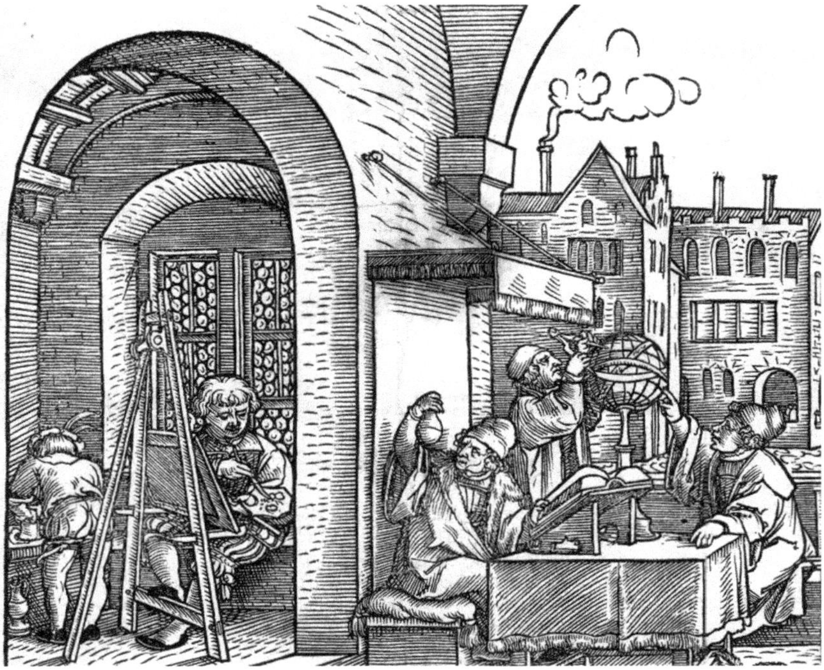

Figure 5.2 Georg Pencz, Children of Mercury (detail), 1531, woodcut, 350 × 218 mm. Image credit: http://www.zeno.org – Henricus – Edition Deutsche Klassik GmbH

the Evangelist Luke, where the two professions of the patron saint are made visible.[15] Around 1625, for example, the painter Orsola Maddalena Caccia placed a series of medical books in the artistic workshop of the Evangelist, including names such as Aulus Cornelius Celsus, Avicenna, Galen, and Pedanios Dioscorides (the author of the widely circulated *Materia medica*).[16] Toward the middle of the sixteenth century, Maerten van Heemskerck painted an image of Saint Luke, possibly for the painter's guild in Delft, which not only places an anatomical work with allusions to Galen and Vesalius on the floor of his fictive workshop, but also includes a bookshelf with two volumes identified as pharmacological works by the Greek physicians Nikandros of Kolophon and, again, Pedanios Discorides.[17]

More frequent than such written references, however, is an iconographic detail indicating the medical expertise of the patron saint of the painters. In numerous depictions of Luke, cylindrical wicker baskets – sometimes with a glass vessel peeking out – can be seen in close proximity to his easel (Figures 5.3–5.7). While understandable that these containers have occasionally been interpreted as containers for oil and other painting materials, early modern observers would have recognised the baskets

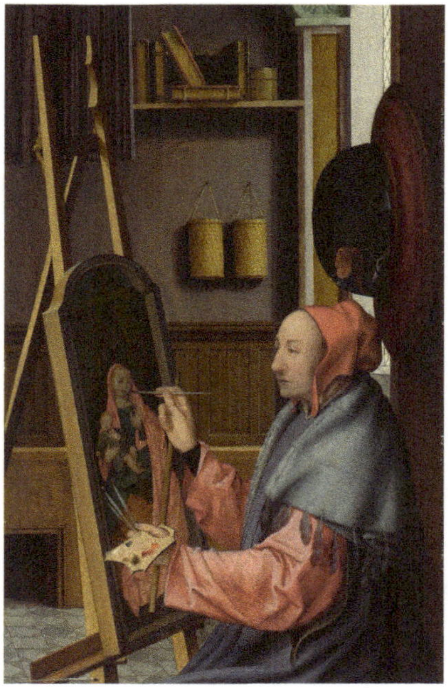

Figure 5.3 Workshop of Quentin Massys, St Luke painting the Virgin (detail), c. 1520, oil on oak panel, 114.9 × 35.4 cm. London, National Gallery, inv. NG3902. Image credit: Wikipedia Commons

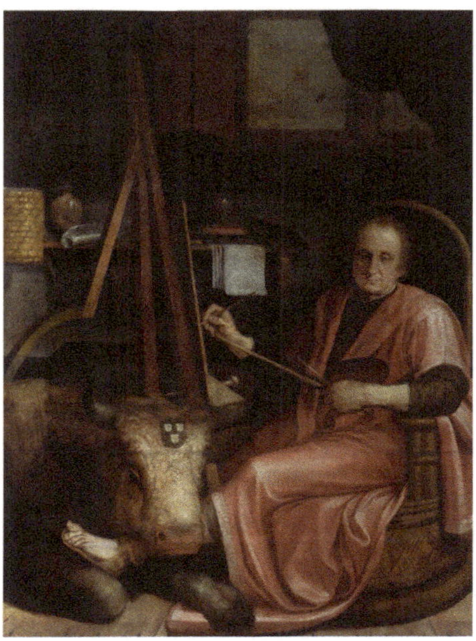

Figure 5.4 Frans Floris, St Luke at his easel (detail), 1556, oil on panel, 214 × 197 cm (patched). Antwerp, Koninklijk Museum voor Schone Kunsten, inv. 114. Image credit: Collection KMSKA – Flemish Community

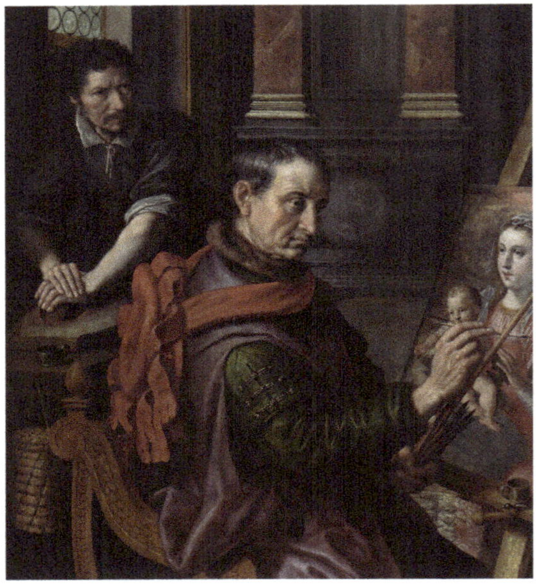

Figure 5.5 Maerten de Vos, St Luke painting the Virgin (detail), 1602, oil on panel, 270 × 217 cm. Antwerp, Koninklijk Museum voor Schone Kunsten, inv. 88. Image credit: Collection KMSKA – Flemish Community

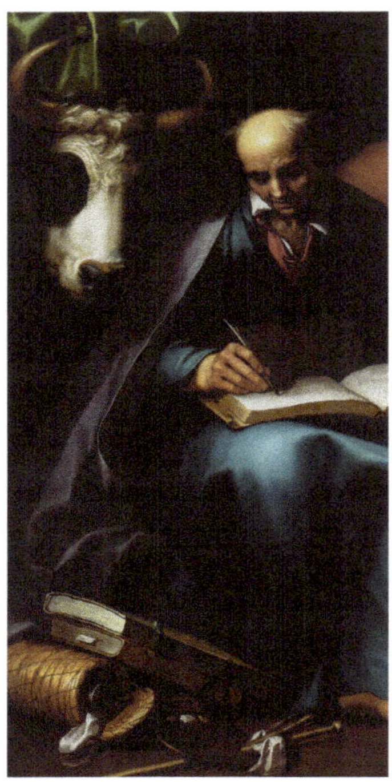

Figure 5.6 Abraham Bloemaert, Four Evangelists (detail), c. 1612/15, oil on canvas, 179 × 227.3 cm. Princeton, Princeton University Art Museum, object no. y1991-41. Image credit: Princeton University Art Museum

Figure 5.7 Joachim Antonisz. Wtewael, St Luke, 1616, oil on oak panel, 77.8 × 60.5 cm. Stuttgart, Staatsgalerie, inv. 3451. Image credit: PubHist.com

as typical means of transport for the glass containers or *matula*, in which patients brought urine to the doctor, and protected it along the way from the influence of light and any danger of breaking.[18]

Although the function and meaning of these baskets has often been ignored in discussions of Luke's iconography,[19] some interest in urinalysis has occasionally turned up in art historical research. Above all, three issues have been addressed: first, the use of the *matula* as an attribute of the physician, which was only later replaced by the head mirror and stethoscope; second, the genre of urinalysis imagery, which also reflects the decline of this diagnostic method, as it began to be associated with quackery from the seventeenth century onward; and third, the urinary colour scales and wheels (*rotae urinarum*), whose appearance in Europe can be traced back to illustrations in medieval Arabic manuscripts.[20]

In classic works on the history of colour, these visually appealing schemata are frequently mentioned and illustrated; however, a comprehensive, comparative analysis has yet to be undertaken.[21] Indeed, little is known about the production and use of colour scales and urine wheels. For example, it has never been proven that these scales were actually used in practice as diagnostic instruments for colour matching, as scholars such as John Gage, Michael Stolberg, and Michel Pastoureau have suggested.[22] Only at the end of the sixteenth century is this specific use described by the physician Pieter van Foreest, but in fact he castigates it as one of the many deceitful methods used by con artists (*alij…chartas vel libros præ manibus & oculis habent, in quibus reperiuntur omnes vrinarū[m] colores ad viuum depicti*).[23]

Such a comprehensive investigation lies beyond the scope of the present study, as it would necessitate a synoptic comparison of a very great number of coloured manuscripts and variants of the twenty names for colour tones usually differentiated in early modern medical teachings. Here, I will briefly touch upon just two particularly significant and well-known printed book illustrations: first, the *Fasciculus medicinae*, a book incorrectly – but persistently – attributed to Johannes Kellner von Kirchheim (Johannes de Ketham), first printed in 1491 with six woodcuts, among them a *Rota urinarum*, and frequently reprinted after 1494 with new illustrations and translations into numerous languages;[24] second, Ulrich Pinder's *Epiphanie medicorum: Speculum videndi urinas hominum*, published in Nuremberg in 1506.[25]

The frequent reproduction of Pinder's uroscopic woodcuts in scholarly literature obscures the fact that his publication had a far narrower distribution and impact than the *Fasciculus*. To date, knowledge of the production and practical uses of these texts and illustrations remains entirely hypothetical. Occasionally it has been assumed that physicians themselves coloured the woodcuts, and several sloppily painted exemplars do indeed indicate an inexpert hand. In most woodcut illustrations of the *Fasciculus medicinae*, there is a twenty-first *matula* that lacks an inscription – a gap that could in fact be interpreted as an option or as an invitation to practicing physicians to expand upon the canonical twenty tones through their own, innovative observations (Figure 5.8).

If in some cases physicians did take up the task of colouring themselves, this must nevertheless have been an exceptional occurrence. The colouration of editions of Pinder's *Epiphanie medicorum* (1506), such as that in the Folger Shakespeare Library as well as an exemplar auctioned at Christie's in 2002, resemble one another so strongly that one must assume the serial work of a professional illustrator, who coloured the prints on commission from a book dealer or salesperson.[26] In the two aforementioned cases, not only is the choice of colours nearly identical, but also the coloured decoration of the rounded middle scene and the ring of ornamentation around the border of the woodcut. A contrasting approach to colouring the contents of the *matula* can be seen in an exemplar at the Staatsbibliothek in Berlin: for example, in the white tones in the upper right quarter of the urine wheel, the correct green colour for the type 'viridis' (which, surprisingly, appears yellow in the other two copies) or the general lack of blue in this copy (Figure 5.9).[27]

Scepticism is thus warranted towards the foundational assumption that colour illustrations in medical works were intended to help the early

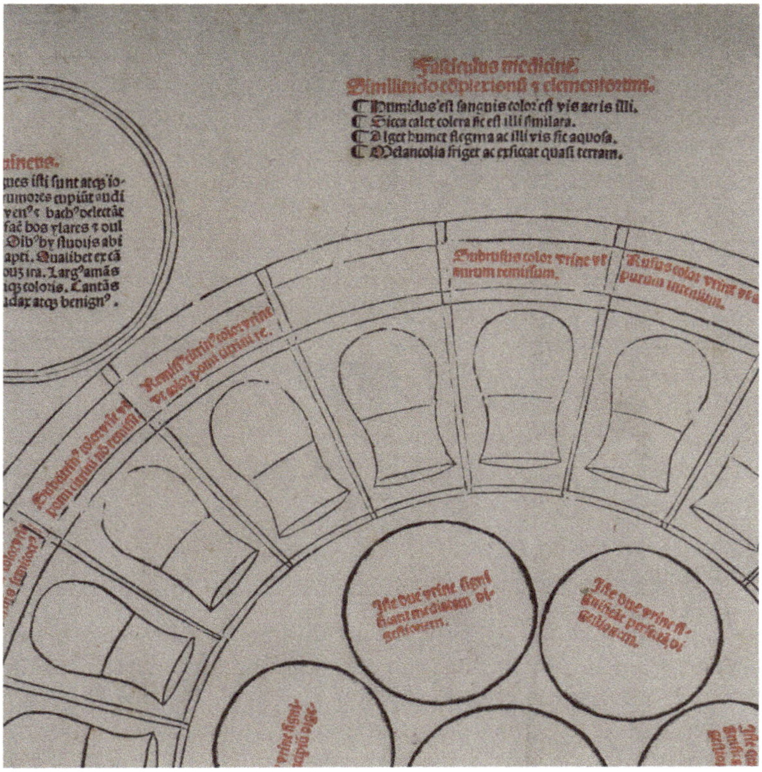

Figure 5.8 Detail showing the unlabeled *matula* of the *Rota urinarum* included in the *Fasciculus medicinae* (ed. Venice 1491). Munich, Bayerische Staatsbibliothek, Sign. Rar. 749. Image credit: Bayerische Staatsbibliothek

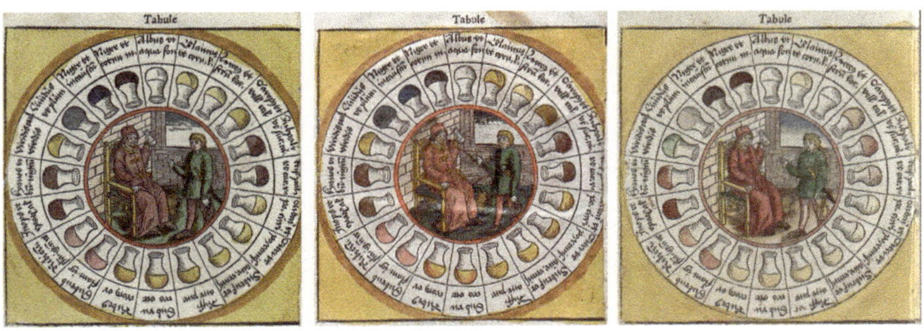

Figure 5.9 Comparison of the colouring of the *Rota urinarum* in three copies of Ulrich Pinder's *Epiphanie medicorum* in Washington, D.C., Folger Shakespeare Library, Call. no. R128.6 .P6 1506 Cage (left), Christie's London, 20 November 2002 | Live Auction 6642: Valuable Illuminated Manuscripts, Printed Books, Lot 55 (middle), and Berlin, Staatsbibliothek, Sign. Jf 660 (right). Image credit: Fabian Jonietz

modern reader. Felice Valgrisi, the editor of Pietro Andrea Mattioli's commentaries on the aforementioned pharmacological *Materia medica*, noted in 1585 that he had printed twenty-five copies of the large format, two-volume work including around eight hundred woodcut illustrations on especially thick paper, in order that owners could introduce coloured illustrations without them bleeding through onto the underlying page. However, it is doubtful that a scientific or didactic purpose was intended, since Valgrisi comments only that physicians and intellectuals could decorate their *studioli* with such splendid copies of the book and send them as gifts to princely patrons.[28] Caution must of course be exercised before one reads Valgrisi's comment as a general statement on the role of colour in early modern epistemological and evidentiary practices. Nevertheless, it is certainly significant that when discussing a book created with such effort and expenditure for a specialised readership, the sixteenth-century editor makes no mention of such practices, instead viewing the value of colour solely as an aesthetic attribute for a bibliophilic luxury edition.

Knowledge transfer in the time of plague

What value, then, would a physician attribute to colour in such a text? As virtually nothing is known about the production and use of colour scales in uroscopic treatises, a source hitherto overlooked by art historians is of great significance. The manuscript in question, attributed to the physician Dominicus de Ragusa (also known as Domenico di Rolando Galeotti), is now part of the collection at the New York Academy of Medicine.

Little biographical evidence is known about the author, who was likely born in the 1360s or 1370s.[29] Dominicus studied in Bologna, earning a doctorate in 1394, and in subsequent years held lectures in astrology. A gap in his biography exists between 1400 and the period from 1415 to 1421, when he resumed teaching in Bologna. He then moved to Siena, where he remained until 1425, before returning to Bologna in 1426 and 1427. By June 1427, his wife was recorded as a widow. It is believed he was buried in the Church of San Francesco.

The manuscript, produced between December 1424 and April 1425, coincides with Dominicus's work on an unfinished uroscopic treatise in Siena. The foundation of his studies can be reconstructed reasonably well from the sources he consults and the literature he cites. Alongside the predictable ancient classics like Hippocrates and Galen, Dominicus consulted Latin translations of medical writings in Arabic: the *Liber Continens* of Rhazes, the treatise *De urinis* by Isaac Judaeus (who co-founded a school in the Tunisian city of Kairouan in the tenth century), the seventh book of the *Liber Regalis* by Haly Abbas, and the first book of Avicenna's *Canon medicinae*.

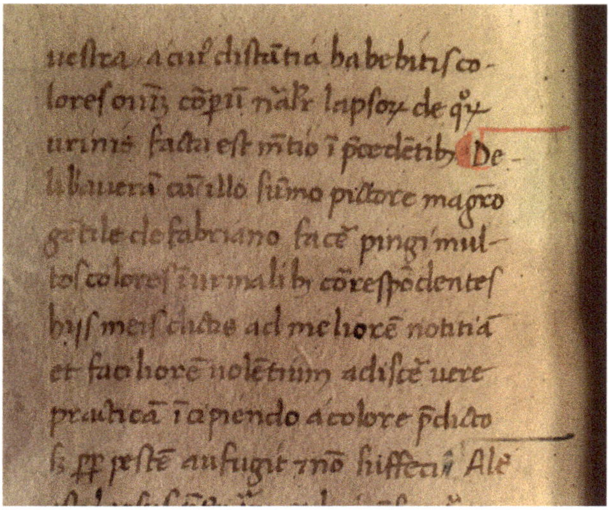

Figure 5.10 Dominicus de Ragusa, *Medical Miscellanea*, fol. 96v. New York Academy of Medicine Library, acq. no. 166860, 15c (Kr V 325b, q.v.). Image credit: Fabian Jonietz

In the context of this study, however, what makes Dominicus' treatise so important is his mention of plans for its artistic design (Figure 5.10):

> Delib[er]auera[m] cu[m] illo su[m]mo pictore magi[st]ro ge[n]tile de fabriano face[re] pingi multos colores i[n] urinalib[us] co[r]respondentes hijs meis dictis ad meliore[m] notitia[m] et faciliore[m] uole[n]tium adisce[re] uere practica[m] i[n]cipiendo a colore p[re]dicto s[ed] p[ro]p[ter] peste[m] aufugit & no[n] suffeci.[30]

> I had decided to have the most eminent painter, Master Gentile da Fabriano, paint many colours of urine, in correspondence with my statements, for the sake of better understanding and to facilitate the learning of those who wish to acquire the true practice, beginning with the aforesaid colours. But he fled due to the plague, and I did not succeed.

Three aspects of this note are of great importance. First, Dominicus indicates unequivocally that he recognises the didactic value of colouring for the education of medical practitioners. Second, he underlines the significance that he attributes to these colours by virtue of the unusual, and crucially important fact that he has not simply entrusted the task to any illuminator or illustrator, but rather to a leading painter of his time. Third, by mentioning a precisely determined correspondence between his description of the colours and their appearance, Dominicus indicates concrete conversations between the author and the painter, Gentile. Taken together, we find here rare historical evidence of a concrete exchange between a learned professor of medicine and a visual artist in the early Quattrocento. By extension, this passage from Dominicus' treatise also offers the reader an opportunity to retrace the paths by which Arabic theories of medicine were transferred into the daily practice of painters – a process that can be verified almost simultaneously by the writings of Lorenzo Ghiberti, which indirectly adapt the optical theories of Rhazes, Alhazen, Avicenna, and Averroes.[31]

It is unclear where exactly Dominicus and Gentile met. The poorly documented Venetian painter is not known to have made a stay in Bologna, whereas he certainly travelled to Florence and Siena for various commissions.[32] There is also some ambiguity surrounding the precise time period to which the written note refers: that is, between the end of 1424 and early 1425. From 1400 onward there were many short outbreaks of plague in Italy (e.g., in summer 1411 and 1420), but Dominicus surely refers to the particularly devastating phase from 1422 to 1425.[33] This wave of outbreaks first swept through Northern Italy: in 1423, the Council of Pavia was moved to Siena, and Bologna was hit that summer, while Siena was struck in the spring of the following year. By this time Emilia was again safe, so much so that, for example, the poet Antonio Beccadelli (il Panormita) fled from Siena to Bologna, where he arrived in 1424 and mourned several of the victims of the Sienese plague in his treatise *Hermaphroditus*, completed in the following year.[34] Gentile was by no means the only artist who dropped everything to leave central Tuscany. In March 1425, Ghiberti, too, had to explain to a patron that he had interrupted his work on the reliefs of the Baptismal Font in Siena, fleeing to Venice due to the plague.[35] Such incidents suggest that the plague had the indirect effect of catalysing the movement of artists and thus accelerating the transfer of knowledge.[36]

Expertise in filthy workshops

This unusual collaboration of a physician with a famous painter on the illustration of an uroscopic treatise raises the question of whether Dominicus de Ragusa might have expected a reciprocal exchange rather than just the straightforward execution of a commission. Might artists like Gentile da Fabriano have even been regarded as knowledgeable about urine beyond their ability to simply match colours against medical doctrines?

At first glance, it seems unlikely, as it is commonly assumed that painters consulted medical authorities without the pretension of adding anything essential to the latter's knowledge. Admittedly, some Quattrocento sources testify to an ancient connection between arcane medical knowledge and practitioners of the visual arts. The aforementioned physician Giovanni d'Arezzo reports a suggestive rumour that ancient books of medical secrets were found not only in the burial grounds of the healing god, Apollo, but also in the tomb of Phidias, the name of the most important ancient sculptor (*alii vero in suis arcanis libellis. quorum quidam suum invenisse ferunt in arca Fidiae, alli* [*sic*: *alii*] *in sepulchro Apollinis*).[37] However, an early writer of art theory in Giovanni's time, the sculptor Lorenzo Ghiberti, readily grants that artists need not develop their medical knowledge to the same degree as professional practitioners, let alone figures like Hippocrates, Avicenna, or Galen (*non bisognia esser medico come Ypocrate et Auicenna et Galieno*).[38] Likewise, Leonardo da Vinci consulted only standard medical texts to inform himself about urine, probably relying in particular on the two treatises that he owned, Bartolomeo Montagnana's *De urinarum iudiciis* and the *Fasciculus medicinae*.[39]

And yet, Leonardo's own written references also demonstrate practical experience gained in the context of artistic practice that goes far beyond the information found in such written works. According to Leonardo, painters used the chemical properties of urine at the start of a new project, before making preliminary drawings, to clean the wooden panel they would paint on (*poi laua con orina*).[40] This note is anything but a curious unicum. In *The Body of the Artisan*, Pamela H. Smith draws attention to recipes in Theophilus Presbyter and Cennino Cennini's books that – alongside other materials, like saliva or earwax – make use of urine for producing artworks. Included among these methods is the preparation of pigments: Theophilus recognises possibilities for producing white, sapphire-blue, green, red, and reddish purple. Urine was also used for applying gold grounds and cleaning instruments. The authors of such recipe books – which in the Cinquecento increasingly came to include sculptors – differentiate the effect of urine from animals and humans according to age, gender, hair colour, or the consumption of beer and wine.[41] Even the physician Girolamo Cardano explains in his treatise *De Subtilitate* and elsewhere how sculptors, metalsmiths, and goldsmiths use urine to colour and experiment with metals – providing a recipe for producing white lead using urine.[42] In the popular genre of 'books of secrets', which circulated widely in numerous editions, translations, and new genres such as the *Dreckapotheke*, lay people were also given recipes for producing green or a blue similar to ultramarine that used urine.[43] Likewise, painters who specialised in the restoration of old paintings and the removal of overpainting and varnishes were familiar with urine-based methods.[44] This use of urine as a material for colouration cuts across modern boundaries between artisans and artists – a point to which I will return in what follows – for not only painters, but also medieval and early modern dyers continually employed it to colour textiles and other materials.[45]

Alongside the widespread use of urine as a material, the artist's workshop made use of many raw materials that could only be traded by members of the pharmacy guilds.[46] For this reason some painters who wished to import or trade pigments, paint media, or products like coloured wax for commercial gain were also licensed pharmacists belonging to the respective guild: this was the case with Lukas Cranach in Wittenberg around 1520, and also Adam Elsheimer and Pierantonio Stiattesi in the early seventeenth century (the latter still only recognised by contemporary scholarship as the cuckolded husband of Artemisia Gentileschi). Stiattesi is characterised as a pharmacist (*aromatarium*) in 1621, and in the following year as a painter; Elsheimer is identified as a 'pharmacist and painter' (*spetiale et pittore*) in a letter to the physician Johannes Faber.[47] The knowledge of artists was not limited to the use of such products in their workshops: as is well known, Pliny already mentions the pharmacological effects of natural pigments on numerous occasions.[48] Around 1651, Salvator Rosa treated his scabies – whose form he interestingly compared with ingenious grotesque paintings (*la rogna vi dipinge a grottesche le più belle attitudini che fabbricò mai ingegnosa invenzione*) – with a mixture of rose ointment, white lead, and lead oxide: that is, materials that he would partially have had stocked in his pigment drawer.[49] At the same time, the Bolognese painter Giovanni Andrea Sirani was also regarded as an authority on medicine, the pharmacological effects of plants, and the production of healing essences (*discorreva benissimo di medicina, che rendea bon conto dell'erbe, de' fiori, de' semi, de gli estratti*).[50]

In several cases, accounts describe painters sharing the dual expertise of Saint Luke or increasingly dedicating themselves to the study of medicine over the course of their careers, sometimes to the point of suspending their artistic activity. In Florence, a 'Mercatino di maestro Bartolo di Mercatino' enrolled as a painter (*pictor*) in the Arte dei Medici e Speziali in 1377 but paid his dues in 1404 as a physician (*medicus*). In 1385, Iacopo di Gherardo entered the guild in both capacities (*pictor sive medicus*) and in 1404 Giovanni di Bandino paid dues as a painter and physician (*dipintore e medico*).[51] Equally revealing cases can also be found in later periods. For example, in the seventeenth century the physician Francesco Cesi, son of the painter Bartolomeo, practiced his father's profession as a hobby.[52] In the early eighteenth century, the abbot Nunziante de Laurentiis, a student of Francesco Solimena, is said to have given up painting entirely, shifting his primary specialisation into chemical-pharmaceutical products.[53] It is worth noting, albeit briefly, how in these centuries the painter's newly elevated noble status fundamentally altered the relationship between the two disciplines. While in the late Middle Ages, visual artists could still benefit from social proximity to the *Medici e Speziali*, by the mid-seventeenth century, the Roman Academy of Saint Luke had grown so proud of its status that it rejected an exceptionally gifted painter merely because he was 'only' a surgeon.[54]

In any case, even in the earlier period, professional physicians occasionally took recourse to the pharmaceutical knowledge of artists. For example, in the second half of the sixteenth century, the Czech physician Georg Handsch, who had studied in Italy, sought information about the effects of alum from a painter in Trento who, like Sirani, was well versed in esoteric pharmacological traditions.[55] Other sources record praise for exceptional individual artists on account of their contribution to the discipline of medicine, and in particular anatomy – at least according to certain writers who stood at the margins of the field, such as the controversial medical autodidact, alchemist, metallurgist, and goldsmith Leonhard Thurneysser zum Thurn, the private physician of the Brandenburg prince. In his *Βεβαίωσις ἀγωνίσμου* of 1576 – his second comprehensive publication on urinalysis, whose title announces itself as a response to the controversy surrounding his first book – Thurneysser relates the achievements of Erhard Schön, Sebald Beham, Michelangelo, Dürer, Jacob [*sic*] Holbein, Maerten van Heemskerck, and Frans Floris in the fields of anatomy and the theory of proportions.[56] A true authority in medicine like Girolamo Cardano, by contrast, acknowledges Leonardo's anatomical studies in his 1550 treatise, *De Subtilitate*, but simultaneously indicates that his ambitions fell short of the work of a learned anatomist like Vesalius.[57] In his 1553 commentary on Mondino's *Anatomia*, Cardano is even more frank: Leonardo was merely a painter, and his studies in this area were beautiful, but worthless.[58]

'Quid enim pictori cum urinis commune est?'

While this disapproval has been met with much scepticism in Leonardo scholarship,[59] passages like those above – where early modern physicians highlight the contributions of painters to medicine – are actually quite rare. By contrast, what predominates among medical writers is a general emphasis on the usefulness of drawing, in much the same way as observed above in Thurneysser zum Thurn's uroscopic treatise. A comparable example can be found in the work of Georg Bartisch, a Saxon eye doctor and surgeon as well as a dilettante draughtsman and painter, who made illustrations as part of his own medical research. In a 1583 work titled *Οφθαλμοδουλεια* (a treatise on eye treatments), Bartisch explicitly postulates the usefulness of drawing and painting for physicians and vaguely attributes this to an alleged tradition that stems back to ancient Greece.[60]

One of the most comprehensive expositions of the mutual usefulness of the two fields was set forth by Pier Antonio Fucini, a physician active in Florence and Pisa who composed a treatise on painting in the early seventeenth century. In this text, Fucini appeals to ancient tradition and introduces into art literature a passage purportedly written by a medical authority, probably known to few painters but familiar to many of Fucini's colleagues in medicine throughout the Cinquecento. The passage Fucini cites is from Galen's often reprinted and translated text, *De sanitate tuenda* (*Ὑγιεινῶν λόγοι*):

> [...] questa arte [i.e. painting] [...] ha convenienza con la medicina, atteso che da Galeno vien detto, che la Pittura è necessaria a' medici mediante crediamo noi al cognoscere la qualità dei colori per haver cognizione dell'essenza, e qualità delli escrementi, si come insegnò nel libro dell'arte medicinale, dal colore del corpo humano, et in particolare del volto, potersi cognoscere le complessioni degli huomini. Onde dal medesimo fù accettata l'opinione di Quinto mentre disse, che fino al Pittore si aspetta cognoscere ancora le urine.[61]
>
> The art of painting has a use for physicians, as Galen says that painter is necessary to physicians, through which they, as we believe, understand the essence and characteristics of excrement with the help of the quality of colours, as he teaches in the Book of the Art of Medicine that one can know the complexion of men from the colour of the human body and especially the face. Furthermore he [Galen] accepts the view of Quintus, who says that one expects painters to know and recognise urine.

Here, then, is an unmistakable reference to the expertise of painters with urine, which benefits physicians. The source for this passage is to be found in Chapter 13, Book 3 of *De sanitate tuenda*, where Galen – the most important transmitter of the teachings of the physician and anatomist Quintus (Κοίντος) – cites a series of often comical aphorisms. Quintus, apparently from Pergamon and trained in Alexandria by the Hippocratean teacher Marinus, can be considered one of the most significant pre-Galenic physicians in Rome, although his views and theories have been passed down only in a few indirect quotations and fragments.[62] His central role in the ancient canon of medical knowledge is, however, not to be underestimated, and was well known to readers of Galen: Quintus himself had inherited the anatomical studies of his teacher, Marinus, and thus could at least pass them down orally to the next generation. The fact that Quintus's competitors drove him out of the city at the time of the Emperor Hadrian complicated the transmission of his teachings, and only after extensive efforts could Galen obtain texts like his now-lost commentary on Hippocrates, which Galen occasionally cites. He specifically sought out four students of Quintus – the 'best doctor of his generation' – in Alexandria, Corinth, Pergamon, and Smyrna (Iphicanus, Numisianus, Satyrus, and Pelops), in order to study with them and glean further information about Quintus' knowledge and views.[63]

Every early modern medical student thus knew Quintus's aphorism on the painter's knowledge of urine. The first appearance of this passage in print was the earliest Latin edition of *De sanitate tuenda*, published in Paris in 1517, and edited by Thomas Linacre, a physician educated in Italy. This edition laid the groundwork for countless new editions into modern times. Meanwhile, Greek editions such as that published in Basel in 1538 (1539, according to the colophon) preserved the reference to the 'γραφέως' – that is, the painter.[64]

Nevertheless, the reception of Quintus split into two groups shortly thereafter. One, including Fucini, continued to cite and circulate the remark about painters into the seventeenth century, whereas the other consulted a second family of corrected editions of Galen. Still in his 1541 edition, Leonhart Fuchs refrained from any commentary on the passage in his publication;[65] yet Fuchs, though a great intellectual, had overlooked the fact that Quintus had not actually spoken of a painter (*γραφεύς*; lat. *pictor*), but rather a fuller (*γναφεύς*; lat. *fullo*) – an error which can be explained by the erroneous substitution of a single letter in the Greek manuscript.

Already in 1542, the physician Agostino Ricchi noticed the confusion of the two letters, ν and ρ, while editing a complete, commented edition of Galen's works in Venice for the publisher Farri. Ricchi marks Thomas Linacre's erroneous choice of the word *pictor* with an asterisk, and amends it in a marginal note (Figure 5.11).[66] The Giunti edition, published simultaneously, did not yet recognise the mistake, but the editor, Girolamo Donzelli, added a corresponding marginal note in the second edition of 1550.[67] In 1548, Ricchi's observation was reproduced verbatim in a single edition of *De sanitate tuenda*, published in Lyon.[68] The mistake was also noticed independently, it seems, by the physician Janus Cornarius, who systematically studied the medical writings of Greek authors throughout Europe. He corrects the passage from *De sanitate tuenda* in his 1556 book about the legacy of the seventh-century physician Paul of Aegina and wonders why one would attribute knowledge of urine to painters, of all people (*Quid enim pictori cum urinis commune est? aut inde colorum rationem collegerit scilicet?*).[69]

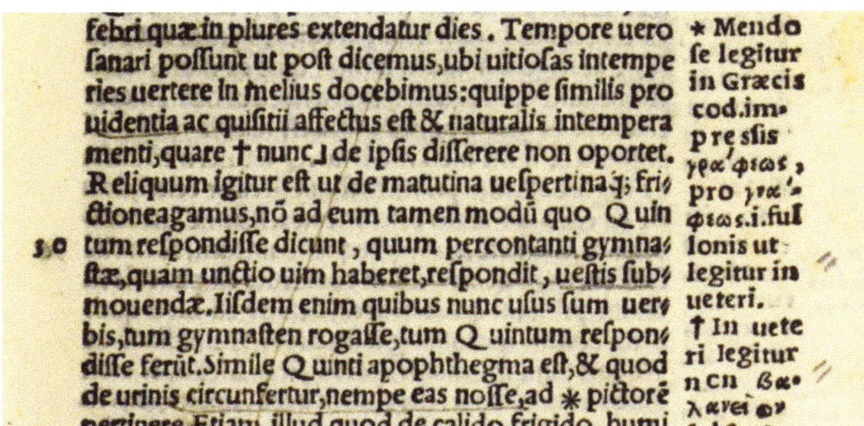
febri quæ in plures extendatur dies. Tempore uero
ſanari poſſunt ut poſt dicemus, ubi uitioſas intempe
ries uertere in melius docebimus: quippe ſimilis pro
uidentia ac quiſitii affectus eſt & naturalis intempera
menti, quare † nunc de ipſis diſſerere non oportet.
Reliquum igitur eſt ut de matutina ueſpertinaq; fri-
ctione agamus, nō ad eum tamen modū quo Quin
tum reſpondiſſe dicunt, quum percontanti gymna-
ſtæ, quam unctio uim haberet, reſpondit, ueſtis ſub-
mouendæ. Iiſdem enim quibus nunc uſus ſum uer-
bis, tum gymnaſten rogaſſe, tum Quintum reſpon-
diſſe ferūt. Simile Quinti apophthegma eſt, & quod
de urinis circunfertur, nempe eas noſſe, ad * pictorē
pertinere. Etiam illud quod de calido, frigido, humi

* Mendo
ſe legitur
in Græcis
cod. im-
preſſis
γραφεως,
pro γνα-
φεως. i. ful
lonis ut
legitur in
ueteri.
† In uete
ri legitur
ncn βα-
λανει ον
ſed βαλα

Figure 5.11 *Galeni operum onmium*, ed. by Agostino Ricchi, 8 vols, Venice 1541–1545, vol. 2, p. 425. Munich, Bayerische Staatsbibliothek, Sign. A.gr.b. 1501-2. Image credit: Bayerische Staatsbibliothek

However, although the correction found more and more acceptance in a variety of editions, it often passed unnoticed, particularly when the word *pictor* remained in the main text, allowing the marginal commentary to be easily overlooked, as can be seen in Fucini's case. Anyone who looked in the highly successful keyword index to the work of Galen, first published in 1556 and frequently reprinted into the seventeenth century, would immediately find the unredacted Quintus quotation (*VRINAS nosse ad pictorem pertinere dicebat Quintus*) as the first entry under the word 'urine'.[70] Similarly, whoever read *De sanitate tuenda* in the Italian edition of Giovanni Tarcagnota would never know that Quintus and Galen had not attributed the painter with competence in uroscopy.[71]

Still, in the mid-eighteenth century, in a medical lecture that was, in fact, first edited in the second half of the twentieth century, the influential physician Giambattista Morgagni fulminated against those who perpetuated the 'uneducated' statement of Quintus.[72] Morgagni not only knows the correct version of the text, but also recognises (as Cornarius had before him) the connection with Suetonius' characterisation of the fullers whose revenue was taxed by the emperor Vespasian based on the urine that they collected; from this Suetonius famously concludes that money does not stink (*pecunia non olet*). Plinius' explanation of why the washers who used ammoniac preserved in urine did not suffer from gout – that is, because they spent the whole day in urine basins – was also connected with this practice, and continued to be discussed well into the eighteenth century.[73] As late as 1700, when Bernardino Ramazzini reported on the working conditions of ancient fullers in a chapter, *De morbis fullonum*, of his often translated work on work-related diseases, knowledge about the effects of human urine as a material that cleans and colours, and that can be either harmful or conducive to health, remained available to a wide readership.[74]

Philologies of colour (and fur)

For two reasons, all these observations were only made known to a fraction of the readership of *De sanitate tuenda*. First, many of the early modern corrections and commentaries on Quintus's passage were published in relatively remote passages of scientific treatises. Ulisse Aldrovandi, for example, points out the error of Galen's editors in a sub-chapter on the use of camel urine in his posthumously published book of 1621 on hoofed animals.[75] Second, learned, critical philological analyses of Galen began to lose steam over time. In the Greek-Latin edition of Galen's work published in Paris in 1679, as also in the nineteenth-century bilingual edition of the complete works by Karl Gottlob Kühn, both the Greek (*γραφέως*) and Latin text (*ad pictorem pertinere*) once again speak only of the painter.[76] For modern readers, who rarely consult these editions in old languages, the situation is even more precarious. In the mid-twentieth century, the editor of a widely distributed English edition translates the erroneous word as 'writer', working from a corrupt source text, since *γραφέως* / *γραφεύς* can mean 'writer' as well as 'painter'.[77] Just as grotesque is the Greek-English reference edition in the *Loeb Classical Library*, first published in 2018, where the original text correctly reads *γναφέως*, but the translation is nevertheless 'scribe'![78]

Moving away from these lapses of early modern (and subsequent) interdisciplinary scholarship, this chapter concludes by laying out the wider significance of uroscopic treatises for colour nomenclature and the need for future research that draws together the skills and methods of art history, medical history, and philology.[79] Without question, colour terminology often proves highly problematic in the transmission of textual sources. A good example is the so-called *Kurzer Harntraktat*, which seems to have emerged in the twelfth century, and was translated from Latin to Middle German and then back again into Latin. Along the way, the passage 'citrinus vel subrubeus' was transformed into 'serena et flammei coloris', while in other passages, 'rubeus' becomes 'ruffus'.[80] However, these difficulties should not detract from the fact that, in the field of uroscopic writings, a genuine engagement with vocabulary and the vernacular translation of nuanced colour terms worked its way from antiquity well into the early modern period. It is no coincidence that one of the most significant early modern investigations of colour, *De coloribus liber* by the humanist Antonio Telesio, was repeatedly printed from 1529 onward as an appendix to a medieval treatise on urine by Johannes Actuarius (Figure 5.12). Tellingly, Telesio begins his text with a lengthy justification, which affirms the right to engage with colour not only to painters (*pictores*) but also to philosophers and philologists.

However, as this final example illustrates, physicians were not alone in seeking to fix their visual observations in a linguistically exacting fashion. Aldrovandi's commentary on the passage by Quintus in the chapter on camels can perhaps be explained by the fact that in his engagement with the terminology surrounding a particular colour of urine, he had come upon a specialised term from medical vocabulary.[81] The colour term 'karopos', which probably emerged in late antiquity through a transformation of the Greek word 'charopos' (*χαροπός*), is explained by way of comparison with the colour of camel fur in the treatise *Περὶ Οὔρων* (*De urinis*) by the Byzantine physician Theophilus Protospatharius. This definition made its way into the medical canon of the *Articella*, which served as a foundation for the studies of generations of physicians from the eleventh century onward. It was generally acknowledged that the colour term 'karopos' was specific to medical discourse, and could require clarification in other disciplines, as is confirmed by sources such as Roger Bacon's commentary on Aristotle's *Περὶ αἰσθήσεως καὶ αἰσθητῶν* (*De sensu et sensibilibus*),

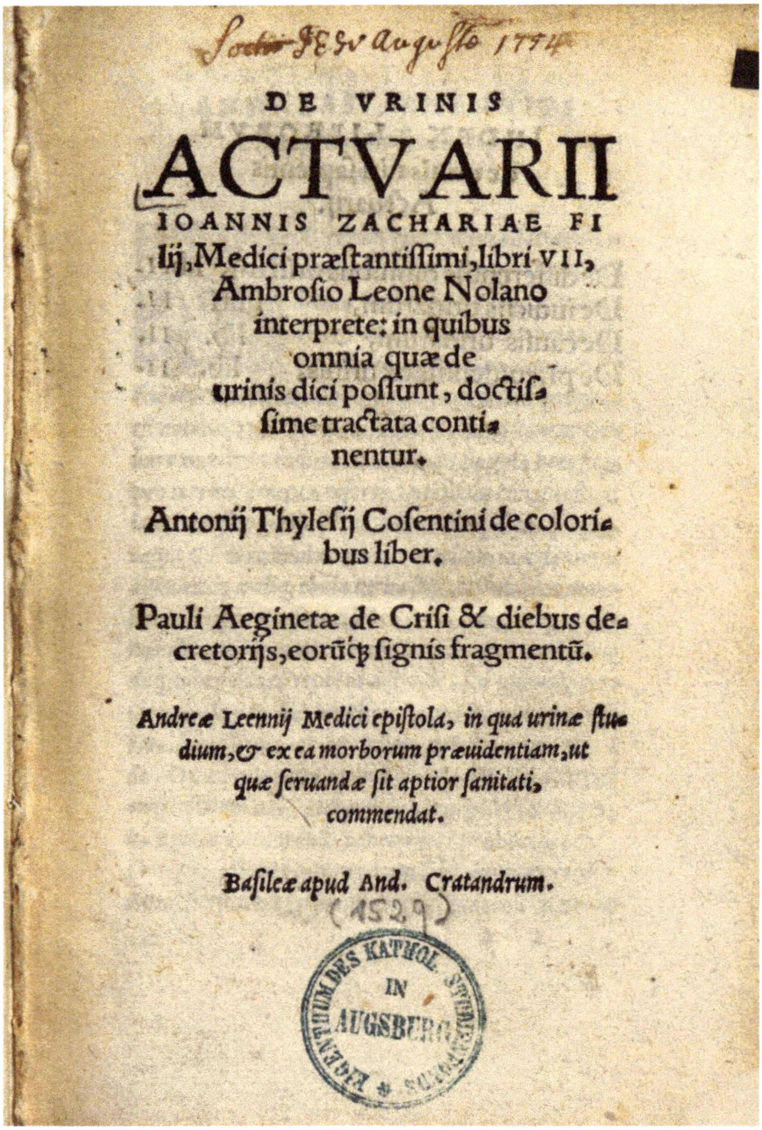
DE VRINIS
ACTVARII
IOANNIS ZACHARIAE FI
lij, Medici præſtantiſſimi, libri VII,
Ambroſio Leone Nolano
interprete: in quibus
omnia quæ de
urinis dici poſſunt, doctiſ-
ſime tractata conti-
nentur.

Antonij Thyleſij Coſentini de colori-
bus liber.

Pauli Aeginetæ de Criſi & diebus de-
cretorijs, eorūq; ſignis fragmentū.

Andreæ Leennij Medici epiſtola, in qua urinæ ſtu-
dium, & ex ea morborum præuidentiam, ut
quæ ſeruandæ ſit aptior ſanitati,
commendat.

Baſileæ apud And. Cratandrum.
(1529)

Figure 5.12 Collected volume containing Johannes Actuarius's *De Urinis* and Antonio Telesio's *De coloribus*, Basel 1529 (frontispiece). Augsburg, Staats- und Stadtbibliothek, Sign. LG 6. Image credit: Bayerische Staatsbibliothek

datable to around 1250. In the sixteenth chapter, where Bacon seeks to impose order on the Greek colour terminology of the treatise, he refers to this expression for the chromatic appearance of camel fur as one that is borrowed from medicine (*secundum quod medici dicunt quod 'karopos' est colour qualis est in vellere cameli*).[82]

In recent research and in modern dictionaries, χαροπός is most often interpreted as 'blue-green', in deference to an aesthetic ideal of ancient heroes' eye colour, although there are strong indications that the expression probably characterised a hue that wavered between amber yellow and light brown. For example, in ancient Greek texts, where it is usually applied to eye colour, the term describes the appearance of the yellow-brown eyes of lions, but also their fur; in the Middle Ages the term is clearly compared with a darker brown tone – that of acorns, chestnuts, or prunes.[83] Lisa Devriese has recently brought to light a 1339 commentary on the Pseudo-Aristotelian *Physiognomica*, in which 'karopos' is described as a mixture of white and red, with reference to Theophilus (*color camelinus et est color mixtus ex albo et rubeo*); the commentator here translates the term as 'meat juice' by way of an absurd etymological argument.[84]

This lively discourse around the appearance of the urinary colour 'karapos' not only relativises the presumed precision of science with respect to the arts; it also invites us to consider such uncertainties as a reason for differences in the design of uroscopic colour scales and urine wheels, in which blue and green tones often crop up, among other confusing hues.[85] Furthermore, these questions can inform longstanding debates concerning art historical, material, and technical problems. For example, it remains unexplained what exactly is meant by the seemingly yellow-brown colour that Leonard da Vinci and others call 'cam(m)elino'. It is worth considering more carefully whether these writers really relate to early modern botany as has previously been proposed, or rather indicate a relation to the tradition of camel fur analogies. In any case, 'cam(m)elino' is another example of a connection that has received far too little attention in the past between the workshops of Renaissance masters like Leonardo and craft producers who relied on the same colour vocabulary.[86] Like all human beings, painters, artisans, and learned physicians were not only born 'between feces and urine' (*inter faeces et urinam nascimur*), as the theological tradition puts it,[87] but also combined practical and theoretical engagement with the appearance and effects of human waste as a part of their professional life, whether *opifex* or *medicus*, *doctus* or *artifex*.

Acknowledgement

My sincere thanks go to Robert Brennan for translating this chapter from German into English, as well as for the valuable intellectual exchange and many important comments. I have presented parts of this project in New York (2014), Göttingen (2015), Chicago (2017), and Salzburg

(2021). Special thanks are due to Arlene Shaner, who generously supported my research in the historical collection of the New York Academy of Medicine.

Notes

1 *La disputa delle arti*, 1947, pp. 35–101, here p. 52.

2 Zerbi, *Über die Kautelen der Ärzte*, 2019, p. 158: 'Sed differat precipue si dispositio de qua petitur dat inducias, et iubeat illi ut in crastinum deserat urinam, ut videatur velle maturius incedere'.

3 De Villanova, 'De cautelis medicorum', 1504 (the attribution to Arnaldus is presumably incorrect). Numerous comparable cases were later discussed, for example, in Van Foreest, *De incerto, fallaci, urinarum iudicio*, 1589; on this, see especially Stolberg, *Uroscopy*, 2015, pp. 132–133.

4 *La disputa delle arti*, 1947, pp. 52–54. On the long-standing tradition of comparing the work of painters, sculptors, or architects with physicians, alongside many characterisations of restoration work or the working of unfavourable materials as 'resurrection of the dead', see for example Marco Boschini's oft-cited metaphor, which cast Titian as a healing surgeon: '[...] e scoprendo alcuna cosa, che non concordasse al delicato suo intendimento, come chirurgo benefico medicava l'infermo, se faceva di bisogno spolpargli qualche gonfiezza, o soprabondaza di carne, radrizzandogli un braccio, si nella forma l'ossatura non fosse così aggiustata, se un piede nella positura avesse presa attitudine disconcia, mettendolo a luogo senza compatir al suo dolore, e cose simili' (Boschini, *Le ricche minere*, 1674, n.p.).

5 For a similar joke between a physician and a jurist, cf. *La disputa delle arti*, 1947, pp. 92–94; generally, for such anecdotes, Land, 'From a Painter to a Doctor', 2018.

6 On the role of sensory perception, see *Medicine and the Five Senses*, 1993.

7 For some standard passages in sixteenth-century sources on the value of anatomy for artists, see for example Vasari, *La vita di Michelangelo*, 1962, vol. 2, pp. 123–127.

8 Ghiberti, *I commentarii*, 1998, p. 46 (I, II.1); on this list, see recently Hessler, 'Et ancora dissono questo più filosaphii', 2019, p. 104. For later theoretical considerations of the use of medicine for artists, see e.g. Zuccari, *L'idea*, 1607, vol. 1, pp. 40–41, 51, and vol. 2, pp. 31–32.

9 Cf. Fehrenbach, *Quasi vivo*, 2021, e.g. pp. 140, 356, 369. On the question of skin colour in painting, see the essay by Robert Brennan earlier in this volume.

10 On this topic, see Jonietz, 'Indecent Creativity', 2023, pp. 214–215.

11 *Historia naturalis* XXXV.71.

12 Baxandall, 'Bartholomaeus Facius on Painting', 1964, pp. 103, 105; Alberti, 'De pictura', 1973, p. 65 (II.37).

13 Chevreau, *Histoire Du Monde*, 1698, vol. 3, p. 287: 'J'ai lû en quelque endroit, que lui [i.e., Titian] & Raphaël avoient peint si parfaitement un homme qui avoit la fiévre, que le Medicin voyant son Portrait, connut qu'il avoit la fiévre quarte'. Around the same time, the physician Giuseppe Francesco Borri is said to have claimed that he would diagnose patients, if not after personal examination, by seeing painted portraits: 'wann er ihn entweder selbst / oder sein eigentliches Contrefait sähe'. Huyssen, *Curieuse und vollständige Reiß-Beschreibung*, 1701, p. 328.

14 'Imagines adeo similitudinis indiscretae pinxit, ut – incredibile dictu – Apio grammaticus scriptum reliquerit, quendam ex facie hominum divinantem, quos metoposcopos vocant, ex iis dixisse aut futurae mortis annos aut praeteritae vitae'. *Historia naturalis* XXXV.36,88.

15 On the cult, legend, and iconography of the saint, see Bacci, *Il pennello dell'Evangelista*, 1998; *San Luca Evangelista*, 2003–2004. An early representation (1368) of his parallel activity as physician and painter occurs in in the *Evangeliar des Johann von Troppau* (ÖNB, Cod. 1182), fol. 91v; an important second case would be Hans Mielich's depicition of St Luke as physician, writer, and painter in the predella of the main altar in Ingolstadt. For an example of anatomical references, see Abraham Janssens's altar for the painter's guild in St Rombouts in Mecheln (1606), where a skeleton in the house of the Evangelist reminded artists that knowledge of anatomy proceeded from medical study; cf. Müller Hofstede, 'Abraham Janssens', 1971, pp. 235–238. Giovanni Lanfranco's painting of around 1620, *The Healing of a Dropsical Boy by St Luke* (Rome, Palazzo Barberini, inv. 4653), represents an iconographical exception and perhaps emerged in connection with the decoration of a chapel for a medical faculty or a physician: see Crispo, 'Un inedito *San Luca*', 2008–2009. The occasional interpretation of this painting as a votive image is highly improbable due to its scale. An little-known eighteenth-century votive painting depicting St Luke as a painter sitting at his easel in a pharmacy can be found in Heidelberg, Deutsches Apotheken-Museum, inv. VII E 0317 (oil on metal, 401 × 253 mm); a comparable painting is preserved in Regensburg, Stadtmuseum, inv. K 1939/63 (oil on wood, 435 × 300 mm): see Habrich, 'Lukas, der Arzt, als Schutzheiliger von Kunst und Heilkunde', 1972.

16 Carbonelli, 'S. Luca medico', 1928; *Orsola Maddalena Caccia*, 2012, pp. 52–53, cat. no. 1 (Paola Caretta).

17 Veldman, 'Maarten van Heemskerck and St Luke's Medical Books', 1974 (substantially identical in Veldman, *Maarten van Heemskerck*, 1977, pp. 113–121); Grosshans, *Maerten van Heemskerck*, 1980, p. 199. The armillary sphere in the picture is not a generic reference to the intellectual, but rather a concrete reference to the astrological and prognostic components of medical diagnosis.

18 For a foundational account, see King, 'National Gallery 3902', 1985.

19 For example, cf. the discussion in Wouk, *Frans Floris*, 2018, pp. 166–169.

20 On uroscopy, see the overviews in Moulinier-Brogi, *L'Uroscopie au Moyen Âge*, 2012; Stolberg, *Uroscopy*, 2015; see also Stolberg, *Learned Physicians*, 2022, pp. 158–167. On the iconography, see Zglinicki, *Die Uroskopie in der bildenden Kunst*, 1982; Stolberg, *Uroscopy*, 2015, pp. 105–121; cf. now also Helas, 'Harnglas und Bahrtuch', 2023, pp. 89–96.

21 Cf. Gage, *Colour and Culture*, 1993, esp. pp. 80 and 274, note 97; Pastoureau, *Jaune*, 2019, pp. 104–108. For less analytical studies without new insights, cf. e.g., Kuehni and Schwarz, *Color Ordered*, 2008, pp. 33–34; Bruhn, 'Harndruck', 2018. See now, however, Boxer, 'Uroscopy diagrams, judgment, and the perception of color', 2022, which appeared in the midst of work on this chapter.

22 Cf. Stolberg, *Uroscopy*, 2015, p. 34 and the references in the preceding footnote.

23 Van Foreest, *De incerto, fallaci, urinarum iudicio*, 1589, pp. 135–136. By contrast, Stolberg, *Uroscopy*, 2015, p. 34, overlooks the criticism expressed by the author on this unscientific comparison of colours.

24 On the *Fasciculus*, see recently Coppens, *De vele levens van eeb boek*, 2009; Coppens, 'For the Benefit of Ordinary People', 2009.

25 On the author, see Zapf, 'Pinder, Ulrich', 2011–2016.

26 Washington, D.C., Folger Shakespeare Library, Call. no. R128.6.P6 1506 Cage (https://digitalcollections.folger.edu/img152966) (accessed 8 August 2025); *Valuable Illuminated Manuscripts, Printed Books*, pp. 101–102, Lot 55. On the question of the professional marketing of coloured books, drawing on the example of Pinder's *Epiphanie medicorum*, see McKitterick, *Print, Manuscript and the Search for Order*, 2003, pp. 79–80.

27 Sign. Jf 660 (http://resolver.staatsbibliothek-berlin.de/SBB0001C4CF00000000) (accessed 8 August 2025).

28 Mattioli, *De i discorsi*, 1585 [1584], vol. 2, p. LLL 2 (*Felice Valgrisi a' Lettori*): 'habbiamo fatto stampare xxu. di questi uolumi in carta reale bellissima, & attissima à riceuere, senza far trasparenza, ciascuna sorte di colore: acciò i Medici, & altri studiosi possino adornare i loro studi; & possino farne anco dono à quei Principi, che si dilettassero d'illustrarne le lor librerie'.

29 On the manuscript in question and the following biographical overview, see above all Kibre, 'Hitherto unnoted medical writings', 1939; Grmek, 'Život i djela Dinka Dubrovčania',1953; Kibre, 'Dominicus de Ragusa', 1971 (Both essays by Pearl Kibre reprinted in Kibre, *Studies in Medieval Science*, 1984); Bónoli and Piliarvu, *I lettori di astronomia*, 2001, pp. 87–88.

30 New York Academy of Medicine Lib. Acq. no. 166860, 15c (Kr V 325b, q.v.), fol. 96v.

31 For an overview, cf. the essays in *Ghiberti teorico*, 2019.

32 For the known sources as well as hypotheses regarding Gentile's travels and patrons in Florence and Siena, see *Gentile da Fabriano*, 2006.

33 On this outbreak of plague, see Corradi, *Annali delle epidemie*, 1865–1894, vol. 1, pp. 264–265. For a generally less precise account, cf. also Sticker, *Abhandlungen aus der Seuchengeschichte*, 1908–1910, vol. 1: *Die Pest*, p. 82.

34 Beccadelli, *The Hermaphrodite*, 2010, p. ix.

35 Krautheimer and Krautheimer-Hess, *Lorenzo Ghiberti*, 1982, p. 399, doc. 154; see recently Jonietz, 'Ghiberti *Viator*', 2019, p. 125. There is a certain irony in the fact that the execution of Dominicus's illustrated treatise on uroscopy did not come to pass due to the plague, because the plague treatises belong to precisely the kind of textual genres that often feature illustrated uroscopic tables; an example is the fifteenth-century *Tractatus de pestilentia* (Prague, University Library), on which see *À travers le verre*, 1989, p. 332, no. 374, and plate XXIX; Pastoreau, *Jaune*, 2019, p. 104.

36 For this thesis and further case studies, see Jonietz, 'Die *Scuole delle arti* als Orte der *aemulatio*', 2011, esp. pp. 776–777.

37 *La disputa delle arti*, 1947, p. 54. The origin of this legend, however, might have indicated the little-known physician Phidias of Rhodes.

38 Ghiberti, *I commentarii*, 1998, p. 50 [I, II.10].

39 According to the list of books in Codex Madrid II, fol. 2v.

40 *The Literary Works of Leonardo da Vinci*, 1939, vol. 2, p. 362, no. 628; on this on the following examples, with further references, see also Jonietz, 'Indecent Creativity', 2023, p. 213.

41 Smith, *The Body of the Artisan*, 2004, pp. 112–113.

42 *The 'De Subtilitate' of Girolamo Cardano*, 2013, vol. 1, pp. 331–332, 345.

43 Wecker, *De secretis libri XVII*, 1582, pp. 886–887.

44 On the use of urine in restoration practices, see the references in Marijnissen, *Dégradation, conservation et restauration*, 1967, vol. 1, p. 72 and vol. 2, p. 361, note 286.

45 See for example Rebora, *Un manuale di tintoria*, 1970, *ad indicem* ('orina'). To date, the role of urine has not played a prominent role in the material history of colours; for example, cf. *The Materiality of Color*, 2012.

46 Although there are local differences, as in Venice, where at a certain point, *spezieri* who sold decidedly medicinal products were distinguished from those who dealt in other types of goods; see DeLancey, 'In the Streets Where They Sell Colors', 2011, here p. 222, note 32.

47 On Cranach, see Schuchardt, *Lucas Cranach*, 1850–1871, vol. 3, pp. 72–75; Heydenreich, *Lucas Cranach the Elder*, 2007, pp. 131 and 418, doc. 98. On Stiattesi, see Cavazzini, *Painting as Business*, 2008, p. 51. On Elsheimer, see Baldriga, *L'occhio della lince*, 2002, p. 175. The denomination of Elsheimer's profession

goes hand in hand with Karin Leonhard's metaphor of the 'painter as apothecary', which itself draws on Elsheimer, but surprisingly does not mention his actual activity as a *spetiale*: see Leonhard, *The Fertile Ground of Painting*, 2020, pp. 123–125. It is unclear whether the apothecary Francesco Urbinelli, who died in 1630, was also active as a painter; in his testament there is reference to a painter's easel, pigments, and several incomplete paintings: see Cavazzini, *Painting as Business*, 2008, pp. 92–93, and 167–168, doc. 26.

48 See e.g. *Historia naturalis* XXXV.13–16.

49 *The Letters of Salvator Rosa*, 2018, vol. 1, p. 230, doc. 93, and the commentary in vol. 2, p. 890, note 4. On the noxious aspect of painting (*Il dipingere per me è diventato veleno*) and inaction as medicine (*non con altra medicina che l'esatezza del vivere e l'ozio del penello, e vi giuro che questo secondo è stato un eficace medicamento…la santissima medicina del non applicare*), see *The Letters of Salvator Rosa*, 2018, p. 688, doc. 336, p. 714, doc. 349, p. 746, doc. 369, and p. 772, doc. 384.

50 Malvasia, *Vite di Pittori Bolognesi*, 1961, p. 123.

51 Jacobsen, *Maler von Florenz*, 2001, pp. 60, 563, 587, and 604. On these physicians, see also Park, *Doctors and Medicine in Early Renaissance Florence*, 1985, *ad indicem*.

52 Malvasia, *Felsina pittrice*, 1678, vol. 1, p. 329.

53 De Dominici, *Vite de' pittori, scultori ed architetti napoletani*, 2003–2014, vol. 3 [III.3], p. 1275: 'Ma perché l'abate Nunziante aveva fatto alcun studio di medicina, pose amore alla chimica, e si diede a lambiccar medicamenti, e olii, e balsami, abbadondando la pittura, e riuscì bravo medico ed ottimo cerusico, […]'. A much later case would be Carl Spitzweg, who was trained and worked as a pharmacist before his decision to become a professional painter.

54 De Dominici, *Vite de' pittori, scultori ed architetti napoletani*, 2003–2014, vol. 2 [III.1], pp. 435–436: 'Aveva Salvatore [Rosa] un amico di professione cerusico ma che per proprio diletto anche dipingeva, ed i suoi dipinti non erano da disprezzarsi, essendo fatti con istudio, e diligenza. Or costui, per quanto si fosse adoperato con sue virtuose fatiche, non poté mai ottenere di essere ammesso tra gli Accademici di San Luca, sol perché non la pittura, ma la chirurgia era la sua professione. […]'; and even earlier in Baldinucci, *Notizie de' professori del disegno*, 1681–1728, vol. 6, 1728, p. 556. In contrast, however, the pharmacist Nicolaas van Haringen ('Mitridaat') is said to have been a member of the artistic company of the Bentvueghels, see Houbraken, *De groote schouburgh*, 1718–1721, vol. 3, p. 101. For the questionable assertion that the painter Jacob van Ruisdael was trained as a physician, see Slive, *Jacob van Ruisdael*, 2001, pp. 693–694.

55 Stolberg, *Learned Physicians*, 2022, p. 311, note 668.

56 Thurneysser zum Thurn, *Βεβαίωσις ἀγωνίσμου*, 1576, pp. 22v–23r (ch. 3). For his idiosyncratic contribution to the method of uroscopy and urine distillation, see Bulang, 'Experte oder Scharlatan?', 2013; Stolberg, *Uroscopy*, 2015, esp. pp. 67–70.

57 Cardano, *De Subtilitate*, 1550, p. 317: 'Est philosophus pictor, architectus, & dissectionis artifex. Argumento est præclara illa totius humani corporis imitatio, quam iam pluribus ante annis inchoatam à Leonardo Vincio Florentino, & penè absolutam, sed deerat operi tantus artifex ac rerū[m] naturæ indagator, quantus est Vessalius'.

58 Cardano, *Opera omnia*, 1663, vol. 10, p. 131: 'Vidimus & Ichnographiam Leonardi Florentini pictoris manu descriptam, pulchram sanè & tam celebri artifice dignam, sed prorsus inutilem: quod eius esset qui nec numerum intestinorum nosceret. Erat enim purus pictor non Medicus nec Philosophus'.

59 For an overview of key research on the reception of Leonardo's anatomical studies, see for example *Leonardo da Vinci's Anatomical World*, 2011.

60 Bartisch, *Οφθαλμοδουλεια*, 1583, p. B iij r (Preface) and 11v: 'Und darzu hat mich vornemlich beweget vnd gebracht der Griechen Exempel / von welchen man schreibet / das sie ihre jugent / als bald sich dieselbige zum *studio Medicinæ* begeben / vnd damit vmbgangen / auch vnverharlich neben ihrem Studiren das Reissen vnd die Malerkunst haben lernen vnd vben lassen / Alls die nach ihrer weisheit wol verstanden / das solches zu der kunst der Artzney hoch nötig vnd nützlich sey. [...] So ist einem jeden Oculisten und Schnitartzte / [...] sehr nötig / das er der kunst des malens und reissens bericht und erfaren sey [...]'. For a comprehensive study, see Berger, 'Georg Bartisch's *Ophthalmodouleia*', 2021, pp. 52–53.

61 Cited from Jonietz, 'Ein unbekannter Kunsttraktat', 2011, p. 159. For ancient views on skin colour, see the sources discussed by Robert Brennan in this volume.

62 Grmek and Gourevitch, 'L'ecole médicinale', 1988; idem, 'Aux sources de la doctrine médicale de Galien', 1994; Mattern, *The Prince of Medicine*, 2013, *ad indicem*. Generally, on ancient medicine, see Nutton, *Ancient Medicine*, 2004.

63 Galen's report on these efforts is found in the fourteenth book of *Περί ανατομικών εγχειρήσεων*, which is known only through its transmission in Arabic translation: Galen, *Sieben Bücher Anatomie*, 1906, vol. 1, p. 232, and vol. 2, p. 168; the praise of Quintus cited here occurs in Galen's book on prognosis (*Περὶ τοῦ προγινώσκειν βιβλίον*): Galen, *De praecognitione*, 1979, pp. 70–73.

64 On Galen's reception in print, see Durling, 'A Chronological Census', 1961; see also notes 67 and 68 below. In what follows, I will quote words and phrases in Greek according to the early modern printed sources, despite occasional inconsistencies (e.g., regarding aspirations and accents) in these publications.

65 Galen, *Medicorvm omnivm facile principis de sanitate tuenda*, 1541, vol. 1, fol. 87v and vol. 2, fol. 98r.

66 Galen, *Operum omnium*, 1541–1545, vol. 2, p. 425: '* Mendose legitur in Græcis cod. impressis γράφεως, pro γνάφεως .i. fullonis ut legitur in ueteri'.

67 Galen, *Omnia Opera*, 1541–1542, vol. 2, fol. 79v and in the following edition (Venedig 1550) vol. 2, fol. 81v. Of course only a selective view of the history of these editions can be offered here; on the 22 published Latin editions of Galen's complete works up to the year 1625, see Fortuna, 'The Latin Editions of Galen's *Opera omnia*', 2012.

68 Galen, *De sanitate tuenda libri sex*, 1548, p. 197: '* Mē[n]dose legitur in græc. codi. impreßis γράφεως, pro γνάφεως. i. fullonis ut legitur in ueteri'. I was not able to locate another edition, which was apparently already published in 1547, according to Durling, 'A Chronological Census', 1961, p. 266 (no. 1547.13); this edition is also not listed in Pettegree and Walsby, *French Books*, 2012 (on the 1548 edition, see Pettegree and Walsby, *French Books*, 2012, vol. 1, p. 842, no. 71404).

69 Cornarius, *Pauli Aeginetae totius rei medicae libri VII*, 1556, p. 74: 'Idem de urinis quid sentiret, cuidam interroganti respondit, ad fullones pertinere ipsarum considerationem. Sed exemplaria Galeni hactenus habuerunt, γραφέως ἐςὶ καταμανθάνειν αὐτὰ, & uerterat interpres, ad pictorem pertinere eas nosse: quum legi debeat γναφέως, & ad fullonem pertinere. Quid enim pictori cum urinis commune est? aut inde colorum rationem collegerit scilicet? fullones autem urinas considerant humanas, & ipsis etiam utuntur, ipsasq[ue] quantò tenuiores ac crudiores sunt, tantò magis probant, id quod etiam Galenus in secundo commentario in prorheticum Hippocratis testatur, ubi Thessalicum quendam urinas numquam inspexisse dicit, & eos qui illas considerarent, fullones appellasse. At uero idem Quintus de calido ac frigido, & sicco ac humido, dicere solebat, balneatorum talia esse uocabula. Hæc Galen. lib. 3. de sanit. tuenda fine'.

70 Brasavola, *Index refertissimus in omnes Galeni libros*, 1556, fol. 522v.

71 Galen, *Delli mezzi*, 1549, fol. 82v: 'Vn simil motto è quello, che delle urine si dice, cioè che la cognitione di loro appartiene à i pittori'.

72 Morgagni, *Opera postuma*, 1964–1966, vol. 3, 1966 (*Lezioni di medicina teorica. Commento a Galeno*), p. 675: 'Expectabam ut pro reliqua (sed non utar Petroniano verbo) libertate, etiam illud Quinti indoctum dictum quod Galenus commemorat 3° de tuenda valetudine refricaret: tractare de urinis non Medico, verùm fulloni convenire Svetonius 7.58'.

73 *Historia naturalis* XXVIII.66; cf. also *Historia naturalis*, XXVIII.91 (*urinam [cameli] fullonibus utilissimam esse tradunt*). On ancient launderers, see the comprehensive work of Flohr, *The World of the Fullo*, 2013. Flohr seeks to relativise the practical role of urine, yet surprisingly makes no reference to important passages such as those in Pliny, discussed here (Flohr, *The World of the Fullo*, 2013, pp. 103–104).

74 Cited here from a later edition: Ramazzini, *De morbis artificum diatriba*, 1703, pp. 85–102 (ch. XV). On the author and further bibliography, see the contribution in this volume by Jana Graul.

75 Aldrovandi, *Quadrupedum omnium bisulcorum historia*, 1621, pp. 902–903: 'Vnde celebre illud Quinti Medici vetustissimi apophthegma apud Galenum. Vbi sic vertit Thomas Linacer Anglus. *Vrinas nosse non ad Medicum, sed ad pictorem pertinere*. falsissimo sane ioco, quid enim Pictori cum vrina, aut quis eius in arte pictoria vsus? nec qui recognouit libros illos, Hieronymus Donzellinus, deprauatam versionem animaduerit, inductus, vt puto, fuerat Interpresa codice malę manus, qui forte habebat γραφέως, quod *pictorem* sonat, cum reuersa γναφέως, quod *fallo* est, legi debuit, & sic argutum est, licet ignorantiæ plenum verbum, *non esse Medici, sed fullonis urinam considerare*'. (Aldrovandi's citation of Donzellini refers to his text of *De sanitate tuenda* in the second printing of the Giunti edition, published in Venice, of the *Opera omnia*; see above, note 67). A further reference to the mistaken transcription of this passage can be found, for example, hidden in Cesare Zarotti's medically oriented commentary on Martial: *M. Valerii Martialis Epigrammatvm*, 1657, p. 337.

76 *Hippocratis Coi, Et Claudii Galeni Pergameni Archiatrōn Opera*, 1679–1689, vol. 6, 1679, p. 113; Galen, *Opera omnia*, 1821–1833, vol. 6, 1823, p. 228. The philologist Carel Gabriel Cobet refers to Kühn's error in two essays: 'Quinti medici dicta', 1878 and Cobet, 'Ad Galenum', 1882, p. 251. The word *γναφέως* is finally corrected once again in Galen, *De sanitate tuenda*, 1923, p. 100.

77 Montraville Green, *A Translation*, 1951, p. 137: 'This statement of Quintus, which is reported, is like that of another famous gymnast about urine, that it is the writer's business to know all about that'.

78 Galen, *Hygiene*, 2018, vol. 1, p. 333: 'This apothegm, put about by Quintus, is rather like that about the urine – it is for the scribe to find out about this – [...]'.

79 In recent years, uroscopic texts are being made more systematically accessible: see e.g., *The Dome of Uryne*, 2019.

80 Keil, *Der 'kurze Harntraktat'*, 1969, pp. 20, 22, 38–41. On the variants and interpreations that arose through vernacular translations of uroscopic texts, see e.g., Moulinier-Brogi, 'L'uroscopie en vulgaire', 2008; Coppens, '"For the Benefit of Ordinary People"', 2009; Zaun and Geisler, 'Die Harnfarbbezeichnungen', 2011.

81 Cf. note 75 above. Aldrovandi certainly knew Pliny's statement (*Historia naturalis* XXXV.91) on the uses of camel urine for launderers; see note 73 above.

82 Bacon, *Liber de sensu et sensato*, 1937, p. 71; cf. Parkhurst, 'Roger Bacon on Color', 1990; generally on colour in ancient medicine, see *Couleur et soins dans les médecines anciennes*, 2021.

83 See especially the highly controversial, philological study by Maxwell-Stuart, *Χαροπός*, 1981; for a contrast example, Dürbeck, *Zur Charakteristik*, 1977, pp. 246–247, note 617. On the medieval reception, see recently Devriese, 'Physiognomy in Context', 2017, pp. 126–128.

84 Devriese, 'Physiognomy in Context', 2017.

85 The assertion in Pastoreau, *Jaune*, 2019, p. 107, that blue never occurs, is untenable.
86 Stefanini, 'Camelino', 2015.
87 The exact derivation of this famous citation is unclear; it is attributed variously to Saint Augustine, Cyprian, or the circle of Bernard of Clairvaux.

6

Crafting surgical expertise in the medical manuals of Jacopo Berengario da Carpi (1518–1523)

Ariella Minden

In his autobiography written in the late 1550s and early 1560s, Benvenuto Cellini recounts that Jacopo Berengario da Carpi (c. 1460–1530), a professor and surgeon, happened upon his workshop in Rome. Cellini recalls the surgeon as having a 'great intelligence for design (*intelligenza del disegno*)' and that:

> One day by chance he was passing by my shop, he cast his eye upon some drawings I had laid out, among which were several sketches of little fanciful vases, drawn for my own pleasure. These vases were entirely different and varied from anything he had ever seen before. Master Jacopo directed me to make them out of silver, which I did willingly and according to my own fancy (*capriccio*).[1]

Cellini uses Berengario to focalise his penchant for imaginative design. The story continues that the surgeon presented the vases to the Duke of Ferrara, stating that they were ancient silverware with a long, illustrious history, given to him by a patient in gratitude for his services. On account of their novelty, the duke believed him. While the anecdote supports Cellini's programme of self-aggrandisement, he does give Berengario some credit in the story: it was through his *intelligenza del disegno* that the surgeon was able to discern from among all the objects in the workshop the drawings that were uniquely demonstrative of the artist's creative capacities.[2] The diagnostic capabilities of the surgeon were just at home in the goldsmith's *bottega* as while assessing a patient.

Another anecdote from Cellini's autobiography provides an inverse situation, where it was the goldsmith's manual dexterity and skill that proved essential to surgical practice. On this occasion, Cellini had summoned a certain Jacopo of Perugia, who he deemed a fine surgeon, to operate on the hand of his fellow goldsmith Raffaello del Moro's daughter. Although Cellini had faith in the surgeon's ability, he was struck by the coarseness of the tools, which were causing the girl immense pain. Literally taking matters into his own hands, the goldsmith rushed back to his shop to make a new tool of the 'finest steel' with which the surgeon purportedly was able to perform a painless procedure.[3] Skilful as the surgeon was, he was nevertheless unable to carry out his own intricate manual labour without tools made with adequate skill by metalworkers.

Reading these two anecdotes together demonstrates how Cellini saw the lives of the goldsmith and surgeon as intertwined both on a material level as well as bound by a series of shared skillsets including manual dexterity, judgement, and discernment. The cultivation of relationships between artists and doctors, enabling the artist to gain a more profound knowledge of the human body, is well documented in the history of Italian Renaissance art. Leonardo da Vinci recorded his time spent at the Hospital of Santa Maria Nuova in Florence and the strong relationship he developed with Marcantonio della Torre in Pavia.[4] Meanwhile, Giorgio Vasari told of how Michelangelo was given rooms to perform dissections at the Church of Santo Spirito, and later in Rome that he was in close contact with the anatomist Realdo Colombo.[5] This focus has largely been unidirectional, investigating and interpreting the role of anatomical knowledge in the figuration of the human body and specific drawing practices of the time; however, Cellini's two anecdotes detail a far more symbiotic relationship between artists and surgeons informed by a shared set of critical categories.

In the second half of the twentieth century, scholars including Charles Singer and James Ackerman proposed that simultaneous 'advances' in the arts and sciences were predicated on a shared worldview that sought to rationalise knowledge across disciplines.[6] This understanding oversimplifies the mechanics of exchange among cognate mechanical practices. Methodological shifts in the intervening decades have since offered new frameworks in which to situate concrete discussions of what Cellini registered as Berengario's *intelligenza del disegno*. Precociously in the realm of art theory, David Summers proposed that the language of Art was not imposed upon practice, but emerged out of it, and dialogue among artists established common terms of engagement.[7] This can be coupled with a more recent shift in attention from final product towards a better understanding of process that has occurred in the context of the material turn and is prescient in this regard. In this vein, Pamela H. Smith has foregrounded embodied knowledge at the intersections of the histories of art and science in which bodily acts of making resulted in the creation and transmission of knowledge in shared artisanal spaces.[8] Alongside Smith's artisanal epistemologies, Pamela Long has demonstrated that in the codification of practical knowledge in artisanal treatises over the course of the fifteenth and sixteenth centuries a translation of embodied, practical knowledge from the workshop and other technical environments into theoretical spheres and discourses occurred.[9] Long introduces into this discussion Peter Galison's concept of 'trading zones', which she uses to describe the creation of a mutually intelligible language for information to be shared between theoreticians and practitioners in the context of early modern architecture.[10]

Building upon this scholarship, this chapter takes the medical texts of Jacopo Berengario da Carpi as a case study to demonstrate how a shared vocabulary between artist and surgeon transcended forms of analogical thinking to inform common criteria used to discuss training, practice, and expertise across forms of manual craft.[11] Berengario's works are perhaps best known for their woodcut illustrations where citations of contemporary monuments, classical sculpture, and other print media demonstrate a profound engagement with the dominant visual culture of sixteenth-century Italy. The images are indicative of how visualisations of the human body and its paradigmatic manifestations, both Christian and classical, came to inform the medical understanding and representation of the anatomised body.[12] In reading the texts it becomes apparent that much as visual culture informs the depiction of the body, the criteria with which to evaluate artistic achievement being established in the realm of practice found common ground with Berengario's legitimisation of his own surgical expertise.

Surgery and dissection were messy, mechanical endeavours. Woodcuts of surgical tools and their accompanying descriptions in Berengario's *Tractatus de fractura calve sive cranei* (1518) (Figure 6.1) offer a glimpse into the requisite craft knowledge surgeons needed to appropriately select and manoeuvre a range of saws, drills, and scalpels. Precisely because surgery was a manual art, two divergent paths could be taken to become a surgeon in fifteenth- and sixteenth-century Italy: the first was an apprenticeship, during which, as in other craft training, from a young age, an apprentice would gain first-hand experience in a master's workshop to eventually qualify as a barber-surgeon; while the second was by way of a university education.[13] The latter appears to have been far less common in the fifteenth century. Despite the first written record of a professor of surgery at Bologna dating to 1388, it was not until 1405 that there appears to have been a regular holder of the chair. Even then, the apprenticeship remained the preferred form of surgical training. Of the sixty-five medical degrees granted at Bologna between 1419 and 1435, only one was in surgery.[14] An annotation in the Bolognese *rotulus* dating between 1503 and 1512 further suggests the pejorative view of surgery in the landscape of academic medicine, with one of the *Riformatori dello Studio*, the communal body responsible for appointing professors, noting that despite surgery not being an honourable discipline, they still had to find a replacement for Berengario while he was on secondment due to the subject's popularity, especially among foreign students.[15]

In this context, Berengario's training was unique. As a young boy he was apprenticed to his father, Faustino, a successful barber-surgeon in

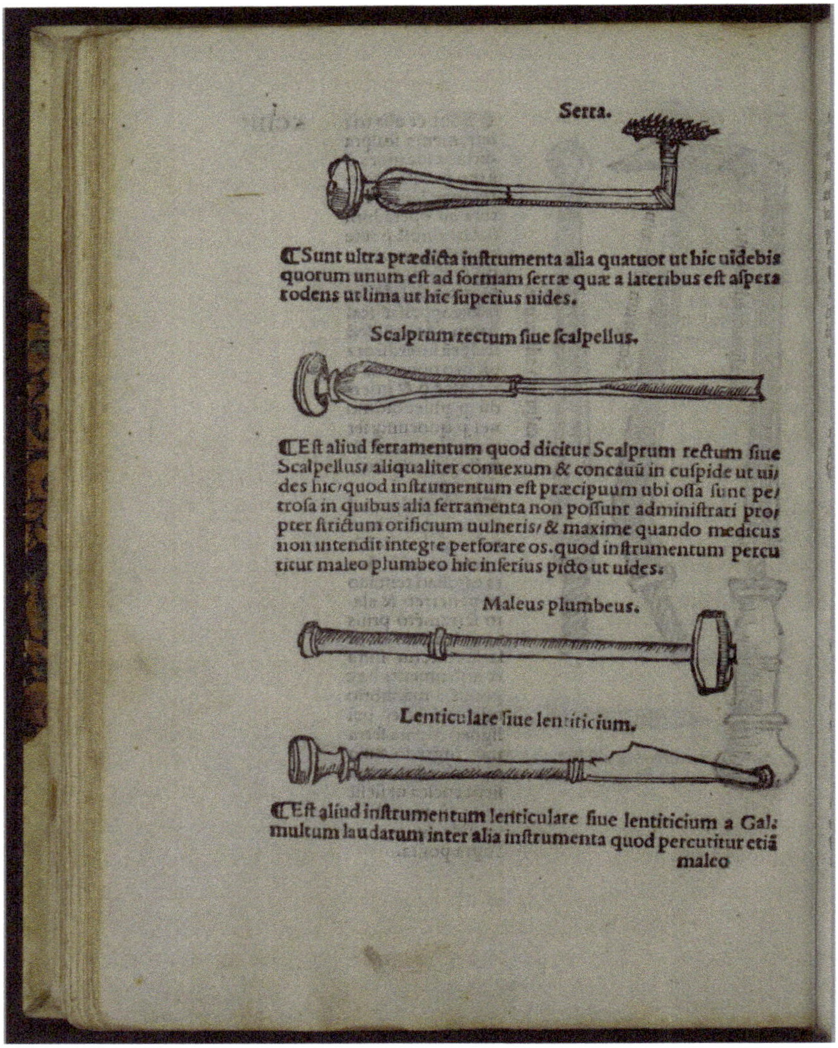

Figure 6.1 Tools for cranial surgery, 94v, Berengario da Carpi, *Tractatus de fractura calve sive cranei*, 1521, woodcut. London, The Wellcome Library. Image credit: Bayerische Staatsbibliothek

Carpi, who worked throughout northern Italy performing difficult operations.[16] Only after his apprenticeship and some Latin schooling did he move to Bologna to undertake a university degree, which he received in 1489. Berengario then returned to Carpi to practice with his father during the 1490s. The 1502 *rotulus* is the first record of Berengario as a *maestro dello studio* at Bologna, a position he held until 1527. During this time, the surgeon maintained an active clinical practice. This was seemingly rare given that in his commentary on Mondino de' Luzzi's *Anatomia,* published in 1521, he was adamant that annual public dissections were insufficient training, countering that anatomy was in the service of the living; therefore, to become a good doctor, it was imperative that students interact with patients, cultivate experience through clinical practice, and perform private dissections, usually at the homes of professors.[17]

Berengario's combined training profoundly impacted his writings, which provide clear insights into his biography and medical approach. In this chapter, I focus on his three most important works: the *Tractatus de fractura calve sive cranei* (1518), the aforementioned *Commentaria super anatomia Mundini* (1521), and the *Isagoge Breves* (1522). The *Tractatus de fractura calve sive cranei,* his treatise on cranial fractures, walks the reader through the process of treating head injuries from initial diagnosis to surgical and non-surgical interventions to post-operative care. The text includes a mix of engagement with classical authorities and anecdotes that record his and his family's experience and success in treating cranial fractures and brain injuries. As his only practical treatise, this work is the most explicit of the three about Berengario's apprenticeship to his father and his father's contributions to surgical practice. Berengario's next book, the *Commentaria super anatomia Mundini,* was a commentary on Mondino de' Luzzi's 1316 anatomical treatise, which sat at the core of the medical curriculum for over two centuries. Printed in 1521, the 1,056 page tome superficially follows the traditional structure of a scholastic commentary; however, the text goes beyond the standard dialectics of the genre and strict adherence to written authorities.[18] Instead, it is filled with clinical case studies and descriptions of experiments and specific dissections that the author himself performed to resolve age-old disputes. Finally, one year later, Berengario published his best-seller, the *Isagoge Breves, A Short Introduction*. The text, organised to follow the sequence of a dissection, clearly and concisely described the process, while signalling what the reader should notice at every cut.

Across these texts, each a different genre, an intertextual portrait of the surgeon and his perceived role in the advancement of the study of the body and its treatment emerges. Berengario advocates for the role of close, manual study in medical education and outlines the professional training and progressive accumulation of skill he deems necessary for successful surgical practice; in doing so, he establishes the terms of his expertise.[19] Sight and touch, '*visus et tactus*', are to be used as the tools by which older authorities can be either verified or challenged, foregrounding the empirical in the cultivation of expertise and experience.[20] In this, Berengario explicitly fashioned himself *artifex* and *operator*, a craftsman and a labourer, one who works with his hands and has cultivated his expertise over a prolonged period of time through extensive hands-on experience.[21] In contrast to Hieronymus Brunschwig's (c. 1430–1530) slightly earlier, vernacular medical writings, which introduced what Tillmann Taape has described as a 'literate – but not Latinate – audience' to complex concepts from theoretical medicine, Berengario, writing in Latin, did the opposite.[22] He presented himself to a university audience as someone whose professional capabilities were predicated on his handiwork and, in so doing, situated himself in a longer tradition of the surgeon as *artifex* able to engage with the craftsmanship of the Divine Creator.

The long visual and literary tradition of God as craftsman traces back at least to the Pythagorean tradition of creation transmitted most cohesively in Plato's *Timaeus*: man is a microcosm – reflecting the beauty and proportion of the universe – the work of a divine craftsman.[23] This imagery, eagerly adopted throughout the Middle Ages, was used to reflect upon acts of creation between human and divine, and as a way to situate the virtuosity of the minutiae of craftwork.[24] The incipit of the book of Genesis was a particularly fecund space to do so, as seen perhaps most famously in the opening miniatures of the *Bible Moralisée*, now in the Austrian National Library in Vienna, in which God as a geometer (Figure 6.2) carefully uses a compass to delineate the world as a perfect circle, while in the roundels on the following page God is shown actively separating light from dark with his own hands (Figure 6.3); in this way the artistic act of creation is tied to the prototypical one.[25]

Surgeons were also keen to assume this kind of relationship with the Creator in so far as it helped to justify the manual component of their labour. Writing in the early fourteenth century, Henri de Mondeville (1260–1320) associated the surgeon with the architect, another common characterisation of God's creation of the universe.[26] Gentile da Foligno, in his commentary on Book Three of Avicenna's *Canon* (1025), the only prescribed text for practical medicine in the Bolognese statutes of 1405, referred to God as *artifex istius mundi*, the craftsman of this world.[27] In his commentary on Mondino, Berengario also takes up the trope of God as divine craftsman to similar effect as his predecessors and other craftsmen, describing God at different points as *primus* and *summus artifex*.[28] Berengario uses *summus artifex*, highest craftsman, in reference to the minutiae of the human body, writing: 'no one can know what is happening with respect to every single limb or nerve except for the highest craftsman, it is only Him who fully understands His work (*opus*)'.[29] In using the same word for the human form as used for a work of art, Berengario clarifies the relationship that the surgeon sought to establish with God and his original act of creation. The medical *artifex* possessed a similar skillset to that which was initially used to construct the human body, and through which it was possible to both explore God's mastery of nature and ultimately, return the body to its original state of perfection.

Already in the *Timaeus* there was a materiality to the facture of the body wherein the creator's sons made humans through a combination of

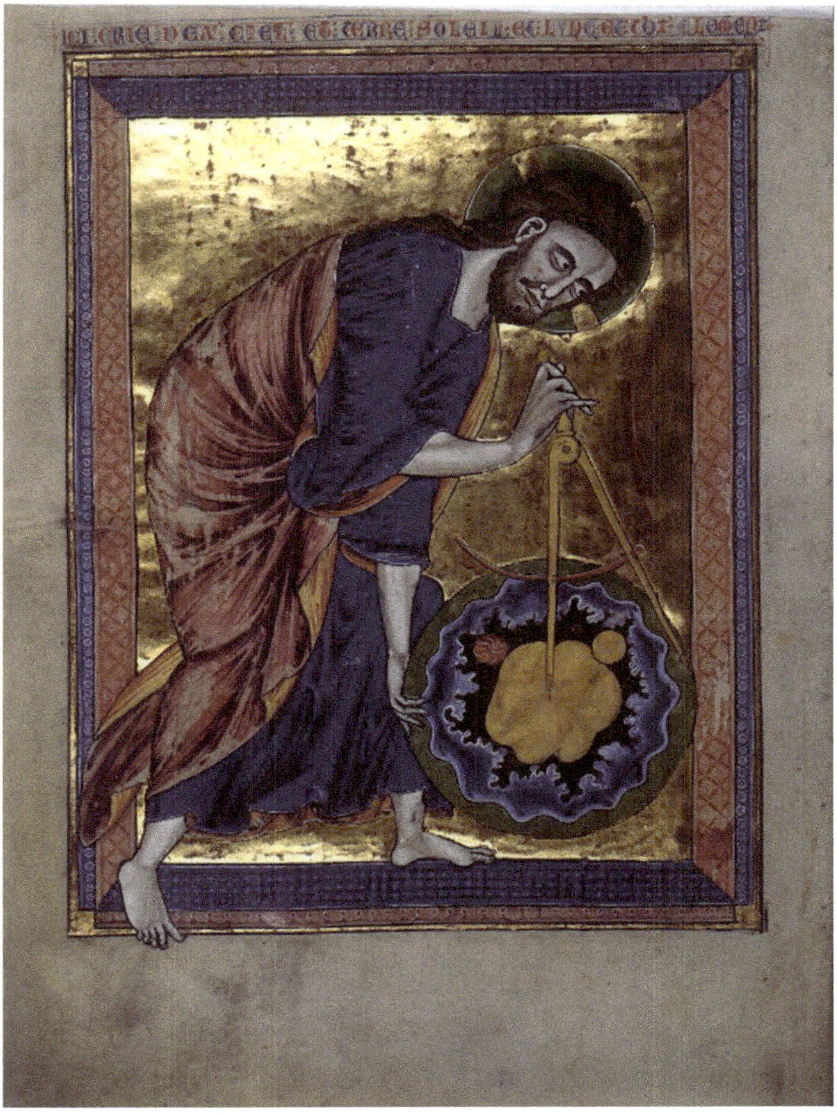

Figure 6.2 God the Geometer, fol. 1v, Bible moralisée, Codex 2554, Paris, c. 1208–1215. Vienna, Österreichische Nationalbibliothek. Image credit: Bild-Archiv, ÖNB, Vienna

the four elements which were welded together 'with a multitude of rivets too small to be seen' and where the bones were made of 'sifted' and 'kneaded' earth 'soaked' with marrow which 'he plunged the stuff into fire, next dipped it in water, and again in fire and once more in water' so that they were 'insoluble by either'.[30] In medicine, the crafted nature of the body was mobilised in the form of analogies to provide readers concrete

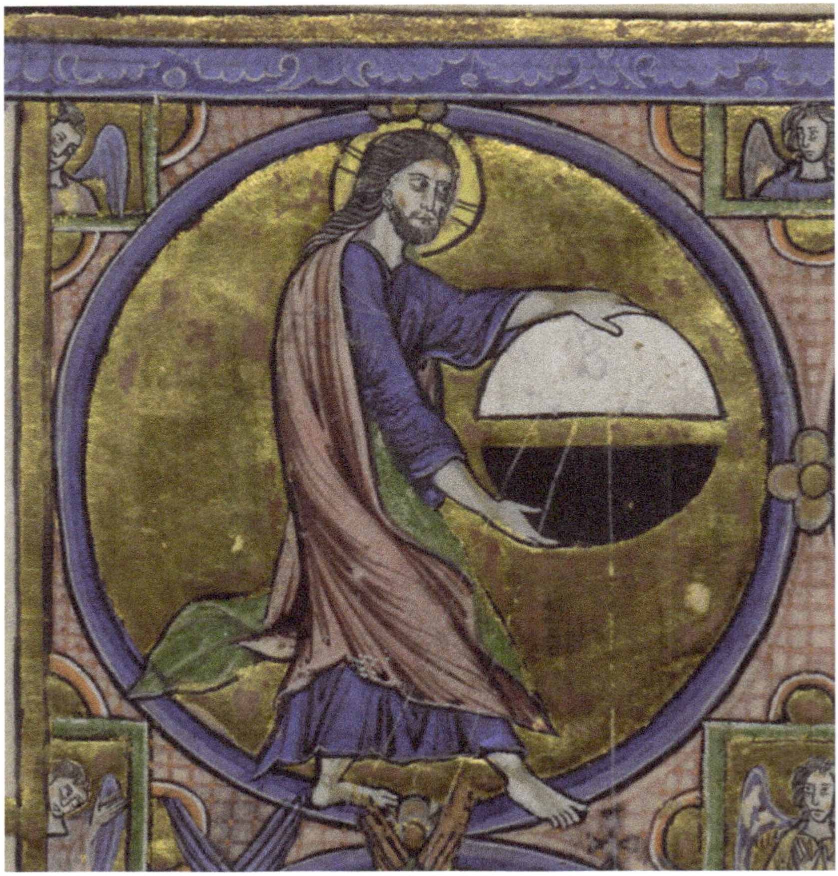

Figure 6.3 Creation of the World, fol. 1r, Bible moralisée, Codex 2554, Paris, c. 1208–1215. Vienna, Österreichische Nationalbibliothek. Image credit: Bild-Archiv, ÖNB, Vienna

reference points to understand the body's innerworkings and systems. In particular, joints and pulleys helped physicians to conceptualise how certain body parts move. Galen, for instance, used the pulley to describe the contraction and expansion of the muscles of the larynx.[31] This type of analogy was pervasive in the medical writing of the Middle Ages. Henri de Mondeville likewise found the pulley a useful comparison to explain the mechanics of the elbow joints, where 'in its lower extremity towards the joint of the elbow has two eminences of which the one is longer than the other; and they are made like a half-wheel with which one draws water from a well, that is a pulley'.[32] For de Mondeville the body was a rich tapestry of materials, likening bones to wood and skin to textile.[33] The body as craftwork even finds visual expression in miniatures made to accompany Roger of Salerno's (before 1140–c. 1195) *Chiurgia* made in Amiens in the first quarter of the fourteenth century (Sloane MS 1977). On folio 6v, amidst a mélange of scenes of surgical treatments and those of the Life of Christ, there is, in the square on the bottom right, an image of a surgeon shown suturing a patient (Figure 6.4).[34] For the sake of visibility, the needle and thread have been enlarged and the gaping wound exaggerated. The way the suturing is depicted inevitably evokes associations with other forms of sewing, including the making of the manuscript itself – a process that also involved the suturing of skin (*vellum*).

Berengario too takes up these kinds of analogies to offer his reader a way to visualise phenomena that are difficult, if not impossible to see. Although when it came to understanding the circulatory system, Berengario was explicitly anti-metaphor, chiding his predecessors for trying to pinpoint

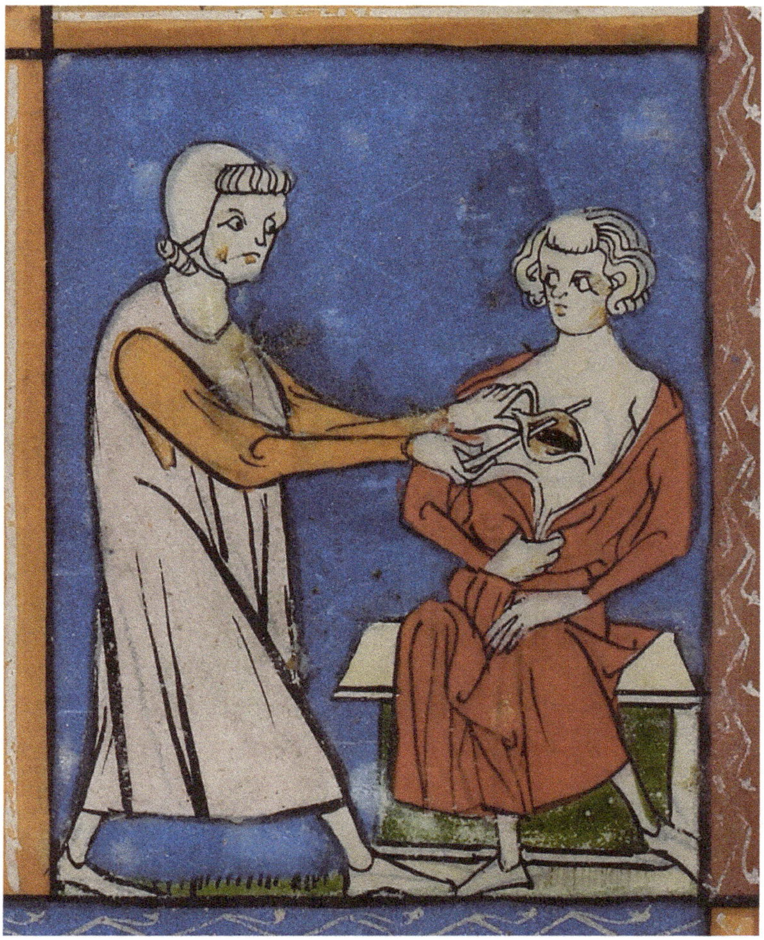

Figure 6.4 Suturing, detail, fol. 6v, Sloane MS 1977, Amiens, c. 1300. London, British Library. Image credit: British Library Collection

an origin for the veins by erroneously comparing them to the source of a river, he found analogy useful.[35] Berengario, in line with his predecessors, saw analogy as practical and didactic.[36] In the *Commentary*, the carpenter's workshop is rich with comparative materials: everyday objects are wrought with a series of techniques not dissimilar to how the bones of the body are joined together. The cranial plates, for instance, fit together with saw-like ridges in the same way that butterfly joints firmly conjoin two pieces of wood so that they hold firm.[37] However, he makes a point to state that not every piece of carpentry, nor every bone in the body was meant to stay fused in place and there were some physiological processes such as birth, that were hard to grasp fully and for which analogy could come in handy. Reproduction, broadly speaking, was a widespread preoccupation across medical disciplines, as such Berengario devotes much space in the *Commentary* to explaining the process of human generation.[38] In the realm of the practical, the surgeon was concerned with how the pubic bones loosen and open during pregnancy to create more space during labour. As a process that would be impossible to observe, Berengario this time explicitly implored physicians to go to a carpenter's workshop to understand how this kind of opening works.[39] Berengario employs verbs like *querere* (to inquire into) and *intellegere* (to understand) to define how the physician ought to approach this observational experience in an analogous sphere of inquiry.

Beyond visual aids offered by craft analogies, surgical techniques too were understood as belonging to a broader artisanal economy, allowing the surgeon to look to other crafts to better understand his own. Such was the case with the drill. At the end of the *Treatise on Cranial Fractures* accompanying a series of woodcuts depicting the tools necessary for performing these types of surgeries, Berengario provides an explanation of each tool and its usage. When it came to the drill, he lays out the longstanding debate over the correct approach to trepanation: is the initial hole to be made with a thicker or finer drill bit? After assessing the different arguments for and against, the surgeon ultimately looks laterally for a resolution. In this case: the sculptor. In doing so, he concludes that the finer drill bit is to be used first because that is how it is done 'in all other mechanical craft or work in wood or stone or any other solid material (*corpore solido*)'.[40] Just as *opus* gets used to describe the body, in using *corpore* to encompass the range of other hard materials that would be worked in the same way, Berengario linguistically inserts his own profession and the medium in which he was working into the same semantic field.

Berengario emphatically uses analogy to situate his practice in the world of craft where there is a specific manual skillset and associated set of tools needed to contend with a wrought body that opens like a window or fuses like butterfly jointing.[41] Where the body is mechanical, the labour of the surgeon is emphatically manual. To Berengario it was wrong for a doctor to transcend a sensorial approach to the body, a direct jab at

theoretical medicine. It is precisely because Berengario is a craftsman and not a natural philosopher – the most prestigious of the academic medical disciplines – that he is not only an author but a translator; and what he is translating is his expertise. He articulates this in the preface to the *Treatise on Cranial Fractures*. Berengario states that due to the nature of the discipline, medical practice cannot be translated in its entirety into writing nor adequately expressed in speech, but comes from years of training and first-hand experience, as such he can only provide a small glimpse into this world and the rest must be acquired on one's own over time.[42] Several pages later he goes on to proclaim: *ego expertus sum* – I am experienced – in reference to his ability to recognise the signs of certain injuries with recourse to the number of men with various head traumas he had personally treated.[43]

Skill could not be cultivated through reading alone but had to be gained through practice over an extended period. This is especially true in the development of a skilled hand which affords primacy to the manual component of anatomy and surgery.[44] Already in the opening of the *Anatomia*, Mondino makes this assertion stating that he is guided by 'the operation of the hand'.[45] In turn, a dissection or surgery could only be as good as the hand used to perform the procedure. In the *Treatise on Cranial Fractures* when Berengario enumerates the surgical interventions that can be performed to treat brain injuries he chides university trained physicians 'who disdain to be called surgeons, but extort lots of money by declaring their knowledge of the craft'.[46] Berengario goes on to defend and advocate for the apprenticeship system and concludes that only by starting at a young age, preferably under the tutelage of one's father, can one acquire the necessary skills. It is for that reason that 'the craft of surgery is performed with the agility of the hand in stitching, grafting, cutting, and burning, alongside many other surgical procedures'.[47] The loaded and knowing language, through the use of *philosophiam* and *doctrina*, equates the training of an apprentice to that of the university-trained *medicus*, while simultaneously reminding the reader that surgery is an *arte* – a skill or craft requiring the *agilitas* of the hand.

In the *Isagoge Breves*, explicitly designed as a teaching tool, Berengario emphasised the critical role of dissection in the medical curriculum, urging students to personally handle the cadaver to develop practical expertise. At several points in the manual, Berengario cautions his readers that a 'learned' (*docta*) or 'practised' hand is required for the sake of precision, so as to not destroy any part of the body intended for study. Such was the case for the guidez vein. Occasionally used in phlebotomy, the surgeon was particular in writing that:

> The incision of the guidez vein is, however, to be made by a learned hand (*docta manu*) with a lancet that has some obstacle near its point lest all the

> sides of the vein be opened, since they are slippery to the touch and since they are not attached to flesh as many other veins are; then also because of the soft and slippery glands that exist under these veins; finally, so that the lancet may not prick a nerve or other members located there.[48]

Berengario envisioned the dead in the service of the living. Dissection was not mere performance, but a practice tool for students to try their hand at delicate procedures without the risk of harming a patient. The author, exacting in the type of tools to be used and explicit about each manoeuvre, warns of the ease with which a misstep can occur at every cut.

In characterising the need for an agile or learned hand in surgery or dissection alongside shared tools and techniques, the criteria used to assess and qualify the talents of a surgeon sit comfortably in line with the language used in an emergent art theory to define artistic achievement. For example, Berengario paired skill and difficulty. The minutiae of the body call for a steady hand in dissection, the ear being a place where,

> To see these items requires a practiced hand, with tentacles, a curved knife, a saw, and a mallet suitable for the task, because the aforesaid items, with the nerve which comes from within as well as the meninge which is towards the foramen of the ear and with the aforesaid little bone, are seen with great difficulty (*cum difficultate*).[49]

In this passage, Berengario presents dissection as progressive. Those with less experience would not yet be equipped to adequately apprehend parts that are both more difficult to access and to see. This is corroborated in how Berengario explains the dissection of the eye. He notes that it is a destructive procedure and to understand the organ both eyes must be broken down. He concludes these instructions with: 'A skilled hand seeks (*perquirit*) ever more difficult things'.[50] Thus, the cumulative nature of anatomy comes to be fully articulated. In these examples there is an appeal to the need for extensive training to successfully study human anatomy, and eventually, perform phlebotomies. The skilled hand is not only capable of carrying out increasingly difficult operations but predetermines a desire to perform these increasingly difficult types of dissections.

This understanding of difficulty predicated on skill closely maps onto *difficultà* as a critical category and as a facet of artistic achievement. This term crystallised in the writings surrounding Michelangelo's practice in the second half of the sixteenth century; however, as David Summers shows, *difficultas* first emerged as a 'broad aesthetic ideal' by which a knowledgeable audience could assess the skill of an artist based on their ability to surpass what were perceived as artistic conventions, elevating their art through identifiable technical conceits. Summers traces this late-Cinquecento term back to the 1480s citing three prominent examples: first, Antonio Manetti's description of the reception of Filippo Brunelleschi's talents, 'Everyone was startled and amazed at the difficulties that he had set before himself [...]'; second, Cristoforo Landino's praise of Andrea del Castagno as 'a lover of the difficulties of art and foreshortening' as part of his exultation of the painters and sculptors of Florence in his preface to the 1481 edition of Dante's *Commedia*;[51] and finally, Antonio Billi's *Libro* written somewhere between 1487 and the 1530s which phrases praise in terms of *difficultà*, *meraviglia*, and *stuppore*.[52] Each of these uses suggests that craftsmen had to be willing to engage with difficult feats in order for them to be registered by a knowledgeable public. In Summers's presentation of *difficultà* in the context of Michelangelo's artistic practice, he recalls Vasari's description of Michelangelo as 'much inclined to the labours of art, having seen that he could succeed in anything, however difficult'.[53] In this usage it becomes clear that the artist saw *difficultà* as intrinsically tied to the manual component of art making rather than the strictly intellectual or conceptual, further confirmed by Michelangelo's letter to Benedetto Varchi in which he states his preference for sculpture precisely because of its higher degree of difficulty.[54]

David Zagoury explores how this mid-Cinquecento Florentine conceptualisation of *difficultà* intertwined with the concepts of *ingegno* (genius) and *fatica* (labour) as understood by the artists themselves. Zagoury uses this triangulation to show how the artist-academicians of the Accademia Fiorentina came into conflict with theoreticians including Varchi alongside Giovan Battista Gelli, both of whom strove to extricate *fatica* from *ingegno* in order to minimise the physicality of artistic practice. One famous anecdote recounts Varchi's compliment to Michelangelo, telling him he has the 'brain of Jove' to which the artist responds, 'but Vulcan's hammer is required to make something come out of it'.[55] The relationship between the hand and the mind, as already seen in the context of academic medicine, had long been a fraught topic and mirrors the anxieties of certain artists. In the final years of the fifteenth century, Leonardo, for instance, elevates the art of painting by denigrating that of sculpture. Leonardo writes, 'The sculptor conducts his work with great bodily fatigue and the painter conducts his work with greater mental fatigue', proceeding vividly to describe the clamour and mess produced by sculpting, even noting that the sculptor had to wear different clothing because he would get so dirty from the dust flying everywhere, whereas the painter was able to dress in elegant attire suitable for the practice of a liberal art.[56]

The conspicuous absence and presence of the hand, and its positioning in practice, strongly resonates with the opposition Berengario confronted in his writings. The only way for the anatomist to see increasingly finer details, was to cultivate the hand over the course of a career. Berengario's presentation of the relationship of difficulty and skill strongly resonates with Billi's constellation of terminology. The pairing of *meraviglia* and *difficultà* in particular appears to go hand in hand in the anatomical context.

By examining the smallest parts of the body – accessible only once the surgeon or anatomist's hand had become more skilled and sought greater difficulty – could the individual approach an understanding of God's initial act of creation.[57] In terms of appraisal it is also hard not to think about the role of spectacle and in turn the performative nature of cutting open a cadaver that attracted throngs of viewers. Skill in anatomy would eventually become about display and public appreciation. Much like in understanding the difficulty of Castagno or Brunelleschi's works, future audiences would be impressed by the skills required and cultivated.[58]

The final critical category that Berengario used to establish his expertise was judgement. Skills of appraisal played a central role in diagnosing and selecting the proper course of treatment, with the face serving as the primary point of reference. In the *Isagoge Breves* Berengario explains:

> Knowledge of the face is much prized by the physiognomist. It is also prized in the physician, since you will make the first prognostication primarily from the face of the sick man; for this it is helpful in the recognition of many diseases, such as leprosy, consumption, yellow jaundice, cachexia, and the time of menstruation in a woman. In the face are also recognized those who pretend illness, but not always.[59]

Judgement, *iudicium*, once again presents itself as a cumulative skill that, viewed through the lens of these texts as translations of experience, cannot entirely be communicated through writing. The more cases one treated, the quicker and more accurately a diagnosis could be made. Berengario identifies a series of signs (*signum*) indicative of certain ailments in the second chapter of the first part of the *Treatise on Cranial Fractures* dedicated to diagnosis. Throughout the chapter, judgement is central, but comes to assume a role of utmost importance when doubt arises in distinguishing one possible condition from another. Here experience and difficulty meet *ingegno*. Berengario writes:

> I deem, however, that the differentiation of such symptoms is very difficult and is only known by experts (or those experienced). These symptoms (*signa*) cannot be described in writing and can only be understood by he who possesses ingenuity (*ingenio*), introspective, analytical, and synthetic capabilities and a long time confronting similar experiences in understanding (*comprehendi*) and judging (*iudicari*) them: there are many things that the doctor knows that are not possible to put into writing.[60]

In a later anecdote, Berengario predicts the exact moment of death of the son of a certain Giacomo Maria de' Lino because of a 'judgement based on an impression' that he was unable to recount in writing.[61] Signs were only accessible to medical practitioners through experience, once again connecting Berengario's diagnostic capabilities to the realm of craft knowledge. The same skills that Berengario tirelessly advocated for, especially in the *Treatise on Cranial Fractures*, align closely to a type of discernment that Cellini acknowledged in describing Berengario as having 'molto intelligenza del disegno'. Judgement served as a prerequisite for experts across craft practices: for physicians, it enabled accurate diagnoses, while for artisans, it guided quality control and empowered discretionary decisions that might have contravened traditional conventions of practice. Elizabeth Sears and Aden Kumler demonstrate that in thirteenth- and fourteenth-century Paris, objects were not only crafted with expertise but also assessed by other experts to ensure quality, prevent deception, and avoid the sale of substandard works.[62] These kinds of regulatory guild measures to prevent fraudulent actions continued to inform art making, with judgement and decorum intimately linked. In the sixteenth century, Michelangelo was seen as representative of this at its apex due to his *giudizio dell'occhio* which permitted him to transcend the prescribed rules of art making in favour of more powerful figures, as Pietro Aretino describes it.[63] Vasari also cites negative examples, warning of what would happen when an artist lacked the appropriate judgement. In the Life of Il Cronaca, he describes Baccio d'Agnolo copying a cornice and placing it over an inappropriately small facade, with his take away being that:

> It is not enough for craftsmen, when they have executed their works, to excuse themselves as many do, by saying that they were taken with exact measurements from the antique and copied from good masters, seeing that good judgment and the eye play a greater part in all such matters than measuring with compasses.[64]

So too in the visual arts was judgement essential, and artistic failure could come down to a lack of discernment, like copying without discretion.

Berengario directly engages with craft judgement in the *Tractatus*, specifically referencing the widespread practices involved in assessing works of *ars*.[65] Shortly after explaining judgement as a requisite skill in the face of doubt, Berengario advises the physician to

> train himself to know these colours so that he knows how to assess them otherwise he won't be able to make a diagnosis. It is only when he is experienced and trained in similar situations in the same way that experts are able to distinguish real gems from fake ones (*fraudatis*) and those of low quality.[66]

He recycles this simile in the *Commentary* with slight modifications: adding an emphasis on duration in the cultivation of expertise and explicitly inserting the verb to judge (*iudicant*) as the way in which the good is separated from the fake (*falsis*).[67] This not only inscribes Berengario's skillset into the realm of craft but is reflective of real craft practice. As Elizabeth Sears has meticulously outlined, there were craftsmen working in Paris who were high-ranking members of their respective corporations, who served as *preud'omes jurez et sermenetez* or *gardes du métier*. It was precisely in their capacity as experts that they protected consumer interests by assessing works before they were allowed to be sold on the market, as the public was not deemed to have the expert knowledge that allowed for these types of appraisals to be made.[68] These examples demonstrate how acts of discernment in both quality control and diagnosis were integral to understanding the role of expertise and the defining the expert across craft practice.

The difficulty of language in encapsulating experience forced Berengario to think about how he wanted to position himself as an expert and to legitimise himself and his training to his reader. In doing so, through a language intended to recall the world of craft, the surgeon made a profound statement on his role in the study of anatomy and practice of surgery to a learned, university audience, taking part in the broader codification of skill contemporaneously taking place in the visual arts and as part of the shift away from theoretical medicine in the university.

Notes

1 All translations are my own unless otherwise noted. Ferrero (ed.), *Opere di Benvenuto Cellini*, 1980, pp. 117–118: 'Aveva questo valente uomo molta intellignezia del disegno. Passando un giorno a caso dalla mia bottega, vidde a sorta certi disegni che io avevo innanzi, infra' quali era parechi bizzarri vasetti, che per mio piacere avevo disegnati. Questo tali vasi erano molto diversi et varrii da tutti quelli che mai s'erano veduti insino a quella età. Volse il ditto maestro Iacomo che io gnene facessi di argento; i quali io feci oltra modo volentieri, per essere sicondo il mio capriccio'.

2 For *disegno* as an intellectual conceit of the goldsmith see: Gasparotto, 'The Power of Invention', 2014, pp. 40–55; Wright, *The Pollaiuolo Brothers*, 2005, pp. 25–34.

3 Ferrero (ed.), *Opere di Benvenuto Cellini*, 1971, p. 173: 'Per la qual cosa preso il ditto maestro Iacopo certi ferri grossi, e veduto che con quelli lui faceva poca opera e grandissimo male alla ditta figliuola, dissi al maestro che si fermassi e che mi aspettassi uno ottavo d'ora. Corso in bottega feci un ferrolino d'accaio finissimo e torto; e radeva. Giunto al maestro, cominciò con tanta gentilezza a lavorare, che lei non sentiva punto di dolore, e in breve di spazio ebbe finito'.

4 Azzolini, 'Leonardo da Vinci's Anatomical Studies in Milan', 2006, pp. 147–176; Laurenza, 'Marcantonio della Torre and Leonardo's Late Anatomical Studies', 2011, pp. 61–77; Bambach, *Leonardo da Vinci*, 2003, p. 253; Vasari, *Vite*, 1966–1987, vol. 4, pp. 27–28.

5 Vasari, *Vite*, 1966–1987, vol. 6, pp. 12–13; Condivi, *Vita di Michelagnolo*, 1998, pp. 57–58.

6 Singer, 'The Confluence of Humanism, Anatomy, and Art', 1957, pp. 266–267; Ackerman, 'The Involvement of Artists', 1985, pp. 94–126.

7 Summers, *Michelangelo and the Language of Art*, 1981, p. 7.

8 Smith, *The Body of the Artisan*, 2004, esp. pp. 95–127.

9 Long, *Artisan/Practitioners*, 2011, esp. pp. 3–6.

10 Galison, *Image and Logic*, 1997, pp. 781–844; Long, *Artisan/Practitioners*, 2011, pp. 94–126; Long, 'Trading Zones', 2015, pp. 840–847.

11 Cf. Nova, 'Valore e limiti del metodo analogico nell'opera di Leonardo', 2016, pp. 25–36.
12 Ciardi, 'Anatomia come allegoria', 2013, pp. 52–59; Stoichita, 'Penello/Scalpello', 2013, pp. 21–25; Kornell 'Rosso Fiorentino and the Anatomical Text', 1989, pp. 842–847; Tordella, 'Raffaello, cemento dell'anatomia e scienza delle cose ultime', 2021, pp. 38–47; Bonsanti, 'Considerazioni sul disegno di Raffaello', 2021; Park, *Secrets of Women*, 2006, esp. pp. 191–226; Park, 'The Criminal and the Saintly Body', pp. 26–29.
13 Siraisi, *Medieval and Early Renaissance Medicine*, 1990, pp. 48–77, 153–186.
14 Siraisi, *Medieval and Early Renaissance Medicine*, 1990, p. 63.
15 Putti, *Berengario da Carpi*, 1937, p. 29.
16 Berengario da Carpi, *Isagoge*, 1522, fol. 2r; Putti, *Berengario da Carpi*, 1937, pp. 12–13.
17 Bernegario da Carpi, *Commentaria*, 1521, fol. 5r: 'Et longe melius cognoscerentur in uiuis que in mortius nisi prae immanitate desisteremus a tali opere. Apparent certe multa in uiuis que non apparent in mortius'.
18 For the relationship between genre and content in the *Commentary* see French, 'Berengario da Carpi and the Use of Commentary', 1985, pp. 49–50.
19 Common words to discuss the expert in Latin were 'peritus' and 'expertus'; while *peritus* is a substantive noun with a meaning closer to our modern understanding, *expertus* is a past participle meaning 'experienced', thus implying cumulative practice rather than necessarily a conferred status. The understanding of the expert in the early modern Europe varies greatly from region to region and profession to profession. However, as Sophus Reinert and Viktoria von Hoffmann have demonstrated there was an established vocabulary for talking about experts in the medical field. Reinert, 'Authority and Expertise', 2016, pp. 114–119; Hoffmann, '*Ingeniosa peritia*', 2021, esp. pp. 107–110. For the historiographical contestation of the expert as an early modern category, see Ash, 'By Any Other Name', 2019, pp. 3–30.
20 Berengario da Carpi, *Commentaria*, 1521, fol. 6r: 'Et non credat aliquis per solam vivam vocem aut per scripturam posse havere hanc discipliam: quia hic requiritur visus et tactus'. On the following page Berengario endows this approach with an epistemological bent describing anatomy as the 'science of understanding individual members'. Berengario da Carpi, *Commentaria*, 1521, fol. 6v: 'Alio modo capitur anatomia pro scientia cognotionis membrorum ubi etiam traditur modus operandi cum manu actu et demonstrandi ipsa membra'. In tracing the formulation 'vidi et tetigi', Viktoria von Hoffmann has presented what she deems 'haptic epistemologies' through which practitioners became 'haptic experts' by way of their skills of assessment, description, and interpretation. Hoffmann, 'Epistemologies of Touch in Early Modern Holy Autopsies', 2022, p. 555.
21 Paolo Savoia has shown that most authors writing surgical tracts in the later sixteenth and seventeenth centuries in Bologna came from craft backgrounds. At the centre of Savoia's article is the professor of surgery, Giovanni Battista Cortesi (1552–1643), the son of a tailor, a profession which analogously required fine motor skills for cutting and stitching. He suggests that this set of professionals was more inclined to use the printing press in order to assert their newfound status and commend their reputation to posterity. Savoia, 'Skills, Knowledge, and Status', 2019, p. 31.
22 Cf. Taape, 'Common Medicine', 2021, pp. 15–16.
23 Østrem, 'Deus Artifex, Homo Creator', 2007, p. 17; Barkan, *Nature's Work of Art*, 1975, pp. 8–14; Kemp, *The Marvellous Works of Nature and Man*, 2006, esp. pp. 71–95.
24 For an overview and bibliography, see Fricke, 'Artifex and Opifex', 2019, pp. 49–52.

25 For a thorough discussion of this iconography see: Tachau, 'God's Compass', 1998. Stoichita also points to a miniature in the Lambeth Bible (Lambeth Palace Library, Ms.3 , fol. 6v) where there is a roundel depicting God sculpting Man our of clay: Stoichita, 'Penello/Scalpello', 2013, p. 10.
26 Pouchelle, *The Body and Surgery*, 1990, p. 103.
27 French, 'Berengario da Carpi and the Use of Commentary', 1985, p. 55.
28 French, 'Berengario da Carpi and the Use of Commentary', 1985, p. 57.
29 Bernegario da Carpi, *Commentaria*, fols 279r–v: 'dicit tamen qua ea quae pertinent ad motus animi sunt obscuriora et altioris rationis tamen quid accidat singulis neruis aut membris nullus scire potest nisi sumus artifex cui soli opus suum notum est'.
30 Quoted in Barkan, *Nature's Work of Art*, 1975, pp. 14, 17.
31 Pouchelle, *The Body and Surgery*, 1990, p. 108.
32 Quoted in Pouchelle, *The Body and Surgery*, 1990.
33 Pouchelle, *The Body and Surgery*, 1990, p. 106.
34 For a more ample discussion of these miniatures, see Whittington, 'Picturing Christ as Surgeon', 2015, esp. pp. 88–96.
35 French, 'Berengario da Carpi and the Use of Commentary', 1985, p. 56 and Berengario da Carpi, *Commentaria*, 1521, fol. 161v: 'quae venae non oriuntur a corde nec ab heptae nisi improrpie et metaphoriae'; Leonardo da Vinci makes this comparison in the Codex Leicester, but does later backtrack on this point: Geddes, *Watermarks*, 2020, p. 105.
36 Berengario cites Galen's description of the uterus having a rough lining so that the spermata can better attach to the lining as analogous to how craftsmen will roughen up wood or stone before applying glue so that the surface is more adherent. Berengario da Carpi, *Commentaria*, 1521, fol. 241v.
37 Berengario da Carpi, *Commentaria*, 1521, 416v–417r: 'sunt igata capitis ossa inuicem mediantibus iuncturis seratilibus [...] ut faciunt carpentari iungendo ligna ut firma maneant licet etiam in capite ossa aliqua sint iuncta non coniunctura seratili: sed cum alia iunctura quae dicitur super apodiata'.
38 For a discussion on the centrality of generation in early modern medicine, see Park, *Secrets of Women*, 2006, esp. pp. 121–160.
39 Berengario da Carpi, *Commentaria*, 1521, fol. 493r: 'qui non comprehendit dicta nostra scilicet qua sit impossibile qua una sola iunctura aperiatur sine alia non est dignus nomine legitimi medici: sed debent ire tales medici ad carpentarios: et querere qualiter potest aperiri ostium seu fenestra composta ex dubus partibus et quae de tribus suis iuncturis non aperiatur nisi una: deinde reddant ad medicinam et intelligent quomodo aperitur os faemoris seu anche ab osse sacro in partu [...]'.
40 Berengario, *Tractatus*, 1518, fol. 97v: 'Quod etiam hoc sit verum .f. quod melius sit incipiendum a subtili quem alato ferramento dum totum os intendimus penetrare patet experientia in omni alio artificio mechanico sive operetur in ligno sive in lapide vel in alio corpore solido: quia semper artifices utuntur terebro subtili & parvo prius deinde lato & deinde latiori: quia etiam sic operando melius & citius perficiunt quicquid intendunt'. Mondeville was also known to have use and modify tools like a carpenter's gouge and a blacksmith's pincers and tongs to perform surgeries. Pouchelle, *The Body and Surgery*, 1990, p. 105. As seen in the Cellini anecdote at the start of this paper, the people making tools were serving a wide range of craftsmen who required similar equipment to carry out their work.
41 For Leonardo and analogy, see Geddes, *Watermarks*, 2020, pp. 103–105; Nova, 'Valore e limiti del metodo analogico nell'opera di Leonardo da Vinci', 2016, pp. 25–36; Kemp, 'Leonardo and the Unity of Knowledge', 2015, pp. 353–367.
42 Berengario da Carpi, *Tractatus*, 1518, fol. 3v: 'Magnifico ego in medico lucidum ac digestum illud iuditium quod nec calamo scribi nec lingua proserri potest hinc honor, hinc labor est, hinc collige grana'.

43 Berengario da Carpi, *Tractatus*, 1518, fol. 10v: 'Ista omnia ego expertus sum et istis signis parum credo vidi pluries homines rumpere testas [...]'.
44 For the role of the senses and 'handwork' in distillation, cf. Taape, 'Distilling Reliable Remedies', 2014, esp. pp. 248–250.
45 'sed magis secundum manualem operationem', quoted in Maurette, 'The Organ of Organs', 2018, pp. 107–108 and Berengario da Carpi, *Commentaria*, 1521, fol. 7v.
46 Berengario da Carpi, *Tractatus*, 1518, fols 29v–30r: 'Hodiernis temporibus medici dedignantur chirugici appellari: sed ut pecunias extorqueant satentur se hanc artem scire. Sed pusillanimes se praedicant in operando et lucre participes secum ducunt chirurgulos et ita cecus cecundit et ambo in soueam cadunt [...] sed ego credo que multi essent de praedicitis medicis qui operarentur si scirent modum operandi. Sed porissima causa ob quam non operantur est: quia nesciunt operari quia non est peritus chirurgicus qui a pueritia non uacauit huic arti [...] quia pueri a patribus progeniem secuti adiscunt philosophiam omni aliarum rerum cura posthabita: ita tum quia a teneris annis in ea doctrina erudiuntur tum quia diuitius in ea perseuerant doctissimi euadunt. Ita dico de arte chirurgica in que cadi tilla agilitas manum suendo, ligando, secando, urendo et alias chirurgicas operationes faciendo'. Cf. Brunschwig, writing in 1512, advises his readership to always pick a 'practicus'. Taape, 'Common Medicine', 2021, p. 48.
47 Taape, 'Common Medicine', 2021.
48 Berengario da Carpi, *A Short Introduction*, 1959, pp. 109–110.
49 Berengario da Carpi, *A Short Introduction*, 1959, p. 154.
50 Berengario da Carpi, *Isagoge Breves*, 1522, fol. 59r: 'Docta tamen manus difficiliora perquirit'.
51 Landino, *Comento Sopra la Comedia*, 2001, p. 241: 'Andreino fu grande disegnatore et di gran rilievo, amatore delle difficultà dell'arte et di scorci, vivo et prompto molto, et assai facile nel fare'; Summers, *Michelangelo and the Language of Art*, 1981, p. 179.
52 Summers, *Michelangelo and the Language of Art*, 1981, pp. 179–181.
53 Summers, *Michelangelo and the Language of Art*, 1981, p. 185. Vasari, 1966–1987, vol. 6, p. 108: 'Fu Michelagnolo molto inclinato alle fatiche dell'arte, veduto che gli riusciva ogni cosa quantunque dificile'.
54 Vasari, 1966–1987, 184.
55 Quoted in Zagoury, '*Ingegno, Fatica,* and Imagination in Early Florentine Art Theory', 2018, p. 70; Jonietz, 'Labor omnia vincit?', 2011, esp. pp. 592–595; Beyer, *Künstler, Leib und Eigensinn*, 2022, pp. 63–76; Löhr, 'Von Gottes "I" zu Giottos "O": Schöpferhand und Künstlerkörper zwischen Mittelalter und Früher Neuzeit', 2011, pp. 51–76. For the place of ingenuity in anatomical practice see: Hoffmann, '*Ingegniosa peritia*', 2021, pp. 94–111.
56 Farago, *Leonardo da Vinci's* Paragone, 1992, pp. 257, 269.
57 Berengario da Carpi, *Commentaria,* 1521, fols 5r, 279r–v.
58 Hoffmann, '*Ingeniosa peritia*', 2021, p. 106: Baldasar Hesler describes watching Vesalius performing a dissection as 'very beautiful to see'. Ferrari ties public dissections to Carnival and through the ludic nature of the period traces its development as public spectacle. Ferrari, 'Public Anatomy Lessons and the Carnival', 1987, pp. 50–106; Klestinec, *Theaters of Anatomy*, 2011, pp. 55–89.
59 Berengario da Carpi, *A Short Introduction*, 1959, p. 113.
60 Berengario *Tractatus*, 1518, fol. 23v: 'Tamen dico que in istis signis distinguendis est magna difficultas et non cognoscuntur nisi a ualde experto qui coniectura aliqua hoc cognoscat. Quia haec signa non possunt integre scribi sed solum a bono ingenio diligenter ruminante diuidente et componente et longo tempore in similibus experto possunt comprehendi et iudicari: quia multa sunt in medico quae non possunt scribi ut continue uidemus'. For the relation of diagnostics and colour perception see: Boxer, 'Uroscopy Diagrams, Judgement, and the Perception of Color in Late Medieval England', 2022, pp. 327–347.

61 Berengario da Carpi, *Tractatus*, 1518, p. 36r: "Iudicio tum existimatiuo et hoc ad plenum non possum tradere in scriptis'.
62 Kumler, '*Periculum* and *Peritia*', 2019, pp. 157–178; Sears, 'Craft Ethics and the Critical Eye', 2006, pp. 221–238.
63 'Guardate dove ha posto la pittura Michelagnolo con lo smisurato de le sue figure, dipinte con maestà del giudizio, non col meschino dell'arte. E perciò fate da uomo naturalone [...]'. Aretino quoted in Klein '"Giudizio' et Gusto"', 1961, p. 112.
64 Quoted in Gregory, 'The unsympathetic exemplar', 2009, p. 15. This admonition of a lack of discernment and in turn good judgement is also thematized in Vasari's brief biography of Amico Aspertini in the lives of artists of the Romagna school. Speaking to the artist's obsession with copying after the antique, he wrote: 'andò per tutta Italia disegnando e ritratendo ogni cosa di pittura e di rilievo, e coì le buone come le cattive', Vasari, *Vite*, 1966–1987, vol. 5, p. 497.
65 Kumler, '*Periculum* and *Peritia*', 2019, pp. 167–173; Sears, 'Craft Ethics and the Critical Eye', 2006, pp. 221–232.
66 Berengario da Carpi, *Tractatus*, 1518, fol. 28r: 'Et oportet qui delectur medicus in cognoscendo istos colores: quia quidlibet non cognoscit: sed tantum ille qui ex expertus & excercitatus: similbus sicut experti cognoscunt gemmas bonas a fraudatis & a non bonis'.
67 Berengario da Carpi, *Commentaria*, 1521, fol. 5v: 'Qui color non cognoscitur in mortius nec a quodcunque: sed a bona extimatiua Medici et longa ipsius experientia hoc etiam cognosci potest: sicut experti circa gemmas iudicant bonas a falsis et illas cognoscunt: similiter experti Medici praenarrata cognoscunt'.
68 Sears, 'Craft Ethics and the Critical Eye', 2006, pp. 227–231.

Source 4

Pier Antonio Fucini, *Trattato della pittura*, c. 1605/21

Fabian Jonietz

Pier Antonio Fucini (1581–1651), born in Castiglion Fiorentino, numbers among the many early modern Italian physicians who – like Michelangelo Biondo, Giulio Mancini, or Francesco Scannelli – had so strong an interest in the visual arts as to write a treatise on the subject. In contrast to the books of the three aforementioned theorists, however, Fucini's text reached few readers and remained relatively unknown. Unlike Mancini's roughly contemporary *Considerazioni*, Fucini's text is known from just a single manuscript, first rediscovered and edited in 2011.

Fucini, who finished his medical studies in Pisa in 1605, dedicated his treatise on painting to the Florentine patrician, academic, and collector Ruberto del Beccuto (1575–1621), to whom he also dedicated a text on fossils and mussels. The single copy of the *Trattato della pittura* that forms the basis of our modern transcription dates from 1723; it is now preserved in the Biblioteca Nazionale in Florence (Fondo Palatino, Ms. 262), and was prepared for the art writer Francesco Maria Niccolò Gabburri (1676–1742).[1] The manuscript also includes two other works: Fucini's aforementioned *Trattato delle Conchiglie* as well as a copy – probably once belonging to Fucini himself – of the early sixteenth-century didactic poem, *Tractato di pictura* (or *Capitolo della pittura*), by the still rather mysterious figure of Francesco Lancilotti.[2]

In terms of content, Fucini's text represents no less than a short universal history of the art of painting. It emphasises the general nobility, relevance, and universal utility of the art; it addresses the theoretical foundations of optics and perspective as well as discrete elements such as lines, colours, and light; it deals with the theme of *Natura naturans* (that is, *Natura pictrix*), and arrives thereby at a treatment of ancient artists from pagan and Old Testament sources. Alongside expected references to famous works of art and to the valuation of art in ancient times, Fucini also devotes attention to non-European practices, such as the body painting of Indigenous peoples, and especially questions concerning idols and the miraculous effects of images. His praise of painting ends with a paraphrased description of its feminine personification, borrowed verbatim from Cesare Ripa's *Iconologia*.

The text thus combines a narration of art historical developments with general observations about the functions and foundations of painting (and less extensively, sculpture). This entirely original approach can be traced back to the scientific training and individual interests of its author. Fucini not only summarises standard works by Vitruvius and especially Pliny's *Natural History* (often accessed by way of the excerpts in Vasari's *Vite*), but also gathers knowledge from widespread works of history by contemporary polymaths, such as Alessandro Sardi (*De moribus et ritibus gentium*, 1557), Francesco Sansovino (*Dell'historia universale dell'origine et imperio de Turchi*, 1560), and Stefano Guazzo (*Dialoghi piacevoli*, 1586). However, as a physician, Fucini relies especially upon the authorities of his own field: above all Galen and Girolamo Cardano, but also for example Soranos of Ephesus, Avicenna, and Levinus Lemnius. In this way, central passages of the *Trattato della pittura*, such as the definition of painting and its scope, come to include surprising citations from canonical medical writers or excurses into the medical field. Fucini also explains optical phenomena through his medical knowledge and speaks exhaustively about the uses of painting for his own profession, as the following excerpt demonstrates:[3]

> [...] Per maggior Nobiltà poi, i Pittori, e per la eloquenza, che devono avere sono stati collocati ancor loro nel seggio appresso di Mercurio, come vole Galeno nell'orazione persuasoria alle bone arti cap: 2., e questi son quelli de' quali parlando il medesimo Galeno, dice che in qualsivoglia sorte di specie fanno quel più di bello, che l'uomo si puole imaginare, e per grandezza di questa arte si scorge, che fino ha convenienza con la medicina, atteso che da Galeno vien detto, che la Pittura è necessaria a' medici mediante crediamo noi al cognoscere la qualità dei colori per haver cognizione dell'essenza, e qualità delli escrementi, si come insegnò nel libro dell'arte medicinale, dal colore del corpo humano, et in particolare del volto, potersi cognoscere le complessioni degli huomini. Onde dal medesimo fù accettata l'opinione di Quinto mentre disse, che fino al Pittore si aspetta cognoscere ancora le urine. Et a corroboratione di ciò per ragione della visione riferisce questo tale Autore, che dai Pittori con i colori cerulei, e fuschi, si giova alli occhi, e si ricrea la visione dicendoci di più dal medesimo, che mentre i soldati di Zenofonte fecero viaggio per le nievi, che è color bianco disgregativo, et estremo, furono offesi nelli occhi; si come di subito perdevano la luce quelli, che da Dionisio Tiranno erano per tempo tenuti in oscurissimo carcere, e poi collocati in una stanza di bianchissimi muri, e così venivano a essere offesi nelli occhi, e così interviene a quelli ancora, che ci hanno qualche malie, come infiammatione detta da' Greci Ophtalmia, mentre però che vedono la luce, per la qual cosa questi tali si devono tenere in loco oscuro, atteso che per lo oscuro, o fusco la visione si rende più perfetta, e meglio li mantiene, come sopra habbiamo detto; il che viene confermato da Tucidide coll'esempio della grande Ecclisse, che fa il Sole, dicendo, che in quel tempo per la tanta oscurità di esso, si vedono alcune stelle in Cielo.

Tengo dunque certissimo, che la Pittura sia una delle più sublime Arti, che l'Huomo possa esercitare, essendo che in essa si scorgano tutte le altre, e che ingrazia di quella è necessario sapere di tutte le Scientie, [...].

[...] For greater nobility and for their necessary eloquence, painters have been placed in a seat next to Mercury, as is stated by Galen in the second chapter of his *Exhortation to Study the Liberal Arts*. These are those of whom the same Galen says that in any kind they produce a greater beauty than what man can imagine. And because of the greatness of this art it can be seen that it is even convenient for medicine, since Galen reports that painting is necessary for physicians because we believe to recognise the quality of the colours in order to have knowledge of the essence and quality of excrements.[4] And he teaches in his book *Of the Art of Medicine* how to understand men's complexion by the colour of the human body, especially that of the face.[5] For this reason he accepted Quintus's opinion who claimed that even the painter is expected to discern urine.[6] As a corroboration of this reasoning about vision, the author reports that painters benefit the eye with bluish and gloomy colours, and – so he continues – that by this way it is possible to recreate eyesight. When Xenophon's soldiers had to march through snow, which has a disruptive and extreme white colour, they were offended in the eyes. Likewise, those men lost their eyesight immediately, who were kept by the tyrant Dionysius for a long time in a very dark dungeon, and subsequently moved to a room with very white walls, because they were offended in the eyes. It happens also to those who have a condition such as the inflammation (which the Greeks call Ophtalmia) while they see light: for this reason they must be kept in a dark place, since for obscurity and gloominess their vision will become better and stay this way, as we said above. This is confirmed by Thucydides with the example of the great eclipse of the sun, by saying that at this time, due to its extreme darkness, some stars can be seen in the sky.

I therefore hold absolutely certain that painting is one of the most sublime arts that man can exercise, being that all the other arts can be detected in it, and for this art it is necessary to know all sciences, [...].

Notes

1 The treatise is noted bibliographically in Palermo, *I Manoscritti*, 1853–1868, vol. 1, p. 450, no. 411; Gentile, *I codici Palatini*, 1889–1950, vol. 1, p. 418. For contextualisation and transcription, see Jonietz, 'Ein unbekannter Kunsttraktat', 2011; the following summary is based on this contribution.

2 The most likely hypothesis identifies this author – whose family name is common throughout Italy – with a painter from Florence who is recorded in Sicily in the early sixteenth century; see Di Marzo, *La pittura in Palermo*, 1899, p. 275; Scarullo, *Dizionario*, 1993, p. 281; Pugliatti, *Pittura del Cinquecento*, 1998, p. 229.

3 The transcription follows Jonietz, 'Ein unbekannter Kunsttraktat', 2011, p. 159; English translation by the author.

4 On the misunderstood passage from Quintus (Κοίντος), see my essay in this volume.

5 On this, see the discussion of sources by Robert Brennan in this volume.

6 See note 4.

7

Slave or *condottiere*? Artists, labour, and occupational health in early modern Italy

Frances Gage

Introduction

In his letter on the *paragone* to the *letterato* Benedetto Varchi, Jacopo Pontormo asserts that the health effects of the arts of painting and sculpture are fundamental consequences of artistic practice and crucial to the distinct identities of the two arts. The sculptor's considerable labour keeps him 'more healthy and with a better complexion', Pontormo explains, whereas the painter's body is 'badly disposed to the toil of art; [painting] rather disturbs the mind than reinforces (*aumento*) life'.[1] Varchi himself articulates the idea that the sculptor possesses a robust body, robustness equating to physical health in the early modern period.[2] Vasari, too, subscribed to the idea that sculptors achieved better health than painters, though he framed it in relation to the physiological conception of complexion rather than in relation to the corporeal strength evoked by the term *robustezza*.[3] All three writers agreed that the positive health status of sculptors derived from the physicality of the sculptural process.

Vasari's famous characterisation of Pontormo as an isolated, mad man, leading an austere and miserable life, overcome by fear of death, long informed modern scholarly treatment of the artist. This discouraged scholars, until recently, from exploring Salvatore Nigro's observation about Pontormo's *Diario* of 1554–1556 (which records Pontormo's observations about his health and records of his diet), that the artist underscored the need for a '*professional* regimen, to neutralize' his health problems.[4] Instead, Pontormo is presented as eccentric and preoccupied with bodily functions such as eating and excretion, the latter of which falls under the Galenic non-naturals category of 'repletion and evacuation', a framework central to early modern medical theory and a subject to which we will return.[5] Pontormo was so extraordinary in this regard that Philip Sohm coined the unique stylistic term 'intestinal' to describe his late compositions in San

Lorenzo.[6] In particular, however, Pontormo's *Prescrizioni e ricordi* strongly argue that the painter understood health to belong squarely within the professional interests and responsibilities of the artist; implicitly the status of the arts (that is, their relative nobility) could not be extricated from this issue. Pontormo himself attested to the fact that practitioners in the arts inevitably negotiated health concerns in order to continue their work.

The scholarly response to Pontormo reflects broader trends within the field of art history, where, with the exception of a considerable body of literature on the question of early modern artists and melancholy, most considerations of artists and illness have occurred within studies of individual masters, typically with little more than passing references to periods of ill health within an artist's career. An exception is the very well-documented Michelangelo, whose health problems constitute a theme of his poetry and his letters and are thus mentioned in scholarly literature with some frequency.[7] With few exceptions, the question of an artist's health has been framed as one of personal accident or fortune, rather than a matter of professional anxiety or method. To what extent, however, might Pontormo's statements in the *paragone* and in his *Diario* illuminate a hitherto neglected facet of early modern professional discourse? For what is striking about this text is the degree to which health concerns are interspersed with remarks about his work, suggesting the degree to which Pontormo managed diet in light of his painting. Put another way, did any antecedents to modern occupational health exist within the context of early modern artistic theory and practice?

Brief as they are, Pontormo's remarks in the section of his *Diario* entitled *Prescrizioni e ricordi*, confirm familiarity with medical theory, while his daily entries demonstrate his application of medical theory to self-care. To what extent other early modern artists shared this knowledge and engaged in similar practices awaits full investigation, but the present essay provides a point of departure for this exploration, aiming to ascertain some of the most acute anxieties amongst artists and within the art world concerning health.[8] In this context, particularly valuable testimony is provided in the writings of the Sienese physician, Giulio Mancini (1559–1630), who, after serving both as one of the four doctors at the Hospital of Santo Spirito in Rome and to several cardinals privately, was elevated under Urban VIII to the position of papal physician. Uniting his profession of medicine with skills in connoisseurship and art criticism, Mancini represents a crucial nexus between the two fields. Indeed, medicine informed the theory of painting articulated in his *Considerazioni sulla pittura* (1619–post-1625).[9]

In this treatise, which Mancini never prepared for publication, he addresses the question of health in various contexts, particularly in the second part, where he provides brief lives of artists, including his contemporaries. Although one might be tempted to conclude that Mancini's attention to health in this treatise was merely a function of his professional expertise and interests, I argue that the sustained and growing attention to health concerns in literature on art across the early modern period, but increasingly in the seventeenth century, demonstrates that it was becoming a matter of professional interest among artists.[10]

Mancini suggests that health was not merely a matter of fortune, but reflected distinct human typologies, one of the most significant being the stage of life. This, in turn, necessarily influenced the practice of the arts. When discussing the effects of old age (with its implicit ill health) in his *vita* of Tommaso Laureti, Mancini provides a brief theoretical declaration about how health necessarily informed artistic practice over a lifetime.[11] He also writes that certain artists intentionally altered their practice in response to this exigency, as painting requires practitioners to possess 'knowledge of the thing [to be imitated] [...] spirit for the invention [of it] and the eye and the hand for execution'.[12] In old age, he goes on to say, suggesting the following constitutes universal experience, 'there is knowledge and judgment to not mar [the work], but there is not the spirit for invention, or the eye and hand for execution'.[13] He nevertheless acknowledges exceptions, such as the Cavaliere d'Arpino, who at the time Mancini was writing was more than fifty years old – that is, in old age – but 'in such health as to be able to work many years [yet]'.[14] Strikingly, too, Mancini suggests that artists who recognise the negative impact of old age upon artistic practice and respond accordingly deserve praise. Michelangelo, ironically one of the Renaissance artists to have lived longest and to have remained most productive in old age, 'knew this very well', Mancini goes on to say, adding that in his late years he devoted himself to architecture, which 'required his judgment', but which did not evidently require the physical labour of eye and hand as in either sculpture or painting.[15] By contrast, Federico Zuccari, as Mancini notes in this same context in his Palatino manuscript, 'did not perceive this [and] wanted to work [in painting] in his old age, but the works did not arrive at their usual excellence'.[16] In doing so, Zuccari cast a shadow over his former glory.[17]

Yet certain artists evidently acknowledged their diminished abilities, even to patrons, while continuing to work in some fashion. In two letters from 1666 to his patron, Leopoldo de' Medici, Pietro da Cortona apologised for the fact that his work would not live up to Leopoldo's expectations due to Cortona's chronic suffering from gout, which prevented him from working more than half of the time.[18] He hoped that Leopoldo would enjoy the two landscape drawings he was sending, described as *domestico* and *selvatico*, 'as made by one who suffers from gout in his feet and hands, and where his force is lacking, he supplements with good will', suggesting Cortona conceived of a distinct form of art criticism conjoining aesthetic judgment and compassion, and perhaps hoped that the Duke may have prized the works as a testament to the artist's dedication to his art, even in disability (Figure 7.1).[19]

Ill health may have been both most acute and persistent in old age, but abundant evidence demonstrates that artists' health anxieties extended across their lives. The increasing attention to health in artistic discourses over the sixteenth and seventeenth centuries may in part have been encouraged by the burgeoning number of printed health manuals in the vernacular from the middle of the sixteenth century into the seventeenth. This in itself demonstrates that Italian men and women avidly sought advice on matters of health in this period, as Sandra Cavallo and Tessa Storey argue.[20] To what extent did artists avail themselves of this growing body of literature addressing both preventive and therapeutic medicine?

With his regular remarks about the health status of individual artists in his short *vite* in the *Considerazioni*, Mancini indicates how health assumed vital importance in the negotiations between artists and patrons. The health of artists even exerted pressure on the art market, since ill health often prevented artists from working, thereby slowing the completion of commissions, or terminating them altogether.[21] This might also have exacerbated potential competition between patrons or collectors. Mancini provides a striking commentary on this issue when writing about the architectural and landscape painter Agostino Tassi, then at the high point of his career, at age forty-three.[22] He was a mature artist, not yet an old one.[23]

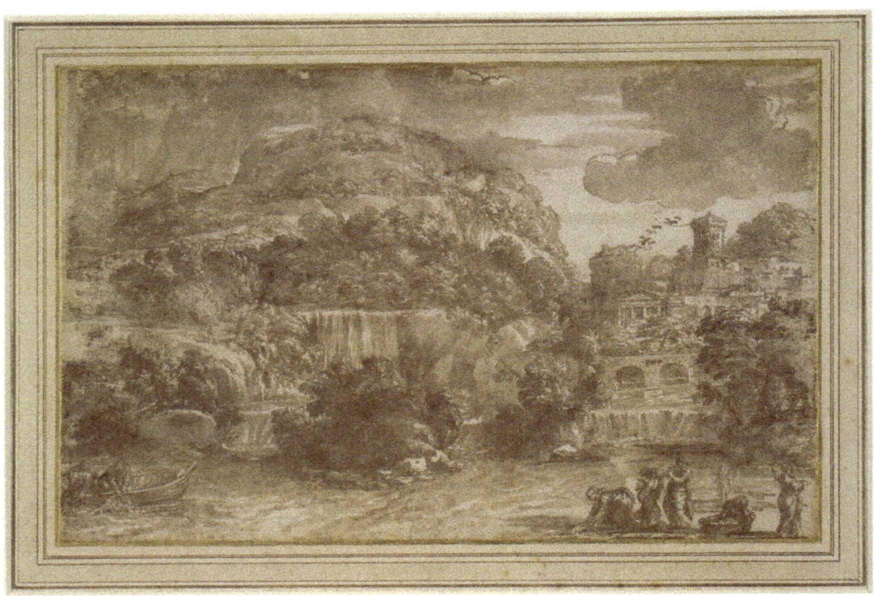

Figure 7.1 Pietro da Cortona, Landscape with Hillside and Waterfall, c. 1660–1669, brown ink and wash over black chalk on Holkam mount, 27.6 × 43.2 cm. London, British Museum. Image credit: The Trustees of the British Museum

> He is at the best stage of working, but he suffers from the pains of gout which often molest him and in particular in the hands and it causes great compassion that this artist and inventor, of so much worth in this sort of painting that one can say [he] is singular, cannot work as much as the world desires.[24]

Francesco Maria II della Rovere, the patron of Barocci, who, according to Giovan Pietro Bellori, suffered acute chronic stomach troubles and could work no more than two hours a day, expressed frustration about the difficulty of seeing Barocci's works to completion.[25] It is difficult to imagine that with patrons clambering for commissions, a prominent artist did not explore available medical technologies in the hopes of a cure or mitigation of symptoms so he or she could produce more works or at least work more rapidly. As evidenced by Mancini's own career, in which he extended the invitation of an apartment in Siena to Antonio Carracci in order to help him recover from illness, patrons offered to facilitate convalescence in the hopes of encouraging the gifting of artwork or the acceptance of a commission.[26]

One of the mechanisms artists employed to negotiate the demands of production in light of chronic illness was, as Mancini observed with respect to Michelangelo, to alter medium, technique, or style. As Mancini noted, Agostino Carracci could not work much in fresco on account of his respiratory problems.[27] This may have contributed to tensions between him and Annibale, who, in apparent marked contrast to Agostino, was described in 1599 as 'working like a horse' for the Farnese in Rome.[28] Could this have constituted a factor in Agostino's earlier decision to pursue printmaking? In Giovanni Baglione's writing about the little-known Bolognese portraitist Antonio Scalvati, who suffered from gout, he describes how Scalvati passed much of his time in bed, producing his papal portraits.[29] Baglione provides no more information, but his commentary raises many questions concerning Scalvati's set-up, and whether he assembled a special bed to constitute his worksite.

Medical theory, *fatica*, and the artist

Given the numerous health challenges faced by early modern artists, there was every reason for them to familiarise themselves with medical theories and practices, though further research is needed to determine which texts on the subject they may have engaged with. As noted, Pontormo's *Diario* attests to his familiarity with the Galenic 'non-naturals', the six conditions or activities that affected health, including air and breathing, eating and drinking, motion or exercise and rest, waking and sleeping, repletion and evacuation, and the passions of the soul.[30] Whether for the sake of health prevention or therapy, early modern physicians recommended the management and regulation of the non-naturals in order to achieve the equilibrium equated with good health. This entailed a consideration of the disposition of the subject, suitable environmental conditions (ideally those native to the subject), and a requisite balance among the physiological substances of the body. Physicians and their patients sought moderation in all of the non-naturals, though how they defined moderation depended in part upon individual disposition as well as typologies according to age, sex, nationality, and profession.[31] Unanticipated or dramatic changes amongst any of the non-naturals, especially environmental conditions, provoked particular anxieties insofar as they altered the balance among the four elementary substances composing the humours.[32]

Among the most pressing concerns for artists was labour, typically viewed by medical writers as corporeal work, linked with motion or exercise, though it could also involve mental effort.[33] The physician Scipione Mercurio associated *fatica* with daily labour, diligence, and industry; a ready figure for this was the peasant's toil.[34] As had Pontormo in writing to Varchi, medical writers generally regarded physical toil and labour as producing similar physical benefits to exercise insofar as it excited natural heat (*calor naturale*), associated with the life force, strengthening the body and its members.[35] However, medical writers recommended moderation in all activities, including labour, cautioning against extremes of either exercise or idleness. As the Portuguese physician Rodrigo Fonseca, who served the Tuscan Grand Duke, reminded his readers, Hippocrates had warned that moderation in labour, food, sleep, and sex was the key to health.[36] Sandra Cavallo and Tessa Storey argue that such expectations of moderation intersected with the demands of civility and with the moralising agenda of the Counter Reformation church.[37] Health care imbricated comportment and artists might be judged on moral grounds for their health or illness. Filippo Baldinucci, for instance, when praising Gian Lorenzo Bernini's health in old age, attributed it at least in part to the artist's 'moderation in food'.[38]

Given the insistence upon moderation and regulation, health contributed to the reputation of an artist. Returning to the question of Tassi's gout, early modern medicine debated the causes of this common illness. The physician Bartolomeo Traffichetti, who surveyed a variety of potential causes in a chapter devoted to the subject of gout in his *L'arte di conservare la sanità* (1565), identified 'disordered living' as a potential culprit, citing excessive sleep, inactivity (*otio*), or sex as the activities most likely giving rise to this condition.[39] Similarly, he argued that excessive labour might also weaken the joints.[40] Although Mancini defended Tassi in his *Considerazioni*, he acknowledged that the painter's free and quick speech led to ruptures with friends, suggesting he was not unaware of Tassi's fiery comportment.[41] The painter's sexual scandals and sexual violence may have led some of the painter's contemporaries to attribute his illness to an indulgent or blameworthy lifestyle.[42] But others may have attributed his illness to overwork. An impediment to labour on account of ill health often threatened an artist's reputation, encouraging practitioners to moderate behaviour, as Pontormo evidently did when restricting his intake of food, or to mitigate the passions, as Bellori noted Barocci customarily did.[43] Not only in the case of Zuccari, but also in those of Laureti and Annibale Carracci, Mancini's writings assert that these artists worked better before succumbing to illness or old age, with the suggestion in his *vita* of the latter that Annibale's last illness and death were caused by *disordini*, a term, as Traffichetti made clear, that indicated immoderate use of one or more of the non-naturals.[44]

Seventeenth-century artists' *vite* take up several thematics concerning artists' illness and in so doing suggest some of the relevant health anxieties of professional painters. The painter and biographer Giovanni Baglione echoed physicians when asserting that *fatica* was easiest to support when it was regular, and when it appropriately corresponded to an individual's disposition. Labour to which an individual was accustomed proved less dangerous and potentially more beneficial than sporadic or variable degrees of toil or effort, particularly in old age.[45] For instance, when Ottavio Leoni endeavoured to etch a series of portraits, a project Baglione admiringly described as a *gran fatica virtuosa*, the enormity of labour caused a serious 'indisposition' that killed Leoni.[46] The implication was that the project far exceeded the labour hitherto customary to Leoni. Not surprisingly, Leoni presented himself in this late self-portrait as a Knight of Malta, not as an artist engaged in labour (Figure 7.2). Other artists, according to Baglione, fell ill because they were unaccustomed to the effort demanded by a particular project or at a certain juncture of their career, with the implication their work life may have been inadequately regulated. For instance, the Bolognese landscape painter Giovanni Battista Viola decided during the pontificate of Gregory XV that he no longer wished to paint and was fortuitously named *guardarobba* to the pope. The pope's untimely death, however, put an end to Viola's good fortunes. Having to return to painting, which required considerably more *fatica* than his courtly position had done and to which he was by then unaccustomed, he became ill on account of 'excess labour' (*troppa fatica*).[47]

Another of the recurring themes in Baglione's *Vite* concerning illness pertains to the intersection of two non-naturals, and in particular to the impact upon corporeal health of what would now be termed psychology, but which people in the early modern period referred to as the passions of the soul. This also reflects a particular theoretical perspective in early modern medicine, which viewed the body and mind as interconnected and mutually influential.[48] As a consequence, early moderns held that changing passions corresponded to corporeal alteration, namely a fluctuation in bodily humours or innate heat.[49] Specific passions might reflect increases or decreases to innate warmth, with the implied positive or negative somatic changes. Traffichetti remarked that whereas *fatica* is unpleasant, exercise, to

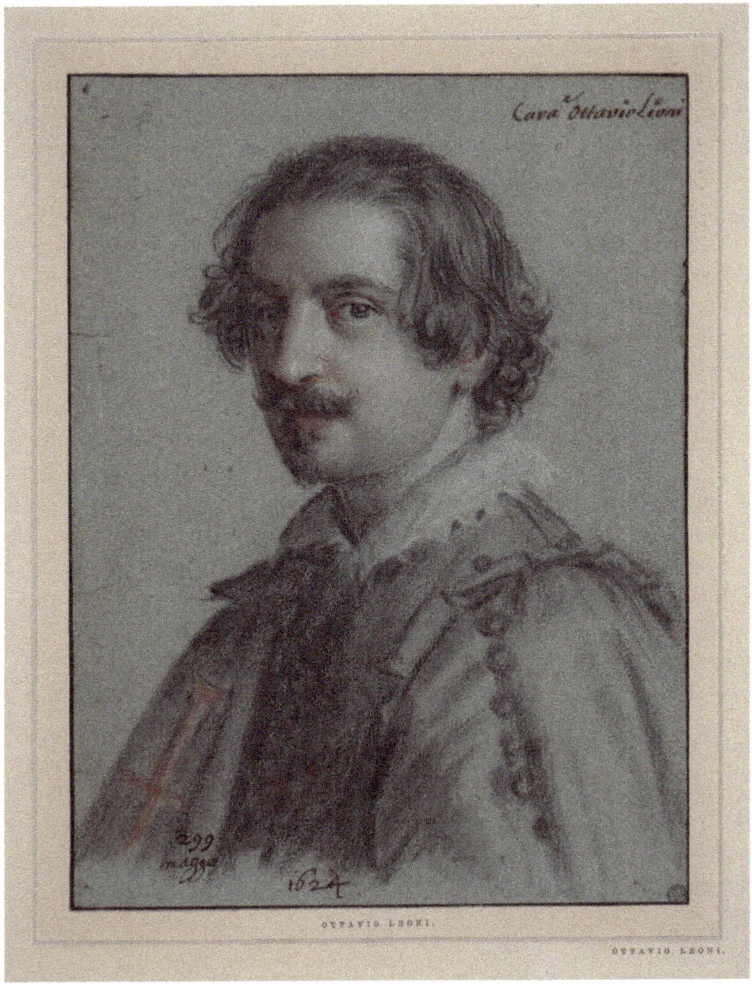

Figure 7.2 Ottavio Leoni, Self-Portrait, 1624, black, red, and white chalk, on blue paper, 22.1 × 15.9 cm. London, British Museum. Image credit: The Trustees of the British Museum

be beneficial, must be delightful, an idea encountered with regularity in early modern treatises on health.[50] Given the association between *fatica* and exercise, one might presume that the same psychological expectations would likewise be sought in relation to work in order to preserve its salubriousness.

In addition to expectations that labour remain at habitual levels, an artist's pleasure or displeasure in the face of work might thereby guarantee health or generate illness. In the case of Agostino Ciampelli, for instance, these factors intertwined, according to Baglione. Ciampelli 'was accustomed to remain comfortable at home, painting according to his own pleasure (*gusto*)'. When Ciampelli received the commission to paint in St Peter's, however, so Baglione goes on to say, he was obliged to work 'rather hard [...] and it was necessary to work both for himself and for others', the implication being that working for others represented much higher expectations and entailed much harder work.[51] This increase in labour, however, led to Ciampelli's last illness and death. Here, Baglione's writings suggest that a high-profile commission, carried out for elevated patrons in the most important edifice in the Catholic world, may not only have required *more* labour, but also may have proved disagreeable to the artist, for, as Baglione writes, Ciampelli could no longer paint for his own pleasure.

The architect Giovanni Fontana formed a striking antithesis to Ciampelli. Fontana took pleasure in exertion; without specifying, Baglione suggests this is a combination of mental and physical toil. When engineering fountains during the pontificate of Sixtus V, Fontana 'moved a mountain, and it appeared that he enjoyed road-blocks so that he could vanquish them, shrugging off any [amount of] labor (*fatica*)'.[52] And there was no less labour involved in Fontana's fountains built for Scipione Borghese's villa.[53] Although Fontana engaged in exceedingly demanding work, Baglione never suggests that Fontana suffered ill health or any negative effects whatsoever as a consequence. Rather, his pleasure in overcoming monumental challenges apparently guaranteed he enjoyed good health.

Having considered the early moderns' view of the passions as contributing to the effects of physical labour on an artist's health, a striking anecdote about Gian Lorenzo Bernini illuminates how they conceived of situations where pleasurable mental labour might nevertheless produce dangerous somatic effects, potentially proving fatal. Both Bernini's biographers – the Florentine biographer and art theorist Filippo Baldinucci and the artist's son Domenico Bernini – relate how the sculptor became enraptured with his work: 'in love', Gian Lorenzo Bernini would say of himself at work, and absorbed in abstract thought.[54] The intensity of his mental labour posed no *immediate* somatic threat, but remained indirectly dangerous insofar as Bernini's distractedness greatly heightened his risk of falling from the scaffolding. In light of this, a young apprentice worked alongside him.[55] This passage affirms that early moderns understood that the passions produced a range of both direct and indirect affects upon the bodies and lives of artists.

If some within the artistic community articulated anxiety concerning the effects of old age and ill health upon both artistic practice and on the finished product, evidently considerable attention was given to the health dangers associated with youthful artists. Seventeenth-century writers on art frequently expressed concern over the tendency of young artists to engage in excessive *fatica*, whether corporeal or mental. Here the issue was not that these artists departed from regular amounts of labour to which they had grown accustomed. Rather, this anxiety echoed medical and philosophical ideas concerning characteristic youthful male behaviour, particularly in the realm of *libidine*.[56] This is not to suggest that youthful sexual pleasure, or indulgence, did not lead to health issues among artists. Nicolas Poussin, for example, contracted *mal francese* (syphilis) shortly after arriving in Rome at age thirty; he was depicted suffering from a 'grave illness' in a drawing around 1630, according to an inscription added later by a well-informed collector (Figure 7.3).[57] When the symptoms of syphilis became debilitating, Poussin benefited from the care extended by the collector Cassiano dal Pozzo, the physician Pierre Poitier, and the Dughet family, until such time as he partially recovered.[58] In a straightforward acknowledgement of the pervasiveness of this illness, Mancini remarks that the loss of the nose, the most visible symptom of syphilis, bestowed dishonour, but compassion was in order for young men who were customarily afflicted by 'venereal perturbations', because 'every man loses his head'.[59]

Yet the majority of remarks concerning young artists and health to emerge in seventeenth-century artists' *vite* centred upon the very opposite tendency: ambitious young artists, eager to study and achieve, not only working too intensively, but also eschewing any natural tendencies towards pleasure characteristic of this age group. However praiseworthy such diligence and devotion to art was, it carried the risk of compromising not only future health but even life itself. When Mancini compiled the *vita* of the young Pietro da Cortona, whom he knew through his artistic exchanges with Cortona's patron Marcello Sacchetti, Mancini praised the artist's rapid progress in the study of life-drawing and in the representation of antiquities, surpassing the achievements of an ordinary artist.[60] 'He draws in pen very well, withstands *fatica* to see [things] from life, and has designed many of these antiquities that he introduces into his works and many nocturnal things'.[61] But his endurance of great labour and effort, which Mancini describes in one of his manuscripts as reflecting Cortona's regulation of his behaviour – 'good habits [...] do not allow him to deviate from art' – leads Mancini to observe that, at twenty-eight, Cortona was 'not too healthy'.[62] In fact, Mancini worried Cortona might not live, though if he did, the physician believed he would reach the first rank among contemporary artists.[63] The early modern artist confronted a terrible double bind: to acquire a reputation he must work exceedingly hard, but this would often lead to illness and reduced production.

A similar intermingling of admiration and anxiety emerged in remarks made by the humanist Constantijn Huygens concerning the painters Jan Lievens and Rembrandt in their youth.

> I can however attest that I have never observed such diligence and application in men of any sort, pursuit, or age. Truly, they are 'redeeming the time', and that is their sole occupation. More remarkably, they regard even the diversions of youth as a waste of time, as if they were already old men burdened with age

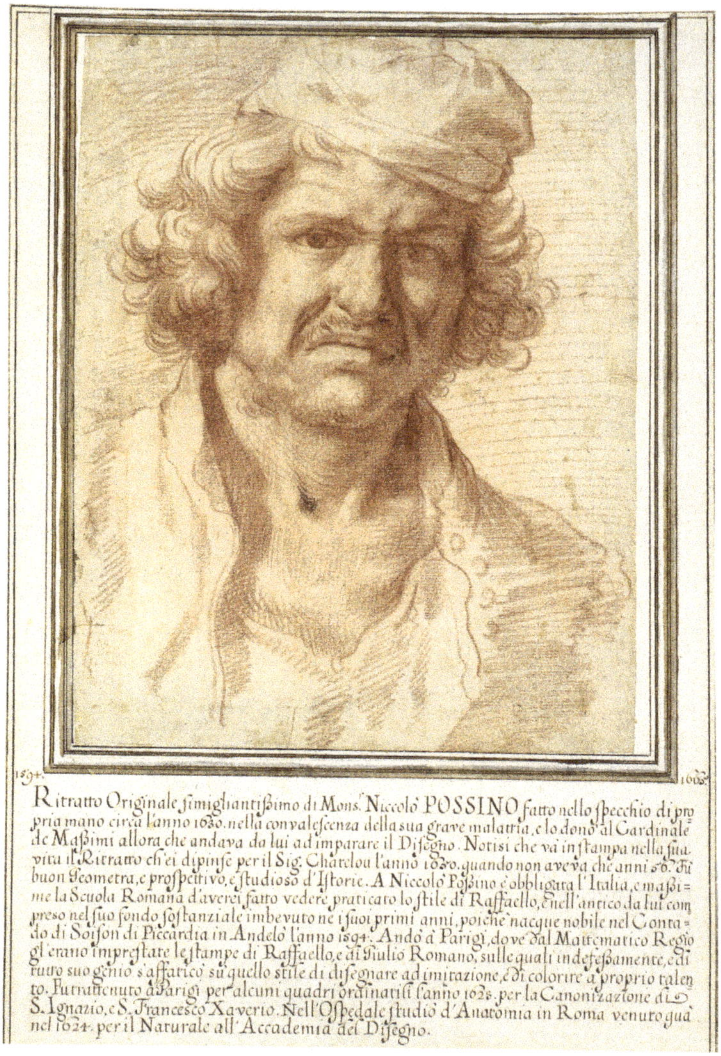
1594.
1665.
Ritratto Originale simigliantissimo di Mons.r Niccolò POSSINO fatto nello specchio di pro
pria mano circa l'anno 1630. nella convalescenza della sua grave malattia, e lo donò al Cardinale
de Massimi allora che andava da lui ad imparare il Disegno. Notisi che va in stampa nella sua
vita il Ritratto ch'ei dipinse per il Sig. Charelou l'anno 1650. quando non aveva che anni 56. Fu
buon Geometra, e prospettivo, e studioso d'Istorie. A Niccolò Possino è obbligata l'Italia, e massi=
me la Scuola Romana d'averci fatto vedere praticato lo stile di Raffaello, e nell'antico da lui com
preso nel suo fondo sostanziale imbevuto ne i suoi primi anni, poiche nacque nobile nel Conta=
do di Soison di Piccardia in Andelò l'anno 1594. Andò a Parigi, dove dal Matematico Regio
gl'erano imprestate le stampe di Raffaello, e di Giulio Romano, sulle quali indefessamente, e di
tutto suo genio s'affaticò su quello stile di disegnare ad imitazione, e di colorire a proprio talen
to. Fu trattenuto a Parigi per alcuni quadri ordinatili l'anno 1628. per la Canonizazione di
S. Ignazio, e S. Francesco Xaverio. Nell'Ospedale studiò d'Anatomia in Roma venuto quà
nel 1624. per il Naturale all'Accademia del Disegno.

Figure 7.3 Attributed to Nicolas Poussin, Self-Portrait, c. 1630, red chalk, 25.6 cm × 19.7 cm. London, British Museum. Image credit: The Trustees of the British Museum

> and long past such follies. Such indefatigable persistence at difficult labor may quickly yield great progress, yet I have often wished that these outstanding youths would practice moderation and consider their constitutions, which a sedentary occupation has already rendered less vigorous and robust.[64]

Huygens' desire that Lievens and Rembrandt practice moderation corresponds precisely to the health recommendations widely articulated by early modern physicians. It also harkens back to the notion that the most healthful mode of living was to respect typological norms. One of the problems for the two Dutch artists was that they transgressed customary behaviour associated with their age group. Additionally, Huygens called attention to one of the paradoxes of artistic production: on the one hand, great physical toil and effort could produce negative health effects associated with excessive exercise; on the other, art-making might give rise to afflictions linked to sedentary behaviour – a concern of the father of occupational health, Bernardino Ramazzini – resulting from idleness and lack of exercise.[65] This passage nonetheless explicitly addresses the issue of the painter's limited bodily movement, a point that will be revisited later in this discussion.

Health and the nobility of art

How did shared anxieties over artists' health inform the early modern debate concerning the nobility of art? Mancini's *Considerazioni* serves as a particularly valuable source, as it addresses the question of the relative nobility of painting. Although Mancini describes painting 'as a history and mute poetry', apparently underscoring its status among the liberal arts, he evaluates its nobility in relation to the health effects of art-making.[66] Mancini classifies painting and sculpture in accordance with the Aristotelian category of arts produced by the factive intellect, resulting in something done or made.[67] In fact, Mancini reveals the degree to which questions of individual honour and rank pertained to everyday practical issues in the art world: when an expert was called in to resolve a dispute about pricing, he should consider the rank of the artist, his merit, and also the labour he 'endured' in a work's creation – a concept previously shown to be intimately tied to medical theory.[68]

Mancini's interest in the question of the nobility of the arts likewise motivated his ambitious treatise *Alcune considerazioni del' honore*, which he was still revising around 1625, and which includes an extended analysis of the professions' relative honour.[69] In this effort (with a view as well to questions of precedence in Rome), Mancini evaluated a vast number of professions in accordance with a five-part framework. This framework considered the knowledge required in that profession, the materials utilised, the nature and processes of execution, the utility of the object, and the effects upon its users or audience.[70] Mancini argues that, in both painting and sculpture, intelligence and wisdom are a prerequisite, specifically the sense that the artist must possess knowledge of the object to be represented and conceived in the intellect.[71]

Harkening back to traditional anxieties about painting being a manual art, Mancini acknowledges the dirty materiality of painting, which soils clothes and potentially discolours the body, and brings to the fore various perils of art-making. As already noted, one of the most serious 'occupational hazards' for the early modern artist – still a concern of occupational medicine today – was the risk of falling, whether involving the fresco painter, the sculptor, or architect who worked on scaffolding.[72] Mancini implies, in fact, that one of the appealing features of the medium of oil painting, and a reason for its widespread use in the sixteenth century, may have been that it did not incur the same risks in this regard as fresco.[73] He notes in his *vita* of the little known painter Lattanzio Bonastri, whom he claims assisted El Greco, that Bonastri fell from a scaffolding to his death when painting in the residence of Cardinal Altemps.[74] Bonastri, he adds, might have made 'the greatest progress if he had lived'.[75] This anxiety over falls and physical danger illuminates the bitter and potentially violent rivalry between the painters Domenichino and Lanfranco in San Andrea della Valle, where each allegedly feared the other might attempt to harm him, either by hurling objects from above or destabilising the scaffolding from below, as they worked on the pendentives and cupola, respectively.[76] Rather than a colourful tale of rivalry, however, this anecdote drives to the heart of the material conditions and dangers of the painter's profession and implicitly to their relative honour within the social order. In assuming great personal risks of bodily harm to undertake their work, artists assumed temporary dishonour in order to prove their virtue and eventually redouble their honour. Yet some might never survive to reap those rewards.

Falls on the work site were among the most serious health risks of the early modern visual artist. However, Mancini, in his treatise, articulates other fears of grave injuries when evaluating the relative honour of the sculptor in particular. In carving marble, the sculptor risked splinters striking the eyes;[77] in modern occupational medicine the sensory organs and extremities are considered to be among the most vulnerable body parts to injury.[78] The perils of bronze casting, however, far outstripped those of marble carving. While Mancini notes that working with various materials such as gesso and lime posed dangers, he argues that the most severe threat arose in founding metal, which exposed the artist to potential fire and explosion. Fleeing and retreating behind a wall, Mancini cautions, was inadequate protection against the attendant dangers of founding.[79]

In another of Mancini's illuminating remarks concerning occupational hazards he drew inspiration from Pliny when censuring the arts on the grounds that painting, tailoring, and some musical performance (among other occupations), entailed occupying confined spaces that restricted voluntary movement.[80] In this context, Mancini alludes to Pliny's anecdote about the painter Amulius (known also as Famulus) who described Nero's Domus Aurea as his 'prison', because, Mancini explains, he continually stayed there to work.[81] Any profession in which the worksite could denote a prison surely risked subverting art's claims to 'liberal' status, but also raised more troubling questions pertaining to the status of the artist.

In the early modern period, the primary function of prisons was to hold those awaiting trial, those in debt or captives.[82] Mancini associates the confined spaces of art-making with both pollution and slavery.[83] These confined spaces 'contaminate the body, rendering it a slave, for the most part enclosing it in a room to work', a connection that reflects his awareness of the conditions of galley slaves in Italy.[84] Livorno, one of the major centres of the slave trade in the Italian peninsula, saw considerable numbers of men from North Africa or the Ottoman Empire, who had been captured by Christians and forced to labour as slaves in the Grand Ducal fleet, held in a prison-like structure termed *Il Bagno*.[85]

The implication that art-making entailed long hours of *concentrated and stationary* activity within a confined space, and which could be likened to imprisonment, is significant, suggesting growing awareness of slavery, a desire to define it and establish boundaries around slave labour, and an anxiety about any potential analogies that could be drawn between the latter and common trades, including art-making.[86] Artists themselves evidently harboured anxieties about the implications of confinement and restricted movement, but also recognised these as necessary conditions of their labour. An anecdote about the early career of the painter Girolamo Muziano, as recounted by Baglione, reveals that Muziano voluntarily fashioned himself with a modified attribute of a galley slave – a shaved head – and vowed not to leave the house before his hair had grown back to its previous length. He aimed to prevent himself from being tempted by potential love affairs (a youthful risk, as previously noted), and to dedicate himself wholly to his art.[87] To the modern reader, this anecdote may not obviously entail a health concern. And yet, Muziano's adoption of an attribute of a slave functioned as a mechanism to control the passions, carnal love being associated with the enervation of the body and dangerous *otium*.[88] Bearing a sign of dishonour associated with servility and slavery, Muziano inflicted bodily discomfort of confinement in order to ensure artistic achievement, thereby presumably acquiring greater honour later.

For Mancini, the physical costs and risks required to paint and sculpt (or engage in other factive professions) risked bestowing dishonour on the practitioner, precisely because they entailed potential injury, illness, and discomfort. Considering such grave dangers, how could writers on art make the claim that painting and sculpture constituted honourable professions? The efforts seventeenth-century writers on art such as Mancini, Baglione, and others took to establish the honour of the visual arts, while negotiating the competing ranks of and associations with intellectual and manual processes, demonstrates the inherent instability of these classifications.[89] The nobility of the visual arts therefore had to be continually negotiated and renegotiated, frequently on the basis of the strategies individual artists adopted to overcome the complications of seemingly competing ontological categories.

Mancini himself turned to this very question in his *Considerazioni*, arguing that painting and sculpture could be ennobled, not *in spite* of the dangers or risks to the lives and health of their practitioners, but precisely *because* of such perils, provided these risks resulted from virtuous and honourable public service. In order to ensure that his claims for the honour of the professions of painting and sculpture were theoretically unassailable, Mancini compared the figure of the artist to the military *condottiere*, who suffered bodily fatigue, pollution, and danger in the service of the prince (or state), and was even sometimes maimed in his service.[90] Provided that artists' objectives remained public honour not private gain, manual labour from this perspective certified the heroic status of the artist instead of casting him into abjection, as such risks and injuries might do if they issued from vice, not virtue. Indeed, considering the ends of physical labour in this way, risk and danger potentially doubled the claims to honour.

This investigation suggests that the energetic reading of health manuals in sixteenth- and seventeenth-century Italy on the part of the lay population extended to the artist community. Early modern treatises on art, biographies, and letters together present a picture of artists confronting shared anxieties very similar to those outlined in early modern medical theory and practice, from questions of excess or moderation in the non-naturals and especially in the restraint of the passions, to cautions about environment. In what way did early modern artists develop professional practices of health care? If the case of Pontormo has generally been construed as an extraordinary instance of an isolated artist obsessed with self-care, the sources considered here largely argue for a different model, one that is explicitly social and collective, rather than individual. One of the most striking aspects of the evidence above is the degree to which the illnesses of artists exerted pressures upon social relationships, demanding or inviting intervention by concerned artists, but also especially from patrons, friends, and critics, as the cases of Poussin, Cortona, and Antonio Carracci demonstrate, with the writings of Mancini and Huygens further amplifying this point. The early modern artist's conjunction of talent, skill, and extraordinary *fatica*, the latter posing potential health problems, gave rise to admiration, alarm, blame, and sometimes compassion within artistic circles, but nevertheless helped develop ideas about occupational health, which would eventually come to fruition in the early eighteenth century in the work of the physician Bernardino Ramazzini.[91]

Notes

1 Varchi, *Due lezzioni*, 1549, p. 133; For Varchi and the *paragone* debate, see especially Mendelsohn, *Paragoni*, 1982, passim, Jonietz, 'Labor omnia vincit', 2011, esp. pp. 587–592.

2 Varchi, *Due lezzioni*, 1549, p. 96. That robustness (*robustezza*) was closely associated with or equated to health can be gleaned from the writings of the physician

Giulio Mancini, whose work will be discussed below. Mancini's association between *robustezza* and *sanità* occurs in his treatise 'Alcune considerationi del'honore fatte da Giulio Mancini per suo trattenimento', (BAV. Barb. Lat. 4314), fols 18v ff. (henceforth *ACDH*).

3 Britton, 'Raphael and the Bad Humours', 2008, p. 179.

4 Vasari, *Le opere*, 1906, vol. 6, p. 270 (henceforth Vasari, *LO*); Nigro, *Pontormo: il libro mio*, 1984, 33 (my emphasis). For Pontormo and literature on hygiene and diet, see Beuzelin, 'Jacopo Pontormo', 2012, pp. 94–95, 101.

5 Pontormo, *Diario*, 2014, pp. 7–36; For Pontormo's *Diario*, see also Nigro, *Pontormo: il libro mio*, ed. Nigro, 1984, passim; Sohm, *The Artist Grows Old*, 2007, pp. 114–119; Jonietz, 'Labor omnia vincit', 2011, p. 589.

6 Sohm, *The Artist Grows Old*, 2007, pp. 120.

7 See most recently, Wallace, *God's Architect*, 2019, pp. 157–159, and below n. 86.

8 For artists' knowledge of the human body, see Fabian Jonietz' essay in this volume.

9 For the role of medicine in Mancini's art theory, see Gage, 'Exercise for Mind and Body', 2008, pp. 1172, 1192, 1201; Gage, *Painting as Medicine*, 2016, pp. 5, 153–155; Frigo, 'Can One Hold a Brush?', 2012, pp. 420–421, 434–435.

10 Significantly, Mancini's concern with the health of artists does not extend to the toxicity of materials, which would become a preoccupation later in the work of Bernardino Ramazzini. See Jana Graul's contribution to this volume.

11 For early modern artists and old-age style, see Sohm, *The Artist Grows Old*, 2007, especially pp. 3–12. See also Campbell, 'The Art of Aging Gracefully', 2002, pp. 321–331, for this passage, as well as p. 322n5, for early modern notions of when old age commenced.

12 Mancini, *Considerazioni sulla pittura*, vol. 1, 1956, p. 233 (subsequently *CSP*). Campbell, 'The Art of Aging Gracefully', 2002, p. 326, interprets Mancini's passage to mean that old artists can still render form. However, as Mancini demonstrated in his treatise on honour, by 'formation', he referred to knowledge and conceptual work, including mental images generated in cognition. In this context, he was not referring to the rendering of images by the hand. This raises the question of Michelangelo's reliance upon assistants in his old age architectural designs. For Michelangelo's working approach and especially his reliance on assistants and his managerial activities, see Wallace, *God's Architect*, 2019, pp. 128–30, and for assistance with writing, pp. 216–217.

13 Mancini, *CSP*, vol. 1, 1956, p. 233.

14 Mancini, *CSP*, 1956, p. 239 for d'Arpino's *vita*. Mancini hereby suggests that fifty years marked an important threshold, and although he did not explicitly say so, implied this represented the commencement of old age, since d'Arpino was exceptional in being in good health and predicted to be able to work many more years. Traffichetti, for instance, defined the period 35–49 as '*prima vecchiezza*'. Traffichetti, *L'arte di conservare la sanità*, 1565, p. 163.

15 Traffichetti, *L'arte di conservare la sanità*, 1565. This was Mancini's opinion, not necessarily Michelangelo's, however. For Michelangelo's old age architectural production, see Wallace, *God's Architect*, 2019, passim.

16 Mancini, *CSP*, vol. 1, 1956, p. 233 apparatus with variant text from Palatino ms.

17 Mancini, *CSP*, vol. 1, 1956.

18 Merz, 'Landscape Drawings by Pietro da Cortona', 2004, pp. 140, 142, 151n62.

19 Merz, 'Landscape Drawings by Pietro da Cortona', 2004. Disability studies scholars might regard this as ableist; however, my interpretation here is strictly historicist, in an attempt to understand how early modern artists considered health care.

20 Cavallo and Storey, *Healthy Living*, 2013, pp. 13–24.

21 See for instance Annibale's methods of coping with his inability to meet demand in Robertson, 'Late Annibale', 2010–2012, p. 272, p. 278.

22 Mancini, *CSP*, vol. 1, 1956, pp. 252–253;

23 See note 14 above.

24 Mancini, *CSP*, vol. 1, 1956, pp. 252–253; for Tassi's illness, see Cavazzini, '*La mala fama*', 2008, pp. 17–18.
25 Bellori, *Le vite*, 2009, p. 199; for della Rovere, see Lingo, *Federico Barocci*, 2008, p. 9.
26 Gage, *Painting as Medicine*, 2016, p. 31.
27 Mancini, *CSP*, vol. 1, p. 217.
28 Martin, *The Farnese Gallery*, 1965, p. 14; Ginzburg Carignani, *Annibale Carracci a Roma*, 2000, p. 83.
29 Baglione, *Le Vite*, 1970 (henceforth *LV*), p. 172.
30 For early modern health advice, see in particular Cavallo and Storey, *Healthy Living*, 2013, pp. 3, 5–6, and Cavallo, 'Conserving Health: The Non-Naturals', 2017, pp. 3, 9–12.
31 For moderation in the non-naturals, especially exercise, see Fonseca, *Del conservare la sanità*, 1603, p. 7; Petroni, *Del viver degli Romani*, 1592, p. 408.
32 Gage, *Painting as Medicine*, 2016, pp. 48–49; Gage, 'Chasing Good Air', 2017, pp. 242–243.
33 For art conjoining mental and physical labour, and art theory of labour, see especially Jonietz, 'Labor omnia vincit', 2011, pp. 593, and passim, and Zagoury, 'Minerva in the Forge', 2018, pp. 62–68. For early modern physicians' treatments of *fatica*, see the following health manuals, Traffichetti, *Del conservare della sanità*, 1565, fol. 109v, who associates *fatica* with both motion and exercise, but distinguishes it slightly from exercise, as we shall see, and who indicated that Hippocrates had classified *fatica* as exercise; Mercurio, *De gli errori popolari*, 1603, p. 236, suggesting that, like exercise, *fatica* strengthens the body; Petronio, *Del viver degli Romani*, 1592, p. 408, affirms the connection between *fatica* and exercise; Fonseca, *Del conservare la sanità*, 1603, p. 25, for the exercise of those in servile occupations. For Renaissance exercise, see Cavallo and Storey, *Healthy Living*, 2013, pp. 151–152, 165–166. For the conception of labour and medical professionals, see the contribution of Ariella Minden to this volume.
34 Mercurio, *De gli errori popolari*, 1603, pp. 10, 58, 171, 361.
35 For the benefits of *fatica* and exercise, see Mercurio, *De gli errori popolari*, 1603, p. 236; Petronio, *Del viver degli Romani*, 1592, p. 408.
36 Fonseca, *Del conservare della sanità*, 1603, p. 7.
37 Cavallo and Storey, *Healthy Living*, 2013, p. 9, pp. 157–158.
38 Baldinucci, *Vita di Gian Lorenzo Bernini*, 1948, p. 138.
39 Traffichetti, *L'arte di conservare la sanità*, 1565, p. 250r.
40 Traffichetti, *L'arte di conservare la sanità*, 1565, p. 248v.
41 Mancini, *CSP*, vol. 1, 1956, p. 252.
42 For his various scandals, Cavazzini, 'La vita e le opera di Agostino Tassi', 2008, pp. 30–33, and Black, *Early Modern Italy*, 2001, pp. 75–76.
43 Pontormo, *Diario*, 2014, pp. 10, 12 for his fasting. Bellori, *Le vite*, 2009, vol. 1, p. 201, noting Barocci's temperance with respect to his passions.
44 For Laureti, see Mancini, *CSP*, vol. 1, 1956, p. 233; for Annibale, Mancini, vol. 1, p. 219. On Annibale's *disordini*, see Summerscale, *Malvasia's Life of the Carracci*, 2000, p. 227. Feigenbaum, 'A Likeness in the Tomb', 2010, p. 21, speculates that Annibale suffered from syphilis. Traffichetti, *L'arte di conservare la sanità*, 1565, p. 250 for early modern *disordini* and *disordinata vita*.
45 Petronio, *Del viver degli Romani*, 1592, p. 280.
46 Baglione, *LV*, 1970, p. 322. For Leoni's portraits, see Robbins, 'Scipione Borghese's Acquisition of Paintings', 1996, pp. 453–458; Sani, *La fatica virtuosa di Ottavio Leoni*, 2005, pp. 161–162. On artists' self-portraits, see Woods-Marsden, *Renaissance Self-Portraiture*, 1998.
47 Baglione, *LV*, 1970, p. 173.
48 See especially Cavallo and Storey, *Healthy Living*, 2013, pp. 179–181.

49 Cavallo and Storey, *Healthy Living*, 2013, p. 180; Hultquist, 'The Passions', 2016, pp. 71–73; Gage, *Painting as Medicine*, 2016, pp. 51–53.
50 Traffichetti, *L'arte di conservare la sanità*, 1565, fol. 110v; see Gage, 'Exercise for Mind and Body', 2008, pp. 1183–1184.
51 Baglione, *LV*, 1970, p. 321.
52 Baglione, *LV*, 1970, p. 130. Baglione uses *disprezzare* to describe Fontana's attitude to intense labour. In English 'to scorn' or 'to despise' does not convey Baglione's sense that Fontana disregarded any amount of labour required.
53 Baglione, *LV*, 1970, p. 131.
54 Baldinucci, *Vita di Gian Lorenzo Bernini*, 1948, p. 139; Bernini, *Vita di Cavaliere Gio. Lorenzo Bernini*, 1713, p. 178.
55 Bernini, *Vita di Cavaliere Gio. Lorenzo Bernini*, 1713.
56 See below.
57 Unglaub, 'Poussin's Reflection', 2004, pp. 520–521, and p. 526n33 for the authorship, identity, and inscription.
58 Unglaub, 'Poussin's Reflection', 2004.
59 Mancini, *ACDH*, fol. 152r.
60 For Mancini's relationship with Sacchetti, see Gage, 'New Documents', 2014, p. 654.
61 Mancini, *CSP*, vol. 1, 1956, p. 262.
62 Mancini, *CSP*, vol. 1, 1956.
63 Mancini, *CSP*, vol. 1, 1956.
64 Huygens, 'Excerpts from *The Autobiography of Constantijn Huygens*', p. 3.
65 See Ramazzini's comments in Jana Graul's contribution in this volume.
66 Mancini, *CSP*, vol. 1, 1956, p. 3.
67 For the factive arts, see Quiviger, 'Varchi and the Visual Arts', 1987, pp. 222–223.
68 Mancini, *CSP*, vol. 1, 1956, p. 11.
69 As attested to in a letter from Cesare Perini of 13 December 1625 (Archivio della Società di Pie Disposizioni).
70 Mancini, *ACDH*, fols 81r–v.
71 Mancini, *ACDH*, fols 120v ff.
72 Wald and Stave, *Physical and Biological Hazards*, 1994, p. 9. For falls and injuries on early modern building sites, see Marconi, *Edificando Roma Barocca*, 2004, pp. 50–52.
73 Mancini, *ACDH*, fol. 121v.
74 Mancini, *CSP*, vol. 1, 1956, p. 230.
75 Mancini, *CSP*, vol. 1, 1956. Vasari articulated the great danger of working on scaffolding in his life of Taddeo Zuccari in the context of Taddeo and Federico painting grotesques in Palazzo Vaticano. Vasari, *LO*, vol. 7, p. 91.
76 Cropper, *The Domenichino Affair*, 2006, p. 8. Condivi tells of another risk in his life of Michelangelo, the angry Julius II threatening to have the artist thrown from the scaffolding because of his delays to completing the Sistine Ceiling. See Condivi, *Life of Michelangelo*, 1999, p. 58.
77 Mancini, *ACDH*, fol 121v.
78 Wald and Stave, *Physical and Biological Hazards*, 1994, p. 9.
79 Mancini, *ACDH*, fols 121v–122r.
80 Mancini, *ACDH*, fol. 120v. Significantly, the issue of spaces of confinement emerges in relation to current debates about labour practices as well as debates concerning vulnerable populations and unjust treatment of particular populations on the basis of race, sex, age.
81 Mancini, *CSP*, vol. 1, 1956, p. 102. For Pliny's anecdote, see Barrett, *Rome Is Burning*, 2022, p. 217.
82 For early modern prisons, see Black, *Early Modern Italy*, 2001, pp. 196–197.
83 For conceptions of early modern pollution, see Rinne, 'Urban Ablutions', 2012, pp. 182–201 and Gentilcore, 'Purging Filth', 2012, pp. 153–168.

84 Mancini, *ACDH*, fol. 96v.
85 Ostrow, 'Pietro Tacca', 2015, pp. 152–153.
86 For the artist and captivity in Michelangelo's art, poetry, and correspondence, see Parker, *Michelangelo*, 2010, esp. pp. 110–115. For slavery's definition, see Bales, *Disposable People*, 1999, pp. 279–280 n. 4.
87 Baglione, *LV*, 1970, p. 50. Baglione's description of Muziano as shaving his head only approximates European representations of early modern Turkish slaves who were typically presented with a topknot, as in Pietro Tacca's *Quattro Mori* (1621–1626) in Livorno, or Cornelis de Wael's series of harbour scenes, etched by Martin Schaep, see Martin and Weiss, *The Sun King at* Sea, 2022, pp. 11–12, 28–29.
88 For early modern love, see Kambaskovic, 'Love', 2016, pp. 53–55.
89 For the sixteenth-century debate concerning labour and the nobility of art, and ambivalence concerning physical labour, see especially Jonietz, 'Labor omnia vincit', 2011, pp. 584–592.
90 Mancini, *CSP*, vol. 1, 1956, p. 161. As Hale argues, image of wounded soldiers and *condottiere* scarcely appeared in Renaissance art and not at all in Italian art. See Hale, 'The Soldier in Germanic Graphic Art', 1986, pp. 95–96. This changed in northern Europe with the publication of Hans von Gersdorff, *Feldtbuch der Wundartzney, newlich getruckt und gebessert*, 1530, the frontispiece of which pictures a wounded soldier.
91 Significantly, Mancini's theory of the visual arts and their relative honour within the professions of Rome raised the issue of occupational health and medicine long before this field began to emerge at the end of the seventeenth century and before. For Rammazini, see Cosmacini, *Storia della medicina del lavoro*, 2022, pp. 9–31, as well as Jana Graul's contribution to this volume.

8

Giulio Mancini and Sebastiano Vannini: medicine and connoisseurship in early Baroque Rome

Fabrizio Federici

This chapter focuses on two physicians, Giulio Mancini and Sebastiano Vannini, active in Rome in the first half of the seventeenth century and linked by a deep relationship, with one being the pupil of the other. Their writings on art represent a significant part of the strong interaction between medical activity and artistic interests, which was common in the early modern period. However, while Giulio Mancini and his *Considerazioni* are very well-known among scholars, the pages written by his pupil Sebastiano Vannini are quite obscure. The aim of this contribution is to underline the interest of Vannini's text *Diporti curiosi*, with its fascinating mixture of analysis of visual and textual sources, medical knowledge and poetic fantasy.

It is not unusual to find, in early modern Italy, physicians who had a strong interest in art, architecture, antiquarianism, and showed that interest in their writings.[1] Sometimes they wrote about medicine with great attention to textual and visual sources of antiquity; other physicians published treatises about art, in which their approach to artists and images was greatly influenced by their medical education. For example, Girolamo Mercuriale's treatise on physical exercise *De Arte Gymnastica*, published in 1569, demonstrates a deep knowledge of ancient authors and visual sources, such as statues and reliefs, and the strong relationship of its author with artists and antiquarians, such as Pirro Ligorio.[2] Mercuriale's interest in images went beyond the appreciation and use of ancient visual sources; it also influenced the production of new images, reflecting a keen engagement with contemporary art. His commission from Ludovico Cardi, il Cigoli, for a painting depicting the *Feast in the House of Levi* as an ancient triclinium – where the tablemates are not sitting but reclining around the table – marks the beginning of a philological approach to the *Coenae Domini*. This representation gained some success in seventeenth- and eighteenth-century painting, especially in Italy and France (Figure 8.1).[3]

Another name worth mentioning is Francesco Scannelli, who, in his *Microcosmo della pittura* (published in 1657), makes numerous references to medical knowledge of his age and even compares the most important Renaissance painters to human organs. Raphael, renowned for his ability to study and transform classical art, is likened to the liver of painting; Titian, to the heart, for the power of his colour; and Correggio, to the brain, for uniting the styles of the other two masters.[4]

We can join to the names of these physicians those of Giulio Mancini and Sebastiano Vannini. The fame of Mancini among art historians greatly developed after 1956, when his treatise *Considerazioni sulla pittura*, written around 1615–1620, was published in an edition by Adriana Marucchi and Luigi Salerno.[5] The text is the expression of Mancini's great interest in contemporary art (it contains many notes and biographies of artists of his days, including one of the first biographies of Caravaggio), but is also an account of his knowledge of Renaissance and even medieval painting.[6] The *Considerazioni* includes instructions addressed to the '*virtuosi*', the art lovers, on issues such as buying paintings, displaying them in the different rooms of the house, the distinction between copies and originals. This led

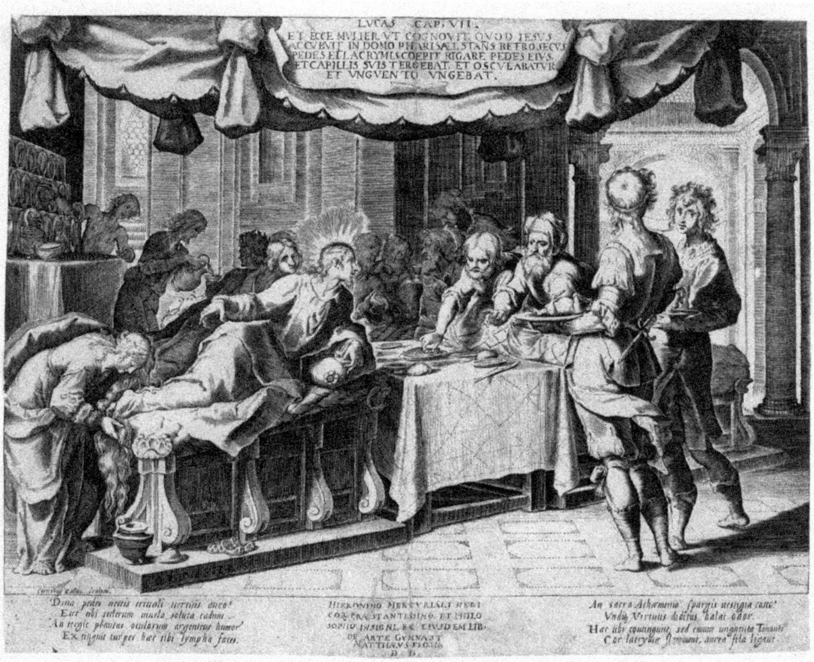

Figure 8.1 Cornelis Galle (after Ludovico Cardi, il Cigoli), *Feast in the House of Levi*, engraving, 1598–1599. Rome, Istituto Centrale per la Grafica, Gabinetto Disegni e Stampe, Fondo Corsini; vol. 35H23. Image credit: Istituto Centrale per la Grafica, by kind permission of the Ministry of Culture

some scholars, in particular Carlo Ginzburg, to see Mancini as the prototype of the connoisseur, the non-artist expert in analysis and attribution of artworks, whose figure would fully take shape only in the eighteenth century.

In a famous 1979 article, Ginzburg presents a compelling analogy between aspects of Mancini's writings and the painting attribution method developed later, at the end of the nineteenth century, by Giovanni Morelli (known as the Morellian method). Morelli, as is well known, identified the characteristic 'hands' of painters through the analysis of minor details such as ears, nails, hair curls, that revealed artists' scarcely conscious shorthand and conventions. In this way the connoisseur operates in the manner of a detective, each discovering from clues unnoticed by others, the author in one case of a crime, in the other of a painting.[7] The Italian historian finds the same attention for clues and minor details of paintings in Mancini, especially when he speaks about the distinction between copies and originals. Ginzburg refers in particular to this passage by Mancini:

> [One must ask if] there is to be seen that frankness of the master, and in particular in those parts that are necessarily made with resolution, nor that can be conducted well through imitation, as, in particular, are the hair, beard and eyes. So that when the ringlets of hair have to be imitated they are made with painful toil, which then appears in the copy, and if the copyist does not want to imitate them, then they do not have the perfection of the master.[8]

Why, then, Ginzburg wonders, are there such similarities between Mancini and Morelli? He suggests that the answer lies in the fact that Mancini was a physician and Morelli – in his youth – had studied medicine. Their method, Ginzburg argues, likely derives from the approach of a doctor who diagnoses by gathering and analysing clues – minor details unnoticed by others – that reveal the nature of a patient's illness. The eye of the physician and the eye of the connoisseur, then, are not so different.

This view of Mancini as the first connoisseur has been questioned in a contribution published in 2008 by Donatella Sparti, who in particular has underlined that painters and not art lovers were seen as the only authorities in the judgment of paintings in the seventeenth century.[9] Mancini, furthermore, talks about the distinction between copies and originals and not about attributions, which are the core of connoisseurship (or, better, we could say, of modern connoisseurship). More recently, scholars such as Frances Gage and Stefano Pierguidi have reaffirmed the interpretation of Mancini's writings as a fundamental step towards the birth of connoisseurship. It is necessary to consider in the right perspective what meaning should be assigned to this word for the seventeenth century:

> Far from being a science of the eye alone, early connoisseurship, as Mancini outlined it, entailed a lengthy process of gathering, sorting and cross-checking both visual and textual information in order to establish and refine the history

> of art. This lengthy process involved an initial examination of the paintings in Roman monuments and churches, the tracking of relevant documentation concerning the monuments, patrons and periods in which objects were produced, and an analysis of stylistic characteristics, gathered and analysed over time against related objects and styles, in order to establish a correspondence between historical documentation and visual evidence.[10]

The relationship between Mancini's activity as physician and that of the connoisseur, however, is not limited to the link between his approaches to human bodies and to paintings but has a broader dimension. Mancini thinks that, as a whole, painting is a form of medicine, as Frances Gage has underlined.[11] In general terms, looking at paintings constitutes an activity that gives benefits both to body and soul: Mancini follows the long-standing medical commonplace that artworks, like music and fables, promote health by affording distraction and delight. Landscape painting, for example, comforts the eye with greenish hues and gentle incitement to ocular movement.[12] More specifically, images are provided with a great power that can affect certain moments and aspects of human life, such as that of conception, operating on the onlooker's imagination.[13]

Pierguidi has underlined that Mancini acts like a connoisseur in his trips around Rome, reconstructing the *corpora* of fifteenth- and sixteenth-century painters not even mentioned by Vasari, such as Jacopo Ripanda or Antonio del Massaro, il Pastura, through the direct observation, analysis, and comparison of paintings.[14]

While Mancini has garnered significant scholarly attention, Sebastiano Vannini has attracted far less interest. Both born in Siena, the young Vannini moved to Rome in 1618, where he became Mancini's pupil in both medicine and art appreciation. At Mancini's death in 1630 he succeeded his master in the illustrious charge of '*archiatra pontificio*', that is, the physician of Pope Urban VIII Barberini. Vannini underlines his status as the 'only pupil' (*solus alumnus*) of Mancini in some Latin verses that he dedicated to him.[15] Vannini praises the ability of Mancini the physician, who healed the future Urban VIII during the conclave of 1623 and then cared for his health for the following seven years. In other verses, Vannini extols his master, saying that Nature provided him with the best qualities of body and soul: saving countless people from death through both his writings and spoken words, and being honest, constant, and sincere, even in the court. The religiosity of Mancini, Vannini affirms, was authentic, not false:[16] these words seem to be a defence against accusations of atheism addressed to Mancini. Mancini was unlikely an atheist; as Sparti notes, he was more likely deeply influenced by the 'Paduan Aristotelism' he encountered as a young medical student in Padua.[17] This philosophical movement usually gave natural explanations of phenomena thought to be supernatural, linked for example to miracles or witchcraft. Mancini more than once showed this same approach both in his medical activity and his art history writings: for example, in his reconstruction of the development of medieval painting in Rome, he takes into account and tries to date also those images and icons that were generally considered *acheiropoieta*, of divine origin, or painted by Saint Luke. It is possible that the naturalistic approach of Paduan Aristotelianism had an influence, through Mancini, also on Vannini, as will be seen later.

Vannini knew very well Mancini's *Considerazioni sulla pittura*: as research by Michele Maccherini has revealed, the young Sebastiano was employed by Mancini as a copyist of the treatise in 1619–1620.[18] Vannini inherited from Mancini an interest in medieval art, which is witnessed by his main text, *Diporti curiosi circa sagre antiche pitture*, written in 1641–1642 in order to answer some questions and doubts about artworks, artists and patrons, that Cardinal Francesco Barberini had expressed to him. Due to the variety of the questions and to Vannini's taste for digressions, the discourse has a very non-linear structure. Many sites, monuments and churches of Rome are discussed or only briefly mentioned, but focus is on four main complexes: Saint Peter's, Saint Paul outside the Walls, Saint John Lateran and Santa Maria in Trastevere. Among many artworks of the Due and Trecento which are carefully analysed, there are great masterpieces such as Giotto's Navicella or the mosaics by Pietro Cavallini in Santa Maria in Trastevere (Figure 8.2).[19]

Mancini's *Considerazioni* plays an important role for Vannini's *Diporti curiosi*. In some passages Vannini echoes his master, thus replicating some of Mancini's errors.[20] However, in the case of Pietro Cavallini, Vannini avoids Mancini's mistake and correctly dates the activity of the Roman painter, following the guidance that Vasari had already pointed out.[21] Under the central scene of the mosaics in Santa Maria in Trastevere there was still visible in the seventeenth century the fragment of an inscription with the name *PETRVS* (Figure 8.3). Both Mancini and Vannini interpret it not as a reference to the name of the artist, as is done today, but to that of the patron, perhaps under the influence of contemporary usage. Mancini thought that the patron Petrus was Cardinal Pietro Stefaneschi, who died in 1417 and was buried in the church; therefore, he wrote that Vasari was wrong and that Cavallini lived in the fifteenth century.[22] For Vannini, Petrus stands for the senator Pietro Stefaneschi, who lived between the thirteenth and fourteenth centuries; so his dating of the mosaics and of the activity of Cavallini is quite correct. In fact, he does not think that Cavallini is the real author of the mosaics: he compares this work with the lost frescoes by Cavallini in Santa Cecilia in Trastevere and in San Francesco a Ripa, and concludes that the mosaics must have been conceived by a much better artist. Hereby one can see in action, not only the erudite that reads and interprets the inscriptions, but also the connoisseur that compares the images, judges them and tries to make attributions. Vannini's concludes '*per salvare il Vasari*', that is, in order to save at least part of what Vasari had written, he accepts part of what Vasari wrote, particularly his attribution of the mosaics to Cavallini. According to Vasari, a great artist active in Rome at the time, such as Giotto

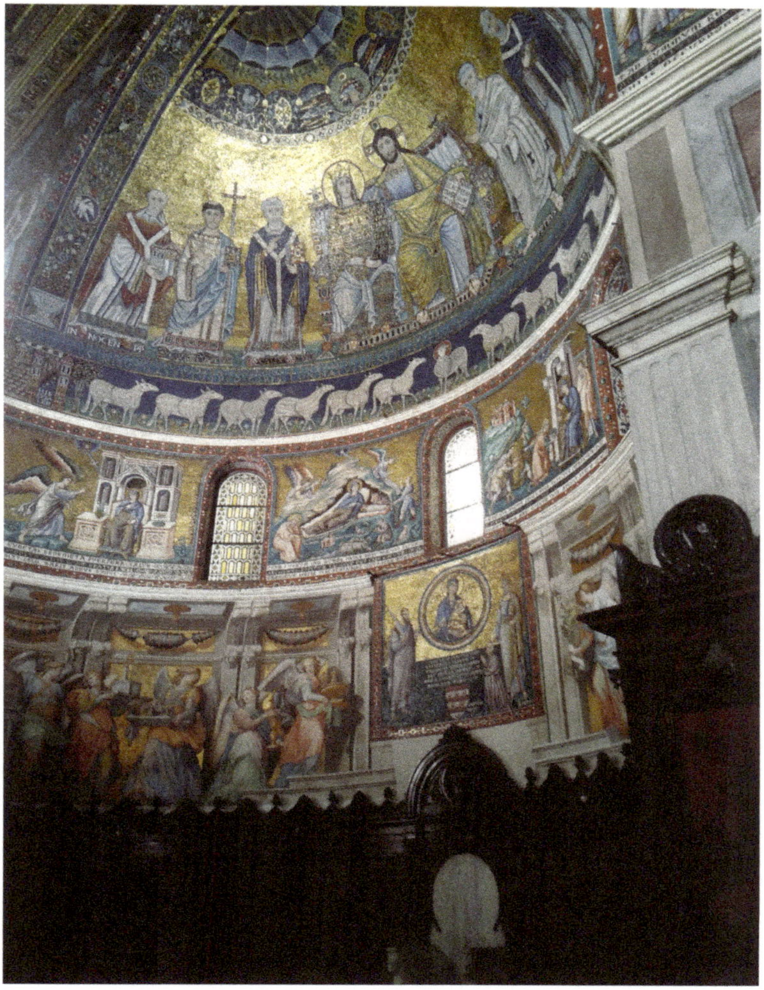

Figure 8.2 Rome, Santa Maria in Trastevere, view of the apse, with some of the mosaic scenes by Pietro Cavallini. Image credit: Wikipedia Commons

or Simone Martini, had designed the sacred scenes, while Cavallini was merely the material executor of the mosaics.[23]

Two moments of Vannini's vast discourse in particular show a connection between his interest in art and his medical profession.[24] Addressing Giotto's *Navicella*, Vannini writes regarding the original position of the mosaic (which stood on the wall of the quadriportico in front of the basilica, east of the church and facing west) (Figure 8.4). Some authors had written that the *Navicella*, and especially other sacred images in previous times, had been placed there because people entering the basilica would turn towards east and quickly pray in that direction as a remnant of paganism and of the

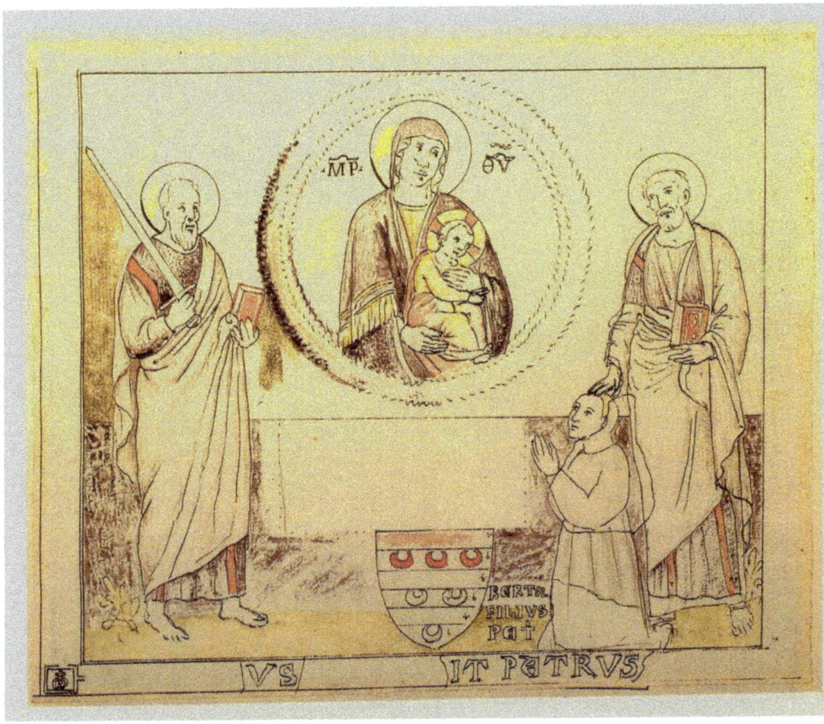

Figure 8.3 Antonio Eclissi, drawing for Cassiano dal Pozzo's *Museo Cartaceo* reproducing the central scene of the mosaics by Pietro Cavallini in Santa Maria in Trastevere, around 1630–1640. Windsor, Royal Library, RL 9041. Image credit: Royal Collection Enterprises Limited 2024 | Royal Collection Trust

veneration of the Sun. Thus, putting sacred images there was thought to represent the Christianisation of a very old and pagan habit. Vannini rejects this hypothesis with various arguments, but particularly interesting is the fact that he decides to make a sort of little experiment, studying the reactions of modern visitors to the church. Turning back before entering the basilica, Vannini says, is a natural behaviour, a pause and a contemplative moment before the entrance into such an important place.[25] This empirical approach testifies to Vannini's professional activity as a physician and the naturalistic explanation of this phenomenon is perhaps a sign of the influence on him of the 'Paduan Aristotelism' that influenced his master Giulio Mancini. It is interesting also what Vannini states immediately after, on the obelisks re-erected by Pope Sixtus V in front of Saint Peter's and in other squares of Rome. Here too, the explanation of the physician-observer avoids any connection between Christianity and Paganism: the obelisks were put there '*per mero, e solo ornamento*', in order to embellish the squares.[26] This point of view is quite striking, if one considers how important it is in Sistine propaganda, on the one hand, and in modern literature, on the other, that

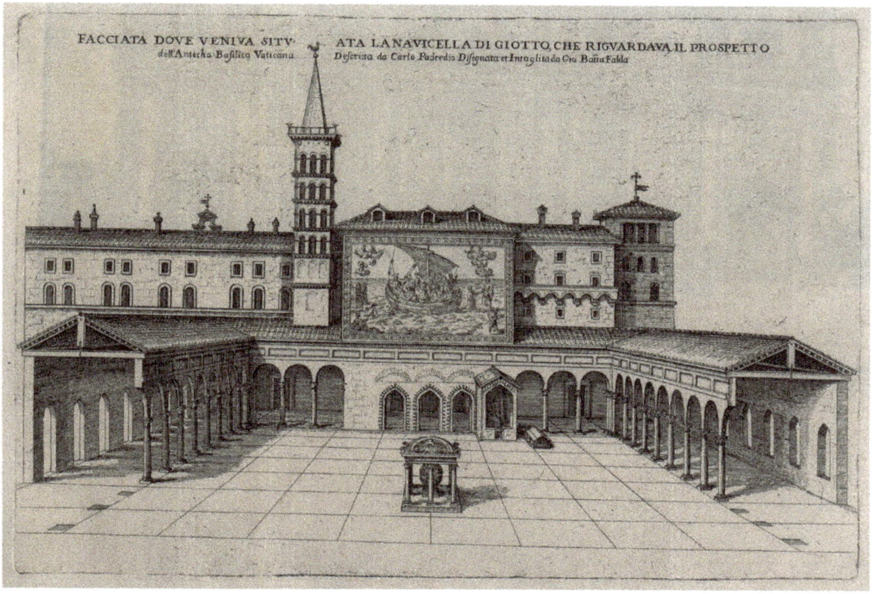
FACCIATA DOVE VENIVA SITV ATA LANAVICELLA DI GIOTTO, CHE RIGVARDAVA IL PROSPETTO
dell'Anticha Basilica Vaticana
Descritta da Carlo Padredio Dissignata et Intaglita da Gio Batta Falda

Figure 8.4 Giovanni Battista Falda, Engraving showing the original position of Giotto's *Navicella* in St Peter's quadriportico, from Giovanni Giacomo de' Rossi, *Insignium Romae templorum prospectus exteriores interioresque* [...], Rome 1683. Image credit: Fabrizio Federici

the re-erection of the obelisks surmounted by crosses is interpreted as a symbol of Christ's victory over Paganism.

At the very end of the *Discorsi curiosi*, one finds another passage that clearly demonstrates the medical activity of the author. Vannini focuses his attention on the gesture of the Pantocrator as represented in two medieval mosaics: one in the apse of Saint Paul outside the Walls and the other in the Grotte Vaticane (Figure 8.5). The way the thumb and ring finger join together in the right hand of Christ was old and strange already for the seventeenth-century observer, used to a much simpler gesture of blessing. Vannini's explanation is quite imaginary, and he admits it: the four Latin verses that he composes about this topic '*se non esplicano a pieno il misterio, mostrano almeno la mia voglia di intenderlo da altri*' (if they do not clearly explain this mystery at least show my desire of knowing the reason from other people). Vannini states that the folded thumb was used already in antiquity to stop fights, and so it represents peace, while the ring finger is directly linked to the heart by arteries.[27] Therefore, Christ's gesture symbolises his mission on earth to bring peace to all people, reflecting God's goodwill and offering peace to all who receive it with an open heart.[28]

Through this final example one can observe how far the explanations and thoughts of Vannini can be from truth, or at least from a plausible

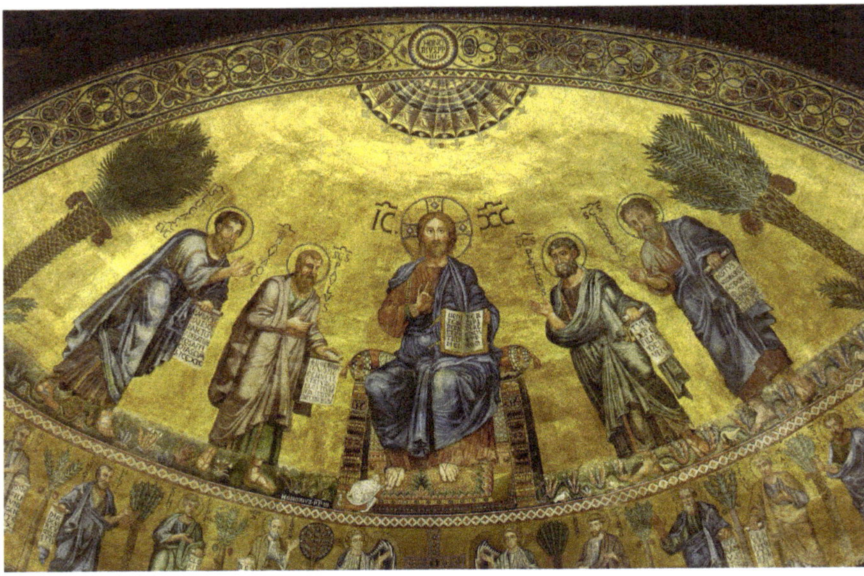

Figure 8.5 Rome, San Paolo fuori le Mura, detail of the mosaics of the apse with Christ Pantocrator, 1220–1227, with later restorations. Image credit: Fabrizio Federici

hypothesis. His text, however, must be esteemed as it testifies to the desire to know more about long-forgotten images, and for the way in which analysis of visual and textual sources, medical knowledge and poetic fantasy contribute to his answers. Even though Vannini's knowledge of medieval art and connoisseurship skills are certainly more limited than those of Mancini, he and his writings deserve greater attention and further research, in order to clarify his place in the relationship between interest in art and medical practice in the seventeenth century. A crucial step in evaluating Vannini's role is a new critical edition of his main text on art, the *Diporti curiosi*. Such an edition would provide scholars with an accurate version of the text and generate interest in its author, much like the 1956 publication of Mancini's *Considerazioni*.

Notes

1 See on this topic, together with the contributions mentioned in the following footnotes, Frigo, 'Can One Speak', 2012.
2 Siraisi, 'History', 2003; Vagenheim, 'Una collaborazione', 2008.
3 Federici, 'Girolamo Mercuriale', 2007. The painting by Cigoli, executed in 1596, is now preserved in the Galleria Doria Pamphilj in Rome.
4 Pericolo, 'The Liver', 2019. Two other seventeenth-century physicians, active in Rome, who greatly appreciated art were Giovan Giacomo Baldini (see Serafinelli, 'Patronage', 2022, pp. 38–50) and James Alban Gibbes, who was also a celebrated poet (Bertolotti, *Un professore*, 1886; Langdon, 'Two Book', 1976).

5 Mancini, *Considerazioni*, 1956–1957.
6 Cateni, *Giulio Mancini*, 2021.
7 Ginzburg, 'Spie', 1979.
8 I quote this passage in the translation by Frances Gage, in Gage, 'It Is not so Easy', 2020, p. 65.
9 Sparti, 'Novità su Giulio Mancini', 2008.
10 Gage, 'It Is not so Easy', 2020, p. 80.
11 Gage, *Painting as Medicine*, 2016.
12 On the effects of the green colour on the beholder, see the contribution by Katharine Stahlbuhk in this volume.
13 Mancini, *Considerazioni*, vol. 1, 1956, p. 143.
14 Pierguidi, 'Giulio Mancini', 2016.
15 Vannini is the author of a *corpus* of poems in Latin which have a certain importance from an art historical point of view, because in some of them he celebrates famous works that Bernini made for Urban VIII, such as the Baldacchino, the tombs of the Barberini pope himself and of Countess Matilda, the now lost bust of Charles I of England. See Federici, 'Bernini artificis', 2017.
16 Federici, 'Bernini artificis', 2017, p. 64: 'Integer et frugi, constans, sincerus in aula / et non fucata relligione fruens'.
17 Sparti, 'Novità su Giulio Mancini', 2008, pp. 54–57. In Padua he was in contact with the abovementioned physician and antiquarian Girolamo Mercuriale, see Sparti, 'Novità su Giulio Mancini', 2008, p. 53.
18 Maccherini, *Caravaggio*, 1993–1994, pp. 335–342.
19 The manuscripts that contain Vannini's *Diporti curiosi* are preserved at the Vatican Library (Federici, 'Bernini artificis', 2017, pp. 63, 78). In the 1970s the text had been published in a very disappointing edition (De Benedictis, 'La vita', 1976), therefore, a new and more correct edition is necessary to make the discourse available to all those interested in the baroque reception of medieval art and in artistic production in Rome in late Middle Ages and Renaissance.
20 For example, Vannini dates at the time of Pope Innocent III, at the beginning of the thirteenth century, just as Mancini had done before him, the beautiful illuminated manuscript with the rule of the hospital of Santo Spirito in Sassia, which is actually of the mid-fourteenth century, just because this pope gave the rule to the hospital and his name is written at the beginning of the text (see Vatican Apostolic Library, Cod. Barb. Lat. 4875, f. 25v).
21 See Federici, 'La riscoperta', 2019, pp. 31–32.
22 Mancini, *Considerazioni*, 1956–1957, I, pp. 179–180. This idea had some success in the Barberini circle, as it is witnessed by a copy of a lost fresco of 1452 in Santa Maria in Trastevere, made for Cardinal Barberini, accompanied by an attribution to Cavallini (see Waetzoldt, *Kopien*, 1964, cat. 523, pp. 52–53).
23 'E per tal rispetto non sarebbe forsi alieno dal vero, tener questo musaico per fattura, se non di Giotto (il che tace il Vasari), di Simone Memmi prima d'andare in Avignone [...] Per salvare il Vasari, che del Cavallini siano i musaici di Santa Maria, et altri, che gl'ascrive, si potrebbe dire, haverli lui lavorati con disegni di Giotto, o del Memmi, e così verificarsi esser riuscito perfettissimo maestro di musaici, et illustratore di quest'arte, cioè in mettere insieme, e lavorare in tal modo l'opere, dategli, già disegnate da altri, havendosi esempij a' dì nostri, di chi esquisitamente lavora musaici, ma non inventa, o dissegna pensieri, da sé inventati'; see Federici, 'La riscoperta', 2019, p. 32.
24 The two passages discussed here are the only two in Vannini's *Diporti* that clearly show a strong connection with the author's medical activity. Further research on Vannini (whose life and work still remain obscure in many respects: for example, none of his letters are known) may lead to the identification of other moments in which he makes artistic interests interact with medical knowledge of his time.

25 Vatican Apostolic Library, Cod. Barb. Lat. 4875, ff. 19r–v: 'Confesso ingenuamente, che fatta reflessione all'antidetto costume, e natami curiosità d'osservare quello, che a' dì nostri, per gratia divina, liberi da simili superstitioni, naturalmente nei forastieri avvenga, ho moltissime volte con mio gran piacere notato, che molti, salite le scale, subito si voltano alla piazza, et ammirata la veduta, e vastità sua, s'inviano al portico, dicendo: 'Veramente è una bella piazza, et questa facciata è una gran machina'; et, contemplatala un poco, soggiungono ai compagni, chi verso la piazza, chi altrove, rivolti: 'Andiamo in chiesa'. Hor non sarebbe un bell'humore colui, che, non considerando ciò essere naturalezza, et curioso diletto degl'huomini, havesse questi d'hoggidì per superstitiosi, e gentili, per voltarsi, salite le scale, a levante?'

26 Vatican Apostolic Library, Cod. Barb. Lat. 4875, f. 19v: 'E molto più, se pensasse, o dicesse, haver Sisto V sopra la guglia posta la croce di metallo indorato, con del Sacratissimo legno del patibulo del Redentore, per abolire questo costume, et fare, che i forastieri, rivolti in tal modo, venerassero la croce? Alla quale ho veduti moltissimi inginocchiarsi, e sopra le scale medeme, et in ogni luogo della piazza indifferentemente, per l'indulgenza, concessavi da quel Pontefice, che non pensò mai a cotesta superstitiosa rivolta, in questa, et altre piazze di chiese di Roma per mero, e solo ornamento d'esse, alzando le guglie'. On the obelisks re-erected by Sixtus V see now Teja and Vespignani, 'Gli obelischi', 2019.

27 Vatican Apostolic Library, Cod. Barb. Lat. 4875, ff. 39r–v: 'Finisco la diceria con adempire la promessa circa al modo di benedire del Salvatore in questo musaico, et in quell'altro, più antico, dal Baronio e da me in proposito della Navicella mentovato, li quali in questo atto tengono il dito pollice, o grosso della mano destra, accostato al quarto, detto anulare della medesima. Che, osservato in infinite simili antiche imagini in pittura, e musaico, ho sempre creduto significhi qualche misterio. [...] Et finalmente il quarto dito, simbolo anco del cuore, esser destinato all'anello, non per vena, o nervo particolare, che ad esso dal cuore, più nella sinistra, che nella destra arrivi; poiché in ambidue le mani, anzi in tutto il corpo le vene hanno origine dal fegato, et i nervi dal cervello. Ma perché, così nel sinistro, come nel destro, quarto dito della mano si ritrovino arterie, in buona anatomia, veramente dal cuore al detto quarto dito, et nell'ambito di tutto il corpo, derivate. Et però credendo potersi dire, il Salvatore con tal gesto di benedittione annunciare la pace, da lui portata in terra (chiamandosi anco 'Angelus pacis') agl'huomini di buona volontà, sincera conscientia, anima, e cuor mondo, mi vennero fatti li seguenti versi, li quali, se non esplicano a pieno il misterio, mostrano almeno la mia voglia d'intenderlo da altri, non havendo finhora veduto in veruno, che m'appaghi a mio modo [...]. Premesse dunque queste parole per espressione, e difesa del pensiero, sottoscrivo li versi: Salvator Digitum Iungens Cum pollice Quartum / Ad bona se pacem Corda Tulisse Docet / Pacis enim signum Pollex Venamque Micantem / Cor quarto digito Mittere Vulgus ait'.

28 Already in Vannini's days other explanations of the gesture were given: thumb and ring finger joined together represented the union of Christ's mercy and justice (see Torrigio, *Le Sacre Grotte*, 1639, p. 75, an interpretation mentioned and criticised by Vannini); or the three folded fingers the Holy Trinity and the two extended ones the double nature, divine and human, of Jesus. Additionally, the gesture derived from that of Greek and Roman orators asking for silence and attention, linking it to the early Christian iconography of Christ as a philosopher. This ancient gesture of people speaking in public was noticed already in seventeenth-century literature, as read in Giovanni Bonifacio's *L'arte de' cenni*, published in 1616, p. 336: 'Spiegar l'indice, et il medio, e restringer l'altre dita. Gli antichi quando volevano parlare al popolo, per chieder silentio, col dito pollice opprimevano l'anullare, e l'auriculare, e spiegavano l'indice, et il medio distendendo il braccio [...] Questo adunque sarà gesto di ricercar silentio per ragionare [...]'.

Source 5

The drawings of Georgius Josephus Camel and their role for the chemical and medical arts between Central Europe and South Asia, c. 1685–1706

Paolo Sanvito

Jesuit medicine, mathematics, and chemistry contributed to the scientific research of many learned and academic institutions in Italy and in the Austrian Empire during the seventeenth century.[1] Even the scientific medical progress in the following centuries, especially in the eighteenth, depended on a number of important discoveries in the natural sciences which members of the Society of Jesus had earlier made in Europe as well as in other continents where Jesuit schools and educational institutions had been founded. The Alpine region had in particular already sent Sigismund Aperger or Apperger SJ from Innsbruck to Paraguay,[2] and around five fathers hailed from Bohemia, as the historian Joseph Gicklhorn observes.[3] This chapter presents the work of Jesuit priest and physician Georgius Josephus Camel or Kamel (Brno/Brünn 1661–Manila, Philippines 1706) who set up a marvellous pharmacy in Böhmisch Krumau/Český Krumlov.[4] Before departing for the missions in 1685, he likely pursued pharmaceutical studies in the college in Neuhaus, Jindřichův Hradec (Bohemia), although no known archival document confirms this. He started his long travel to Manila in 1688 but took the last vows of the order there only on 15 August 1696, long after his arrival.

During his life Camel not only contributed to several medical discoveries, but also bequeathed to both his communities (in Europe and Asia) incredibly rich and detailed descriptions and drawings of plants and biological objects which await new consideration from a graphic and aesthetic point of view. Eventually Camel's discoveries were received by the scholarly communities of Rome and Messina, where earlier researchers had used drawings to document the flora and fauna of the Mediterranean.[5] Camel was the first to describe the *Liana Strychnos Ignatii* or Ignatius bean, which contains the alkaloids brucine and strychnine, isolated by the French chemists Pierre Joseph Pelletier (1788–1842) and Jean Bienaimé Caventou (1795–1877) in 1818. Most of the alkaloids are contained in its seeds, called *Fabae Sancti Ignatii*. When consumed in high concentration, they can cause convulsions, but they can also heal if taken in lower quantity and in combination with other agents.

Camel accurately drew all the plants he knew and produced extensive *herbaria* with a skill which can only be explained by a very sound training as a draftsman, perhaps through his education in the two aforementioned Jesuit schools at Brno and Jindřichův. Baroque painters' skills in the representation of natural objects can and should be seen as related to sophisticated scientific handbooks. Paula Findlen demonstrates this with regard to such handbooks produced in the college of Messina, which hired the Dutch painter and botanist Pietro Castelli for the documentation of the plants in the important botanical garden as early as 1638. Camel had surely been similarly trained in some of the arts of drawing, which were an important part of the Jesuit courses, recognising, in Ofer Gal's words, 'that all empirical knowledge is fundamentally mediated; that nature can only be approached by art'.[6]

Camel, at the same time while investigating plants and pharmacology in Manila, was in close correspondence with the most distinguished scholars of his period, such as the English pharmacologists and botanists John Ray Black (Notley, 1627–1705) and James Petiver (Rugby, 1663–1718), thanks to whom he was able to acquire several of his works published in the *Philosophical Transactions* of London. Two of these works, somewhat more extensive, appeared in 1703 in an appendix to volume III of the *Historia plantarum* by John Ray (1627–1705). Ray and Petiver were members of the distinguished Royal Society of London.

Simultaneously, Samuel Browne, a physician working for the Eastern Indian Company in Madras, India, first collected information about Camel's work on Luzon and subsequently engaged in an intense exchange of materials from and about this island with Camel, including *herbaria* and natural samples. After Brown died around 1699, his successor Edward Bulkley suggested that Camel's drawing collections should be sent to his famous compatriot, the physician and botanist John Ray (1627–1705) for scientific purposes (Figure S5.1 *Citrullus colocynthis* '*Colocynthis pomi rosei, Indis Tabaiyag*', 'called by the Indians *Tabaiyag*').

Another physician and botanist who frequently corresponded with Camel was Willem ter Rhyne (birth and death dates unknown) from Batavia city, the Dutch colonial capital corresponding to present-day Jakarta. Camel's professional affinity with Ray in fact dated back at least to the 1690s. An edition of Ray's *Historia plantarum* was available in the St Ignatius College in Manila and Camel decided to acquire these two volumes privately for himself. On 3 January 1699, he mentions in a letter to Ray that already in 1696 he had sent him some of his plates (some might have been duplicates of the originals, because the ships transporting mail were often attacked by pirates and thus susceptible to loss). In this same letter he included 170 similar drawings prepared for Samuel Browne.

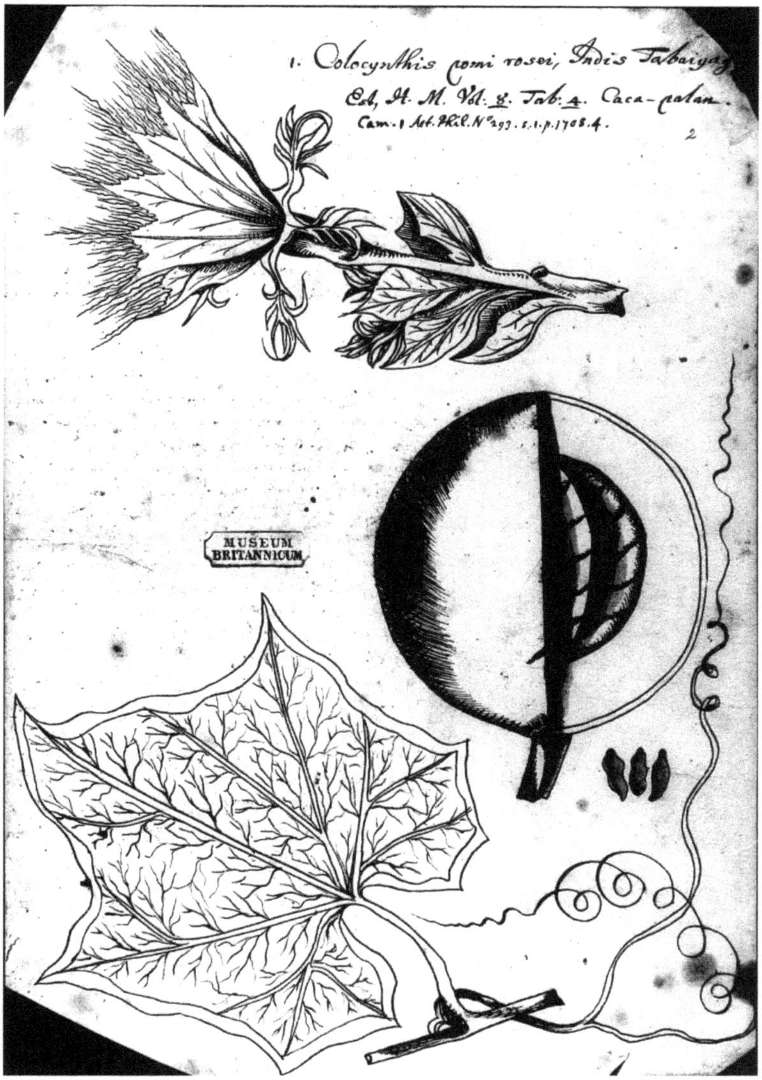

Figure S5.1 'Colocynthis pomi rosei, Indis Tabaiyag' (coloquinte), in: *Gazophylacium naturae et artis*, London medical. The British Library, Sloane MS 4081, fol. 2; 4083B, fol. 20. Image credit: The British Library

In return, on 7 October 1699, Camel in his turn received from Petiver two hundred (*zwei Centurien*) herbarium sheets from the *Museum petiverianum*.[7] From this moment on Camel dedicated himself to studying animals and animal drugs ('Drogen'; cf. Figure S5.2, *Cercopithecus Luzonis minimus*, in profile and with frontal view of the head).

In his *Gazophylacium* of 1704, Petiver reports that Camel offered a high number of integrations to Ray's *Historia plantarum*, which despite

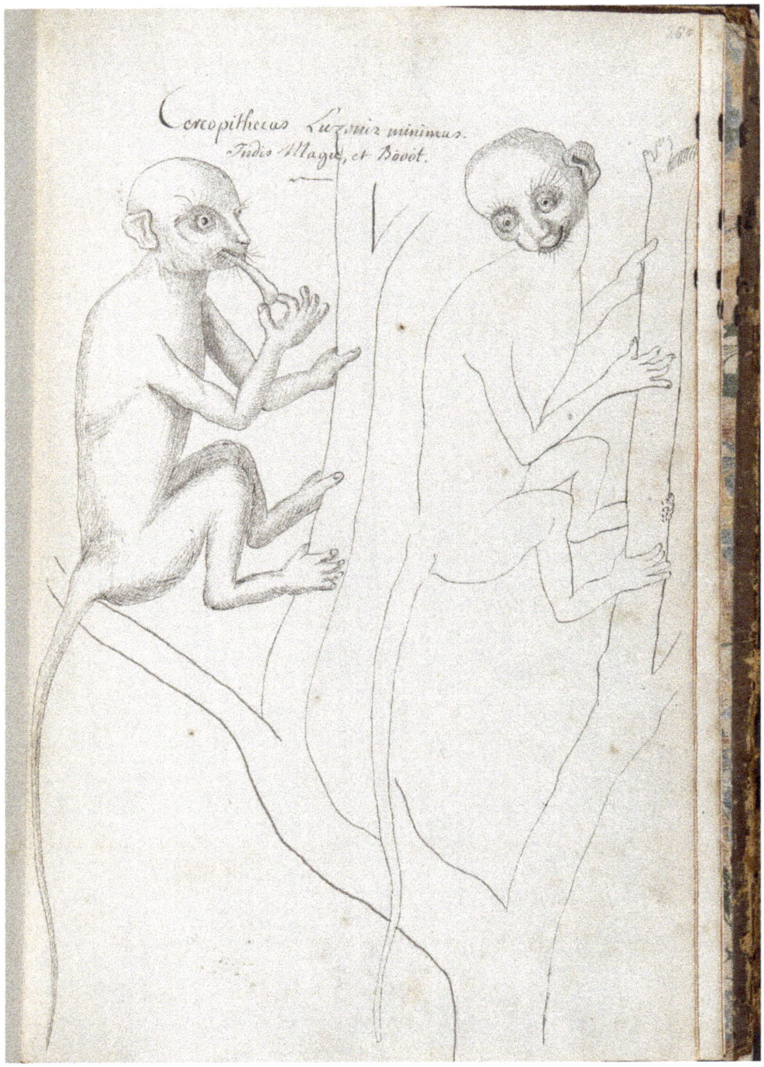

Figure S5.2 Georg Joseph Kamel, *Herbarum aliarumque stirpium*, original autograph manuscript. Leuven, Leuven Libraries, Maurits Sabbe Bibliotheek, shelf mark PM0038/V, fol. 260r. Image credit: KU Leuven Libraries

its enormous extent was still incomplete.[8] Furthermore, in London, the *Herbarium Sloane*, vols 153, 163, 165, 231, 233, and 240, similarly came to be mixed in into other *herbaria*: both with other collections and with his entire volume of *Descriptiones Fruticum et Arborum Luzonis*, now at the Natural History Museum (Bauer Unit, Shelf H7). Both works contain enormous amounts of drawings by Camel, and both were fundamental for botany in Britain. The work was transferred to the Department of Botany of the British Museum in 1884 and became a fundamental reference within the collection.[9]

Camel figured into subsequent histories of science primarily as the inventor or developer of the properties of the *Strychnos Ignatii Berg*, from which Pelletier and Caventou would later extract strychnine. But, in fact,

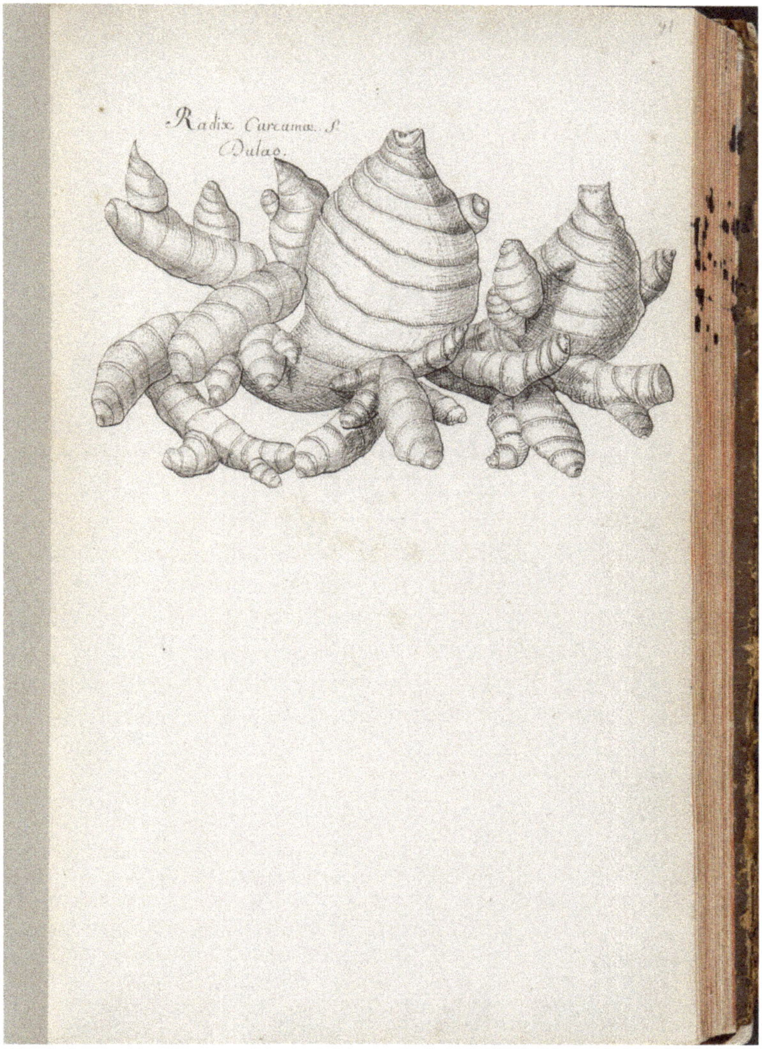

Figure S5.3 Curcuma Root (*Radix curcumae s. Dulao*), from: Georg Joseph Kamel, *Herbarum aliarumque stirpium*, original autograph manuscript. Leuven, Maurits Sabbe Bibliotheek, shelf mark PM0038/V, fol. 91r. Image credit: KU Leuven Libraries

he was engaged in many major activities, working as a practising physician (*pro bono*), and alongside the discovery of specific medical drugs, he also left his lavish drawings and refurbished a pharmacy in Český Krumlov. What is perhaps his most luxurious collection of manuscript drawings is held in the *Herbarium* in Leuven at the Katholieke Universiteit Libraries, Maurits Sabbe Library (Figure S5.3).[10]

One of Camel's major contributions to the history of pharmacy was the refurbishment of the exemplary pharmaceutical workshop in the Český Krumlov *Collegium*; here he began with the first production of drugs, whereas there is, unfortunately, no longer any trace of the pharmacy in Manila.[11] Indeed, the former is mentioned in the *Litterae annuae* for Austria for the period 1600–1617, that is, the reports sent from the *Collegium Crumloviense* to the *Provincialis* in Vienna (at this moment, the Bohemian province did not exist yet and was administered from Vienna).[12]

The basic equipment of the pharmacy exists today in an approximate, posthumous reconstruction at the Regionalni Muzeum. It consists of no less than approximately 200 smaller items – mortars, kettles, ladles, wooden boxes, and glass, wooden, stoneware, and porcelain jars, bottles, and stands, which date from the seventeenth through the nineteenth centuries.

Camel's contribution to public health was indisputable in his time, though he largely fell into oblivion for the history of science. This was certainly his most important achievement, grounding his reputation in the Philippines no less than in Europe, such that his death was not only mourned by the Society, but also regarded in Manila as a serious setback to the state of public health among all Filipinos as well as colonisers. The two large and influential pharmacies that he created represent much more than a routine feature of university infrastructure in this period, whether in Europe or overseas, just as the enormous diffusion of his scientific treatises stand as evidence of his pivotal importance in the global history of science.

Notes

1 The present text is part of a larger project in the context of my investigations of the relevance of Jesuit handbooks and treatises in recent years, which were used in the local Collegia as well as in non-Jesuit universities and came to be exported north and south of the Alps, stimulating scholarly studies all over Europe.

2 For Asperger, see Fechner, *Sigismund Aperger*, 2008, and Anagnostou, 'Missionsmedizin und Missionspharmazie im kolonialen Amerika', 2005, pp. 261–291, here p. 279.

3 Gicklhorn and Gicklhorn, *Georg Joseph Kamel S.J.*, 1954, pp. 13 and 24: their surnames are Haller, Klein, Maisler/Maysler, Riedl, Schenk. And I add Johannes Steinhöffer; and Josef Zeittler (Paraguay).

4 Cesky Krumlov was also the Jesuit College where he last studied, whereas his early time as *novitius* had been in Brünn, Brno.

5 Findlen and Scilla, 'A Baroque Painter in Pursuit of Science', 2013, p. 119.

6 Gal, 'Introduction', 2013, p. 7.

7 Gicklhorn and Gicklhorn, *Georg Joseph Kamel S.J.*, 1954, p. 42.

8 Petiver, *Gazophylacii naturae & artis decades*, 1702–1706 (1704), p. 63.

9 Other descriptions and illustrations by Camel from the Sloane collection are the MSs. 4,078 and 4,081.

10 Dulao is a district from the city of Bago, Negros Province. A possible medical use of the parts of the curcuma tree might be reported in a local tale. In Dulao the local district website – Barangay Dulao – Bago City http://bagocity.gov.ph – reads that 'During the Spanish colonization, the soldiers of Capitan Nicanor Villarosa began to suffer from a disease called "bulao", which symptoms include the yellowish colouration of the skin. The captain summoned a well-known "babaylan" [Filipino shaman] from Panay to heal his men. As it was already dark, the healer noticed a tree covered with fireflies. He stripped a bark of the tree and from it concocted drinking water for the sick people. After several days, the sick began to heal and became stronger. Much later, Capitan Nicanor Villarosa named the place Dulao, after the healing tree, Mandulao'.

11 The Collegium had already settled between the years 1584–1590, which is a quite early date for the Bohemian province. The pharmacy which he curated in Krumlov however might have been existing (contrary to what is sometimes thought), in more primitive shape and with different furnishing and decoration *long before* Camel himself, as pharmacies were usually present in each *collegium*.

The chronicler Václav Brezan describes Alexander Voigt as the earliest contractor and planner for this site, who in his function as Rector of the Prager Collegium Clementinum delivered the first plan of the complex. The principal Jesuit foundation of Bohemia was thus directly involved. The foundation stone of the college was laid on 1 March 1586. Construction works were entrusted to the professional architect Baldassarre Maggi (also called in German May), with stonemasonry executed by the master Antoni[n]o Cometa. The inauguration of the building took place on 10 December 1590. From this time onwards, the new college was quickly developed, inspired by the Roman Gesù. It is worth highlighting the 'Jesuitische Gärten' on the opposite side of the river Moldau/Vltava, which indicates once again a high level of interest in medical and other herbs on the part of Camel and other members of the order already in Bohemia, long before the mission. See Vlcek, ed., *Ceský Krumlov*, 2016, p. 129 (contribution entry signed by Vlcek).

12 For the years 1609–1611, cf. Society of Jesus Archive in Rome (ARSI): *Litterae Annuae. Historiae*: shelf mark *Austria*, 133, Hist. 1600–1617, *Collegium Crumloviense*, fol. 23*v*.

9

1638 – Bones of contention

Katharina Sabernig

Introduction

The year 1638 is the birthyear of several proponents of this chapter. At the time the Thirty Years' War (1618–1648) raged in the heart of Europe. In China the Ming dynasty collapsed before the establishment of the Qing dynasty in 1644 and the Tibetan roof of the world was beset by internal conflicts and external dependencies. Globally, the period is characterised by a decline in temperature, known as the 'Little Ice Age', during which people worldwide suffered from recurrent endemic outbreaks of the plague and smallpox. Nevertheless, in Europe the seventeenth century was a productive time for the advancement of medical knowledge and its visual presentation building on the fruitful development of the earlier Renaissance.

Based on Andreas Vesalius's *De humani corporis fabrica libri septem*, the anatomical text *Anatomie universelle du corps humain* by the French barber surgeon Ambroise Paré (1510–1590) was translated into Chinese by the Jesuits. During that Mission, the Jesuit Father Johann Adam Schall von Bell (1591–1666) played a central role. He stayed in Beijing and served at the imperial court, attracting attention through astronomical calculations, and becoming an advisor for the young Qing Emperor Shunzhi (1638–1661).[1] Politically, his role remains controversial, both in the context of the mission and in the context of the V. Dalai Lama's (Ngawang Lobsang Gyatso, 1617–1682) journey to Beijing in 1652–1653.[2] With the enthronement of the V. Dalai Lama, the 'Great Fifth', the second half of the seventeenth century became a fertile Tibetan era in both political and medical terms. The personal physician of the 'Great Fifth', the physician, surgeon, and anatomist Lobsang Chödrak (called Darmo Menrampa, 1638–1712?) played a decisive role in its anatomical achievements.

Did Lobsang Chödrak develop his insights on his own, or did external influences have a significant impact on this development? To investigate this question, I have looked for similar developments in Tibet's neighbouring countries and for possible transfers of medical knowledge from Europe, finding that at least three European scholars of anatomy were born in the same year as the Tibetan scholar. Even if the life achievements of these researchers were to reach their peak in the second half of the seventeenth century, their common birth year connects them in addition to their passion of exploring the human body. Born in very different circumstances with different religious, social, political, educational, institutional, and economical environments, they became famous for their anatomical and scientific achievements. Their biographies show individual stories of success and failure, but they have independently become the focus of my interest in forms of anatomical representation.

The European scholars in question are Frederik Ruysch (1638–1731) from Amsterdam (Netherlands), Nicolaus Stenonius (alias Niels Stensen or Nico Steno; 1638–1686) from Copenhagen (Denmark), and Crisóstomo Martínez (1638–1694) from Valencia (Spain). In the following, I will look briefly at their early years, as well as the most important medical debates which may have shaped the anatomical approach of young doctors or artists, and highlight the achievements with which they are remembered in history. Finally, the connection and legacy of this anatomical generation will be explored in the context of the so-called *Manchu Anatomy* created by the later Jesuit mission in the early eighteenth century, first created under the Joachim Bouvet (1656–1730) and later brought to fruition by Dominique Parrenin (1665–1741).

Early years

Fernand Meyer's article, *The Golden Century of Tibetan Medicine*, appears in the publication *Lhasa in the Seventeenth Century: The Capital of the Dalai Lamas*.[3] This article's title is true for the second half of the century but a mastermind of this fruitful development, the prominent scholar Lobsang Chödrak,[4] was born in politically unstable times. Born in the same year as the first emperor of the newly rising Qing dynasty, Shunzhi (1638–1661), major political changes were afoot. During that time the region as well as northern China were affected by several endemic smallpox (*vbrum-nad*) outbreaks.[5] Lobsang Chödrak was just four years old when the Fifth Dalai Lama was able to seize power and unify the kingdom in 1642 with the military help of the Koshud Mongols under Gushri Khan. As a physician he became famous by the name of Darmo Menrampa, indicating he was a Physician (*sman rams pa*) from Darmo, his birthplace near the mountain Sham-po-gangs in the eastern part of the historical Yarlung valley. Not much is known about his parents; according to Byams-pa-phrin-las, he received a Buddhist monastic education at Lubukling (*Klu-sbug-gling*). Later on, the medical faculty at the Buddhist Yellow Hat (Gelugpa) school of

Drepung Monastery (*Vbras-spungs dgon-pa*) near Lhasa provided him with comprehensive medical training. Afterwards he was appointed instructive head of the medical school in one of the towers of the Potala Palace where he started to edit, compile, and write medical texts together with his students.[6] It is not entirely clear if he met the Jesuit Johannes Grueber who stayed in Lhasa in 1661 for one month on his return from Beijing where the Austrian missionary stayed for two years at the court of the Emperor Shunzhi. Grueber must have known about various anatomical translations into Chinese by his Jesuit colleagues, and it is likely that they communicated on an informal basis, although an official audience with the Great Fifth did not take place.[7] Could an exchange of medical knowledge with Grueber have sparked an interest in the empirical study of the inside of the body? There is no evidence of such an encounter and as will be explored later in this chapter, it is possible, but again not provable, that the V. Dalai Lama and his entourage also learned of the Christian missionaries and their anatomical knowledge during his trip to Beijing in 1652–1653.

'Frederik Ruysch was born during a period of intellectual change'. Thus begins the article 'Master Anatomist and depictor of the surreality of death' by Mark Kidd and Irvin M. Modlin. Born of a respectable Dutch family in The Hague,[8] little is known about his religious background; he was considered a moralist and was raised in a Protestant environment that had just liberated itself from Spanish Catholicism. Due to the early death of his father in 1654 he was apprenticed in pharmacy and received a licence in 1661 (the year the Jesuit Johannes Grueber arrived in Lhasa). After Ruysch's marriage with Maria Prost he started his medical studies at the University of Leiden in the same year. Graduating in 1664, he received his doctorate on pleurisy entitled *De Pleuritide*. At that time Leiden kept one of the best collections of anatomical objects in Europe. At this early stage of life, he was acquainted with the debates about the work of the philosopher Descartes (1569–1650) and observed the anatomical experiments of his Professor Johannes van Horne (1621–1670), who gathered around his dissection classes a number of later renowned young anatomists. This academic atmosphere of anatomical research allowed him to learn important visualisation techniques. One of his comrades who shared his knowledge was Jan Swammerdan (1637–1689), who would later be remembered more as a microscopist and entomologist; another was Regnier de Graaf (1641–1673), better known for his work on the ovarian follicle named after him.[9] Among his fellow students around Professor Horne were two other future anatomists relevant to this chapter: Thomas Bartholin (1616–1689), son of the anatomist Caspar Bartholin (1585–1629), and Nico Steensen (1638–1686), also known as Nikolas (Nicolaus) Steno, both born in Denmark.[10]

Ruysch's Colleague Nicolas Steno had a completely different biography. According to Frank Sobiech, 'The anatomist Nicolaus Steno (1638–1686), a key figure of the Scientific Revolution and founder of modern geology, engaged in research on human procreation and proved for the first time that women have ovaries and not so-called female testicles'.[11] Nikolas Steno, baptised as a Lutheran in Copenhagen, grew up well cared for and was well educated in various languages from a young age, not only in German but also Latin, Greek, Hebrew, and Arabic. In 1656–1659 he studied medicine at the University of Copenhagen and wrote his dissertation on the parotid gland in 1661. After completing his studies, a period of travelling and lecturing followed, which took him all over Europe and brought him into contact with renowned physicians. Following a call from Thomas Bartholin, the polymath moved to the Netherlands where he met the hard-working medical student and preservator Frederick Ruysch in Leiden.[12]

Little is known about the early ears of the anatomical painter and engraver Crisóstomo Martínez (1638–1694) from Valencia. We know from Nuria Valverde that 'Throughout the seventeenth century the population of the region suffered dramatic changes due to the expulsion of the Morisco community and recurrent outbreaks of the plague'.[13] Though born in a region of rich academic, medical, and anatomical tradition in the sixteenth century, the early seventeenth century was characterised by a decrease of population and prosperity of the region. The break with the Calvinistic Netherlands based on religious liberation initiated by the Calvinists is only one aspect of the situation. Nuria Valverde points out that a growing sensibility toward the fragility of life fostered the social acceptance of the institutionalisation of medical knowledge.[14] Moreover, with Valverde de Hamusco's Atlas *Anatomia del corpo humano* (1560) Valencia was already part of an academic anatomical tradition. Another factor that has been beneficial to Crisóstomo Martínez's career is the professionalisation and institutionalisation of painting in Valencia and other Spanish cities already in the early seventeenth century.[15] José Pardo-Tomás and Àlvar Martínez-Vidal argue that the decades of stagnation could be less than generally assumed as the practice of medicine, dissection, epidemiology, or the study of plants continued.[16] Crisóstomo Martínez did not receive an academic education in medicine, but he began painting at the age of fifteen and became a professional engraver highly influenced by Spanish Catholic baroque art.[17] Based on the longstanding educational and intellectual tradition, Crisóstomo Martínez helped Valencia become an early hotspot of the Spanish *novator* movement in the final quarter of the seventeenth century.[18]

Important medical debates influence the young doctors

With the establishment of a new Government (*ganden phodrang*) under the rule of the V. Dalai Lama, supported by the Koshud Mongol Güshi Khan, rival Buddhist schools were united in 1642. The Great Fifth became a 'medical impresario' and [medicine] 'was a key component of the cosmopolitan spirit in the capital more broadly [...]'.[19] In retrospect, this period is called the 'Golden Age' of Tibetan medicine.[20] Debates on medical issues have a long tradition in Tibet. In the centuries before, profound discussions took place among Buddhist and medical scholars on the topography of the heart or about the existence, meaning, and location of various types of invisible as well as empirically perceptible channels (*rtsa ba*) that may be identified as arteries and veins but also as nerves and tendons.[21] The most vigorous discussion in the seventeenth century did not concern anatomy but materia medica (see short essay 'Visual Culture of Tibetan Materia Medica'). Tibet's most important text, the *Four Tantras* (*rgyud bzhi*) presumably dating back to the twelfth century, are attributed to mythical scholar Yuthok Yonten Gonpo. Consisting of four parts, the second, called the 'Explanatory Tantra', comprises three chapters on anatomy: embryology, bodily metaphors, and component parts. As a metrical text composed to be memorised by prospective physicians, it provides a basic textual fabric that only becomes comprehensible through the commentaries. The examination of the commentaries reveals the medical zeitgeist of the respective time and school of interpretation. The sixteenth-century commentary *Transmission of the Elders* is comprehensive and loaded with religious ideals that are, however, not always clearly applicable to medical practice, while texts from the seventeenth century tend to be characterised by a more empirical approach related to clinical practice.[22]

Lobsang Chödrak encompassed both of these approaches: the clerical tradition and practice-oriented empirical exploration. His anatomical achievements were particularly important because he had the intention to corroborate and question the orthodox anatomical literature through dissection. Around 1670 he performed a public dissection in a park.[23] This is remarkable not because of the opening of the corpse per se, which was not taboo in Tibet, but because he questioned the classical texts. The *Four Tantras* are constructed as if they were Buddha's words, even though this was untenable from the point of view of some historical Tibetan scholars. The very idea of questioning a religiously authorised text could only be carried out successfully if such a process was accepted by the highest state authorities. His commentarial text on anatomical structures organised within tree hierarchies visualised at Labrang Monastery (Figure 9.1, see also the short essay 'Visual Culture of Tibetan Materia Medica')[24] did not touch at all the discussion of invisible or tantric channels; instead, it searched for 'channels of medical practice', that is, empirically perceptible channels. In a nutshell, he meticulously revised the number of bones and smaller articulated joints of the hands and feet, finding twenty-five instead of fifteen small carpal or tarsal joints per extremity. Compared with the *Blue Beryl* he gave more attention to sutures and conjunctions of the neurocranium (braincase) rather than the viscerocranium (facial bones).

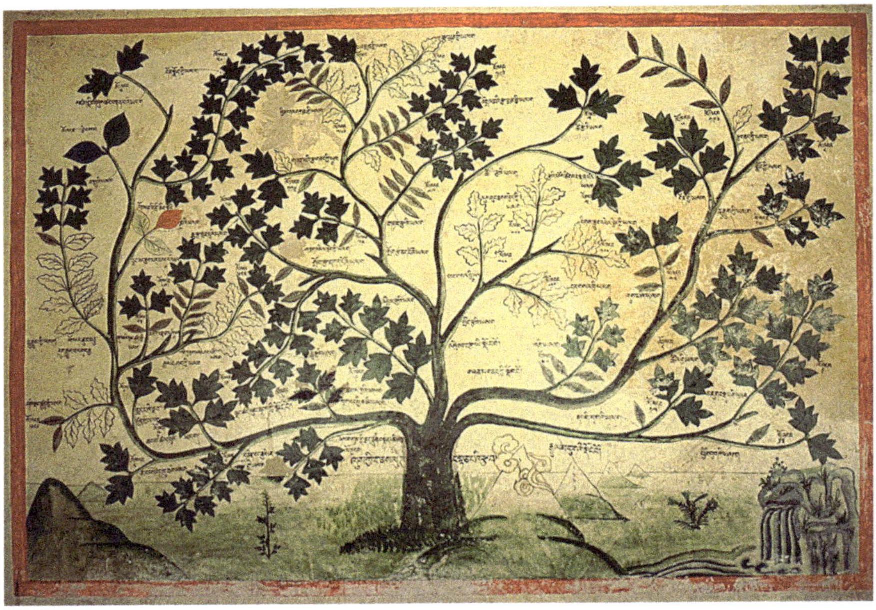

Figure 9.1 Tree of Anatomy in the inner courtyard at Labrang Monastery according to Blo-bzang-chos-grags text, 2005. Image credit: Katharina Sabernig

Through hands-on examination, he also amended the mode of counting vertebra, evident insofar as he regarded the promontory as part of the sacrococcygeal unit. This inevitably resulted in a modification of the topography of the vascular supply of the internal organs in relation to the height of the vertebra. He then investigated the structures of the musculoskeletal system. After he had listed and identified diverse forms of 'tendons', he stated that out of 900 alleged tendons, 580 did not come to light.[25] This may have been considered too progressive, because the immediately following authoritative works by subsequent scholars did not integrate his findings.

Discussions about bones, channels, and the internal motion of fluids were not unique to Tibetan medicine. A major and highly contested development in the seventeenth century was the discovery of blood circulation. In Cairo, Ibn an-Nafīs (born in Damascus 1210–1288) had discussed Galenic ideas and Avicenna's comments on circulation. Today he is regarded as the discoverer of the pulmonary circulation. Based on Ibn an-Nafīs' historical findings, William Harvey (1578–1657) suggested and described the systemic circulation of blood which became one of the most discussed topics among European anatomists in the seventeenth century. Harvey, an Englishman, also examined the flow of the lymphatic fluid in its vessels, and Jean Pecquet (1622–1674), a Frenchman, contributed to the reservoir of chyle of the Ductus thoracicus, which he called the *receptaculum chyli.*

His acquaintance, Thomas Bartholin, named it *cisterna chyli* and following Van Horne the Leiden circle became essential in the controversy and exploration of the lymphatic system and the functional role of the liver.[26] Based on his craftsmanship and this research environment, Ruysch found the best conditions for inventing and developing the technique of injecting blood and lymphatic vessels with which he succeeded to demonstrate finest structures. Due to his elaborate skills he became able to visualise the existence of valvular structures. Although he wrote an article entitled *Dilucidatio valvularum in vasis lymphaticis et lacteis* in 1665, Ruysch's interest shifted more and more towards providing visual evidence of the direction of blood and lymph flow and refining his injection, embalming, and preservation techniques.[27]

Still in Leiden, where he already examined the ovarian tube, Nikolas Steno researched the anatomy of the brain and various smaller structures of the head. The death of his stepfather prompted him to return to Copenhagen in 1663. But after his mother's death soon afterwards, he began to travel throughout Europe again, first to France, then to Italy where the polymath worked as an anatomist as well as a paleontologist and geologist. Perhaps it was his classical philology education that prompted him to engage in profound mystical reflections at a young age. After his experience with Reformed churches in the Netherlands and a moment of epiphany during a procession in Italy he converted to Catholicism in 1667. Conceivably this impression was reinforced by the conflict with Regnier de Graaf, whom he accused of plagiarism for his discovery of the ovarian follicle.[28]

In Valencia the eminent physician Matías García (1640–1691) was appointed head of anatomy at the University. As in other places in Europe, William Harvey's statement on the blood circulation was a keenly debated topic and Garcia was not entirely confident in the theory. He was very much in favour of dissection and even vivisection and fostered the practice of public dissection. Opening up the body to observe the interior structure empirically and gain otherwise invisible knowledge was regarded as an important technique of research and teaching. The question of how to visualise functional processes became increasingly relevant.[29] The creative process from knowledge gained by 'seeing' and 'making' was crucial in anatomical representation over centuries and influenced by culture, art, science and religion.[30] Through Crisóstomo Martínez's contacts with the medical faculty, he was able to attend dissections and imagine the ideal artistic representation. His scientific microscopical examination of bones brought him to develop a mode of gradual presentation of the invisible macroscopical and microscopical interior.

In contrast to the Valencian Matías García's reservation with regard to the blood circulation, Pierre Dionis (1645–1718), '*Demonstrateur anatomique*' at the Royal botanical garden in Paris, was convinced of the newly introduced concepts of blood circulation by William Harvey. He even felt he could not recommend the anatomical work of Thomas Bartholin because he did not describe blood circulation decisively enough.[31] Crisóstomo Martínez managed to get in touch with anatomical techniques in Central Europe and Raúl Velasco Morgado mentions that Martínez stated that he was working hard to study techniques in other European countries and that he started to modernise the static bodily representation of his Valencian predecessor Valverde de Hamusco's based on Vesalian Renaissance anatomy. There is evidence that he kept written correspondence with members of the French academy of science around the famous anatomist Guichard-Joseph Duverney (1648–1730), the successor of Pierre Dionis. This bone specialist was to be of crucial importance for Crisóstomo Martínez and the creation of the atlas during his time in Paris.[32]

Decisive years

Tibet in the late seventeenth century was undoubtedly a fruitful period, marked by prosperity across the upper classes, promoting both the transfer of knowledge and the growth of an intellectual environment fostering the development of Tibetan contributions to medicine. The history of Tibetan medical traditions is replete with external influences from China, India, or the Eastern Mediterranean – regions to which Tibetan philosophical and medical scholars also offered their own interpretations.

Lobsang Chödrak not only had contacts with Indian scholars to create a pharmacopoeia,[33] but also learnt cataract surgery from the Indian physician and ophthalmologist Manaho (Rma-na-ho), who was invited to Lhasa in 1675–1677.[34] His interest in the ability of performing eye surgery was certainly stimulated by the aim to treat the eye problems of the V. Dalai Lama. According to Olaf Czaja he also considered techniques of the 'Upper Tradition' (*stod lugs*) and the eye surgery practice of *Mahāsiddha Mi-tra-dzo-ki*.[35] After the death of the V. Dalai Lama in 1682 he became author and editor of various medical texts. The *Nationwide Collected Ancient Tibetan Medicine Book-Name Catalogue* lists forty different texts stored in ten different libraries attributed to Lobsang Chödrak. Most of them, can be found in the Tibet Autonomous Region Tibetan Medicine Library in Lhasa and the Library at Labrang Monastery.[36] Aside from being the compiler of the aforementioned pharmacopoeia, he served as editor of the blockprint of the hagiography of Yuthok Yonten Gonpo, considered the author of the *Four Tantras*. Lobsang Chödrak carried on several lines in the transmission of the classical texts.[37] Although he completed the commentary initiated and written in large part by Zurkhar Lodrö Gyelpo (Zur-mkhar Blo-gros-rgyal-po, 1509–1579), it was he who urged the Regent of the V. Dalai Lama Desi Sangye Gyatso (1653–1705)[38] to write a new commentary reflecting the medical thoughts of his particular time.[39] Entitled *Blue Beryl*, a milestone in Tibetan medical tradition, it was written with the intention to clarify structure and improve practicability. Under the reign of the Regent Sangye Gyatso, the establishment and standardisation of medical knowledge received great support. Lobsang Chödrak played an important role in this, even though the relationship between the two experienced a marked difference of opinion (see essay on 'Tibetan Materia Medica').

Lobsang Chödrak must have spent much time on medical educational activity and became an astute intellectual teacher. Kurtis Schaeffer translated one of his statements on students: 'Even though some physicians do not understand [the *Four Tantras*], they rashly think that understanding is easy. Some [on the other hand], see the [medical treatises] as difficult to understand, while others become frightened by the mere sight of a book'.[40] A didactic centrepiece of the Tibetan medical tradition is the concept of unfolding trees (*sdong vgrems*) that hierarchically structure large amounts of information into tree metaphors. The classical tradition, however, only refers to the first and very short part of the *Four Tantras* and the regent suspected that the other, much more extensive parts would be too complex to organise with such a thorough itemisation. Notwithstanding this difficult task, the prudent teacher also managed to structure the longer text of the second part, the 'Explanatory Tantra', in the form of tree hierarchies. There is no evidence that his reflections were also incorporated into the medical curriculum in Lhasa, but it did become part of the tradition of the medical college at Labrang Monastery, where the text is visualised by a series of instructive murals in the inner courtyard.[41]

The making of the *Blue Beryl* commentary was accompanied by another prestigious work: the comprehensive set of seventy-nine thangka illustrations (scroll paintings) depicting colourful and vividly selected content for the commentary. Among them, ten thangkas present anatomical knowledge, including embryological development and ideal body proportions in the style of the Vitruvian conception of man.[42] Another ten thangkas present the human body organised on a modular grid for the exact application of minor surgery, such as bloodletting or moxibustion as well as topographical lines providing orientation for the management of wounds. However, it seems Lobsang Chödrak was not officially involved in the creation of the paintings, as his name is not mentioned in the inscriptions; even the anatomical paintings which demonstrate observed knowledge gained via dissection are not connected with him, but instead the reincarnate Tendzin Norbuchen from Lhodrak is mentioned as executive anatomist.[43] Lobsang Chödrak's modified method of counting the vertebral bodies and mapping the corresponding organ topography was also excluded from official recognition, as it deviated from orthodox medical knowledge. Perhaps one reason for this was the incompatibility of his findings with classical therapeutic charts for moxibustion and bloodletting points.

When I examined Lobsang Chödrak's text on tree metaphors to decipher the content of the murals in the medical college at Labrang monastery, I compared the selected content with respective thangkas and noted that they complemented each other in that the content of the 'Explanatory Tantra' was almost completely visualised.[44] This indicates that Lobsang Chödrak was involved in the creation of the didactic concept of the medical education in Lhasa. The culmination of the fruitful development in Lhasa was the establishment of the medical college on top of the Iron Hill directly opposite the Potala palace. Founded by the Regent in 1696, soon after, Lobsang Chödrak became appointed director of the institution. This pleasant progress ended abruptly with the violent death of the regent 1705. Legend has it that Lobsang Chödrak was part of the entourage that accompanied the First Jamyang Zhepa (Vjam-dbyangs-bzhad-pa 1648–1721) on his return to Amdo in 1709, heralding the foundation of Labrang Monastery.[45]

In Europe in 1666, his Dutch colleague Frederick Ruysch cared for the sick affected by an endemic plague outbreak in his hometown. In the same year he became professor of anatomy (Praelector Chirurgiae et Anatomiae) and one year later Chief Anatomist in Amsterdam, where he performed public dissections. He also became teacher of obstetrics (1668) and master of midwivery (1672), later also doctor to the court (1679).[46]

Less well known is his interest in indigenous botany based on his apothecary apprenticeship. By applying his techniques, he conserved and dissected exotic plants provided by sailors in the Dutch commercial fleet. In 1685 he became professor of botany at the city botanical garden.[47]

At least two of his students became famous for the publication of exceptional anatomical atlases in the style of baroque art. The earlier *Anatomia humani corporis* was supervised by Govert Bidloo (1649–1713), who provided the text for 105 ingenious copperplate engravings, artistically implemented by Gerard de Lairesse.[48] The images in the atlas, published in 1685, impressed the Valencian engraver Crisóstomo Martínez who decided to produce comparable images on osteology.[49]

While Bidloo – also a poet, librettist, surgeon, and personal physician of King Wilhelm III of England – ended up in dispute with Ruysch, another student acquired his preservation techniques: the German Bernhard Siegfried Albinus (1697–1770). Albinus published an anatomical atlas on the human locomotive system entitled *Tabulae sceleti et musculorum corporis humani* in 1747. Ruysch not only taught preservation techniques to Albinus, but also taught anatomical illustration to Jan Wandelaer, the artist behind the atlas. Even Guichard-Joseph Duverney, a central anatomical scholar in this chapter, studied his art of preservation.[50]

Although Ruysch did anatomical and pathological research, especially on lymphatic tissue, his greatest achievement was the creation of anatomical visual material through his conservation techniques. His objects were suitable for subject-specific teaching as well as for interested laymen, therefore Ruysch founded a museum to present his comprehensive collection of anatomical specimens to the public. Before his time, only tissues from criminals and suicides were conserved, but Ruysch also preserved body parts from women, children, and the unborn. He was in the position to prepare over two thousand objects, including tableaux with skeletal infants. They presented scenes conveying a deeply Christian message on the morbidity of life better known through engravings by Cornelius Huyberts. Unfortunately, the tableaux have not been preserved for posterity.

Considering the elaborate mode of decoration and presentation of the objects in Ruysch's anatomical cabinet, Gijsbert van de Roemer raised the question of whether Ruysch should be regarded as scientist or rather as an artist.[51] Artistically he was also supported by his daughter Rachel who became a famous Dutch painter of still lifes. A large part of his collection was sold to Tsar Peter the Great during his second visit in 1717 and brought to St Petersburg, in the Kunstkamera where 'the specimen are still preserved in a mint condition'.[52] In 1731 he died of fatal fever in Amsterdam at the ripe old age of ninety-three.[53]

The life of Ruysch's fellow student, Nicolas Steno, developed differently. Despite his broad interest in geology, geometry, paleontology, and the human body, religious studies and thoughts on philosophy of science and a critique of science became the focus.[54] He published a geological treatise, entitled *Prodromus*, describing the principles of crystallography and stratigraphy.

From 1672 to 1674, he followed a call to become 'Royal Anatomist' in Copenhagen, although according to Frank Sobiech, he only did so for pastoral reasons.[55] It is not surprising that he encountered difficulties in Protestant Denmark. Nuria Valverde found a statement in the introduction to his *Proemium demonstrationum anatomicarum in Theatro Hafniensi* (1673), which reveals that he was of the opinion that the task of an anatomist 'is to elevate the minds of the onlookers, giving way to the marvels of the body, to its noble spirit, to the conscience and love of our Creator'.[56] Adolf Faller also refers to Steno's comparison of an anatomist with a pointer or a rod in the hand of God.[57]

After his time as 'Royal Anatomist' in Copenhagen Steno decided to become a priest and was involved in counterrevolutionary activities. His comprehensive education and in-depth engagement with the philosophical and religious aspects of scientific questions did not protect him from disappointments in his lifetime. An early disappointment was the dispute over the plagiarism of Regnier de Graaf on the ovarian follicles. Another disappointment must have been the appointment of the son-in-law of his mentor Thomas Bartholin as an anatomy professor instead of Steno.[58] Finally, he settled in Schwerin, where he died in 1686. In 1988, he received belated recognition in the form of beatification from Pope John Paul II.

Thomas Bartholin, son of the famous Danish anatomist Caspar Bartholin originally studied theology before devoting himself to the study of medicine and anatomy. Bartholin wrote a popular anatomy book which was not only translated into English, but whose accompanying images, as will be discussed in more detail later, were used to create the *Manchu Anatomy*, an anatomy atlas in Manchurian by the Jesuits.

When Crisóstomo Martínez went to Paris at forty-nine years old, he left his wife to remain with their four children in Valencia. Raúl Velasco Morgado investigated the requests for financial support for his stay in Paris to produce or complete the series of microscopic and macroscopic anatomical engravings. Providing for his family finances played a major role in the application. According to Morgado's examination of archival material, the first request was made in 1685 and it seems that he started engraving the corresponding plates, which would make him famous, at least by 1683.[59] Nuria Valverde assumes that plates I–IV, depicting bones of the hands and feet, along with plates XIV, XV, and XVI, were probably already created before his arrival in Paris on 19 July 1687.[60] Plates I–IV depict pure bones in a meticulous manner, but without topographical reference. Plate XVI illustrates the dorsal view of a man in the same pose two different ways: in one the view of the musculature is primarily highlighted, whereas in the other the silhouettes are hatched. The elaborate copperplate engraving is a refinement of the tradition of Andreas Vesalius' (1515–1564) *De Humani Corporis Fabrica* and Valverde de Hamusco, but does not yet show the sort of pictorial composition that would make him famous. Plates XV and XIV present anatomical images within images, showing the pelvis and hipbones in relation to the whole body.

Already under Pierre Dionis, Paris had emerged as a centre for modern anatomy and promised opportunities for Crisóstomo Martínez. Dionis performed public dissections and anatomy lessons from 1673 to 1680 in the Royal botanical garden, the *Jardin du Roi*. He then became personal surgeon to the royal court and published *Anatomie de l'homme, suivant la circulation du sang, & les derniéres découverte* in 1690.[61] This book was translated into several languages and formed the textual basis of the *Manchu Anatomy*.

By the time of Crisóstomo Martínez's arrival in July 1687, the anatomist Joseph Guichard Duverney, successor to Pierre Dionis, held the prestigious post at the *Jardin du Roi*. Duverney was a specialist in otology, osteology, and osteoporosis. His major work on otology included engravings that influenced Martínez's style of anatomical plates and were later incorporated into the *Manchu Anatomy*. Duverney emphasised the sequence of images, ensuring that viewers could identify structures consistently across plates. This provided the Valencian artist with the ideal academic conditions and inspiration to conceptualise the visual architecture of his atlas.

In correspondence with his agent in Valencia, Gil de Castelldases – main chair of the medical faculty in Valencia and likely the visionary behind the atlas project – Martínez mentioned the copperplate engravings accompanying the atlas by Bidloo, as well as works from the group around Frederick Ruysch, including Thomas Bartholin, Nikolas Steno, and Reinier de Graaf.[62] With Steno he shared a passion for geometrics and his first plate he engraved in Paris either at the end of 1687 or at the beginning of 1688 was the marvellous one on the proportions of both the adult and infant, based on the Vitruvian ideal (Figure 9.2). As soon as the work was completed, he sent samples to Italy, Germany, England, and Portugal. It was to remain the only plate that he printed in his lifetime.[63]

What began as a glorious prelude to a future great anatomical masterpiece took a tragic turn with the outbreak of the Nine Years' War in October 1688, in which France and Spain were parties to the conflict. Coincidently he suffered from a painful outbreak of gout which forced him to spend abundant time behind the microscope. The sequence in which his pictures were created is not entirely clear, but the gradual deepening from the macroscopic whole to the microscopic detail by using different types of magnification lenses marks him as the discoverer of the trabecular bone and pioneer of the artistic representation of bone histology.[64]

Martínez was also concerned with embryology and membranes, both in terms of artistic visual composition and with regard to gaining scientific knowledge.[65] In a letter to Gil de Castelldases written on 29 May 1689 he explained that the atlas would 'simulate a letter written by an unknown person to a research director', presumably Duverney.[66] The dimension that this atlas could have taken in peacetime can only be imagined, but he was accused of espionage and fled to Flanders in 1690 where he died in 1694 (Figures 9.2 and 9.3).

The Jesuit mission and the transfer of knowledge

Already before the period of the birth of the 1638 anatomists an active mutual translation activity took place between Europe and China, led by the Jesuits. A central figure was the Jesuit Johann Terrenz Schreck, alias Torrenzius (1567–1630), who translated technical, astronomical, and anatomical texts into Chinese.[67] Due to his premature death he could not complete his anatomical translation *Renshen shuo* (*A Treatise on the Human Body*) which was revised and published as *Taixi renshen shuogai* by the Chinese scholar Bi Gonchen in 1643. Another manuscript belonging to the Beijing University library is the *Renshin tushuo*: the translation is attributed to the Italian Jesuit Giacomo Rho (1592–1638), but also mentions Niccolò Longobardo (1565–1655) and Johann Terrenz Schreck. The text has been identified as a translation of the work *Anatomie universelle du corps humain* by the French barber surgeon Ambroise Paré (1510–1590),

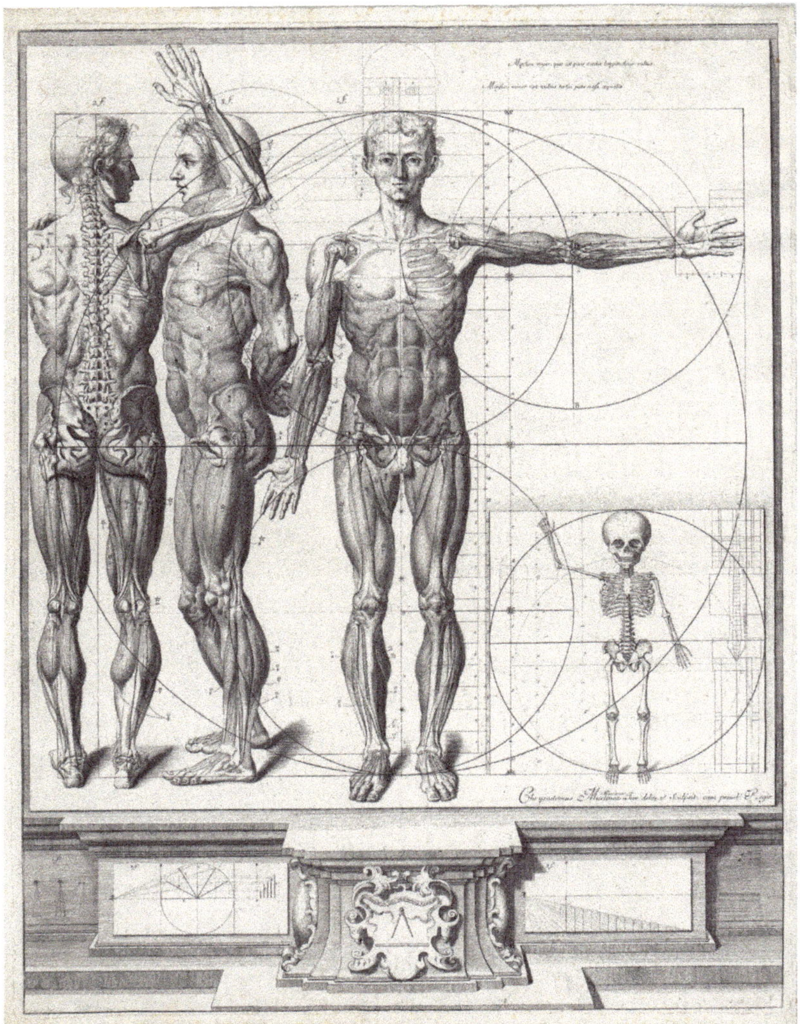

Figure 9.2 Crisóstomo Martínez, Body Proportions, plate c. 1680/1694, printed 1740, unpublished Plate for the *Atlas Anatomico*, Etching, 70.9 × 53.6 cm. The Metropolitan Museum of Art, New York. Image credit: Public domain

based on Andreas Vesalius' *De humani corporis fabrica libri septem*.[68] Not quite clear is the role of Johann Adam Schall von Bell (1591–1666) who stayed in Beijing until his death in 1666 and published several of Schreck's texts post mortem.[69] He certainly knew the translation of the anatomical text into Chinese. Lobsang Yongdan states that it was he who 'prevented the expressions of honour and dignity which the Manchu would have

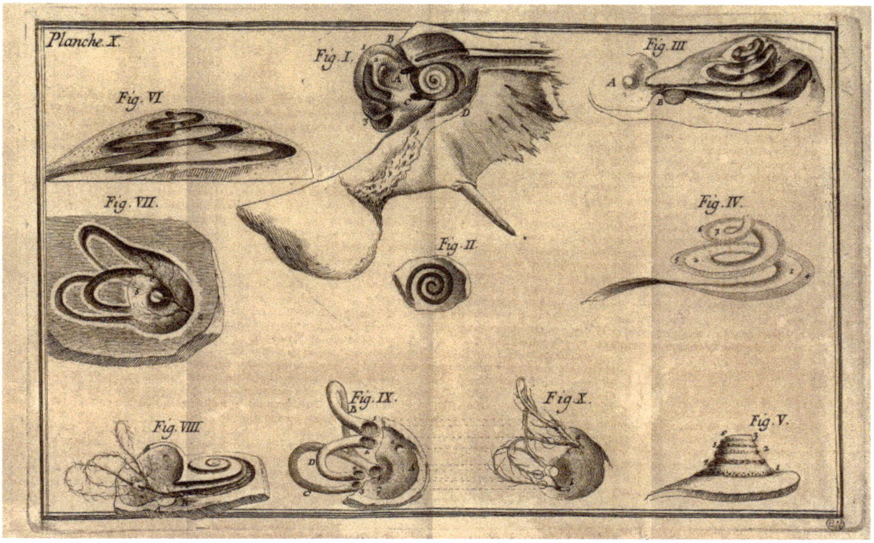

Figure 9.3 Joseph-Guichard Duverney, *Traité de l'organe de l'ouïe*, Paris 1683, Figure X. The image was kindly provided by the French National Library. Image credit: Paris, Bibliothèque nationale de France

reserved for greeting the Dalai Lama' during the Tibetan mission to Beijing in 1652–1653.[70]

After a period of translation of mainly astronomical and geometrical texts there followed at least two attempts at the creation of a *Manchu Anatomy* by French Jesuits.[71] The activities of the Jesuits in the late seventeenth and early eighteenth century were not limited to China and France, as Paolo Sanvito's contribution in this volume on drawings of medicinal plants of the Bohemian Jesuit Georgius Josephus Camel in South Asia demonstrates.

The creation of the *Manchu Anatomy* started in Paris, where King Louis the XIV was at the height of his power in the 1680s. At the time Pierre Dionis was appointed his court surgeon and Duverney held a position titled *Demonstrateur anatomique* at the *Jardin du Roi*. Only four years before the outbreak of the Nine Years' War, a group of French missionaries, including Joachim Bouvet, were sent to the imperial court of China, not least to counter the influence of Portuguese missionaries.[72]

Before their departure in March 1685, the missionaries specifically prepared themselves with the latest scientific achievements. When they arrived in Beijing in March 1688, they had prepared themselves to instruct the Kangxi Emperor in astronomy, mathematics, philosophy and anatomy.[73] Dionis's anatomical atlas was not published until 1690, but his successor Joseph Guichard Duverney had already published a number of texts, especially on the anatomy of bones and on otology. According to Daniel Asen, Bouvet's anatomical explanations to the Kangxi Emperor were mainly based on Duverney's texts.[74]

When Joachim Bouvet left Beijing in 1693, the Kangxi Emperor was impressed by the anatomy lessons he received and requested that the scholar return with other missionaries to continue the medical exchange. Nevertheless, it became clear during this period that the emperor sought more clinical relevance and less structural precision.[75] In Chinese medical culture the exact structure or shape of bones was given little importance; the anatomy of the palpable bones, especially the vertebrae, was of primary interest as a guide to the topography of internal organs. Li-chun Lee describes the resulting Chinese bone maps in terms of a 'cartography of the tactile'.[76]

Chinese medical scholars were generally more interested in the physiology or pathophysiology of living humans or in therapeutic options than in anatomical knowledge of dead bodies.[77] Moreover, it was not easy to convince the Emperor that the anatomical knowledge found on European bodies was also applicable to Asian, respectively Chinese or Manchurian, bodies.[78]

Creation of the *Manchu Anatomy* and the origin of the images

Within a group of French missionaries and with France's most popular anatomical atlas by Pierre Dionis at hand, Dominique Parrenin arrived in Beijing in 1698. He stated that he had chosen the book because among those he knew it would be the 'most clear and exact' one and Parrenin decided to take the images of Thomas Bartholin[79] because they would be the 'biggest and better engraved than the others'.[80] Much has been written about the choice of the included illustrations, as well as about different versions in various European libraries.[81] In this chapter I refer to the manuscripts held in the Bibliothèque nationale de France in Paris, in the following referred as 'Paris Library Manuscript'[82] and The Royal Library in Copenhagen.[83] Superficially, the *Manchu Anatomy* became a translation and fusion of two famous anatomical works: Dionis's text and the compilation of images in Bartholin's atlas. Since the detailed examination by John William Schibby Johnsson[84] of the images of the Copenhagen manuscript in 1928, it is well-known that the image templates are of much more diverse origin than Bartholin's atlas. The later publication of John B. Saunders and Francis R. Lee is based on Johnsson's contribution and the Copenhagen edition.[85] The images in the Copenhagen manuscript, which is rather a fragment, differ considerably from those in the Paris Library Manuscript, especially regarding the presentation of the bones. Walravens suggests that the Copenhagen fragment probably was used as an object of presentation.[86] In terms of details, the more extensive Paris edition is hardly described.

What is the difference between the two manuscripts and is there any relation to the four anatomists mentioned? What was the role of Bidloo's atlas? Dionis and Duverney must have known one of its editions which was celebrated for its images but not for its text.[87] Duverney and Bidloo both learned the art of anatomical preparation from Frederik Ruysch. Martínez was not only impressed by Bidloo's Atlas; it was a major stimulus to the creation of his own osteological atlas. While examining the Paris Library Manuscript and being aware of Bidloo's skeleton, I discovered that the skeleton – one of the most famous images in the *Manchu Anatomy* – is not derived from Bartholin but from Bidloo (Figure 9.4).[88] This galvinased the beginning of my examination of the identification of the images.

Noël Golvers's article 'The Jesuits in China and the Circulation of Western Books in the Sciences' contains a published inventory of titles and authors regarding the anatomical structures and functions of the human body.[89] Among these titles one finds the atlas of Bartholin as well as Bidloo. The early anatomical publications listed, such as Costanzo Varolio (1543–1575) or Adriaan van den Spiegel (1578–1625), contain hardly any illustrations, but the atlases by Ysbrand van Diemerbroeck (1609–1674) or Sieur de Saint Hilaire (first published 1683–1685) contain some images included in the *Manchu Anatomy*, while also referring to earlier publications such as the atlas by Guilio Cesare Casserio (1552–1616).[90] Based on Johnsson's, as well as Saunders's and Lee's publications, and after a closer look at the images in anatomical works such as Dionis, Bidloo, Bartholin, or Valverde de Hamusco, as well as a comparison of the two manuscripts of the *Manchu Anatomy*, I have come to the conclusion that the origin is more diverse than previously thought.

The Copenhagen version does not contain any bones aside from individual skull bones and cervical vertebrae.[91] After I realised that in one of the most famous images of the *Manchu Anatomy* included in the Paris Library Manuscript, the complete skeleton is not taken from Bartholin's Atlas but from Bidloo, I checked other images depicting bones. It became evident that almost all images presenting bones, including tiny ones such as the wrist, tarsal bones, or teeth, are based on details in Bidloo's engravings, but painted with less shadow.[92] The illustrations of the spine and the sacral bone come closest to those in Vesalius' atlas,[93] but the selected vertebral bodies are again identical to those from Bidloo.[94] The Bibliothèque nationale de France Manuscript even contains a contribution of the French otologist Duverney: the illustrations of the middle ear with its ossicles and the inner ear with the cochlea are clearly a copy of his work (Figure 9.3).[95] In turn the Copenhagen manuscript contains not only images based on the Atlas by the Danish Bartholin, but also contains several images of the Danish Catholic Nikolas Steno which are not included in the Paris Library

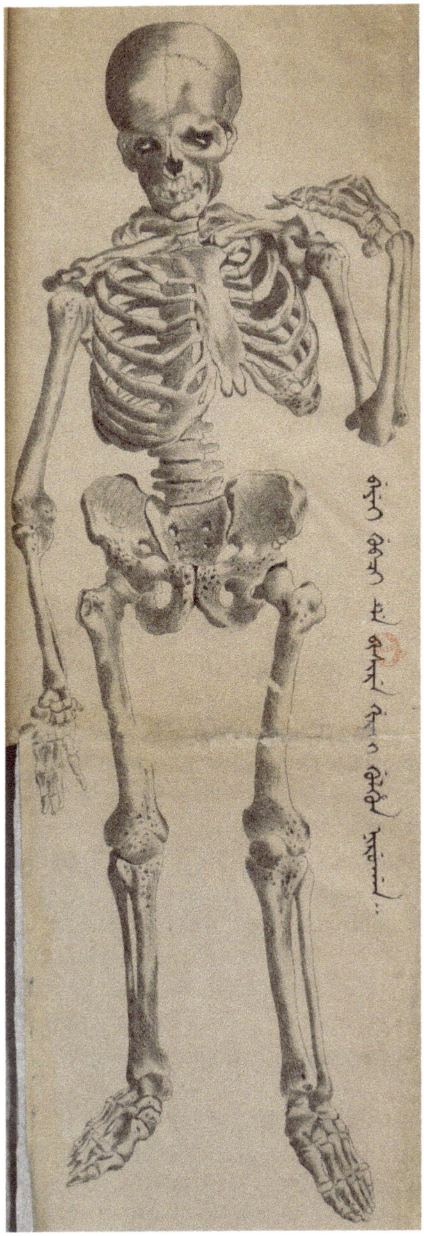

Figure 9.4 The Skeleton from Bidloo's atlas in the *Manchu Anatomy*. Paris, Bibliothèque nationale de France, Mandchou 289/FM 191, book 10, p. 65. The image was kindly provided by the French National Library. Image credit: Paris, Bibliothèque nationale de France

Manuscript.[96] The same applies to two drawings by Frederick Ruysch of the spleen with its vascular supply (Figure 9.5).[97] No direct evidence was available that Spanish Valverde de Hamusco's atlas was brought to China, but several images are included in both manuscripts. Although it is evident that many images in Valverde's atlas are based on their precursor by Vesalius, the images differ in part, as for example in the postures of figures, while in other cases the image is mirrored and correspond in detail to the Jesuit's manuscripts.[98] The images on the superficial venous system below the skin derived from Valverde have no equivalent in Vesalius' atlas but are included in both manuscripts (Figure 9.6).[99] The sketch-like images of the leg muscles in anterior and posterior view display a completely different style. These images appear no less than four times in the Paris Library Manuscript and can be traced directly to Dionis's work, which does not

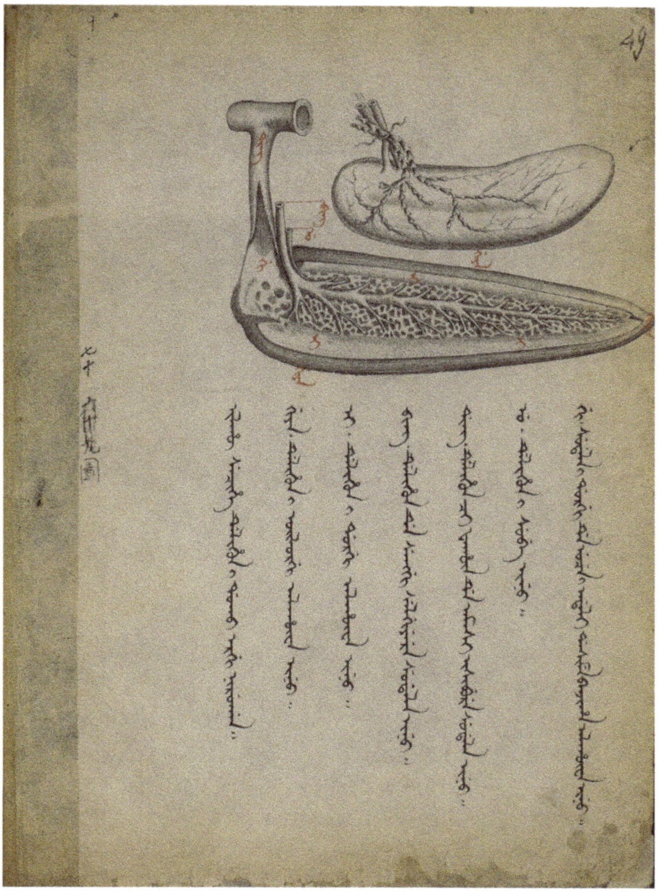

Figure 9.5 Frederick Ruysch, *Spleen*, 1700/1725. Copenhagen, Oriental Collection of Det Kongelige Bibliotek, Manchu 49, Figure 49. Image credit: København, Det Kongelige Bibliotek, CC BY-NC-ND 3.0

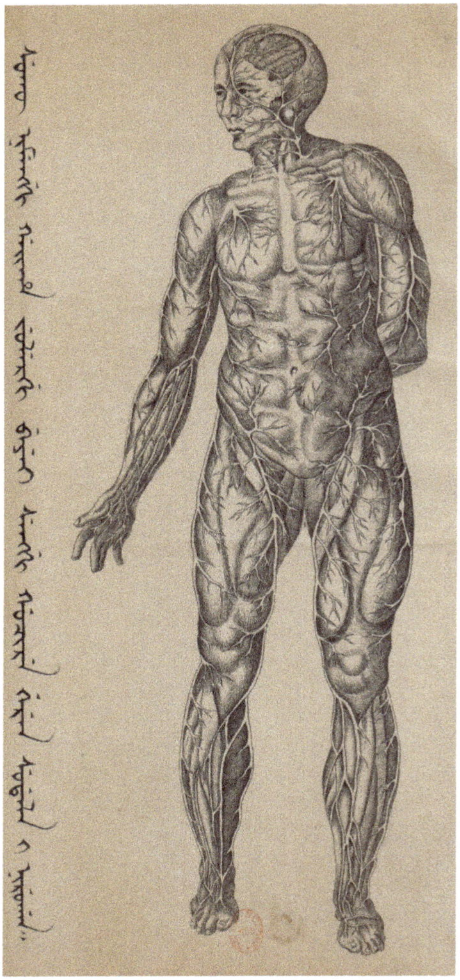

Figure 9.6 Valverde de Hamusco's atlas in the *Manchu Anatomy*. Paris, Bibliothèque nationale de France, Mandchou 289/FM 191, book 10, p. 73. Image credit: Paris, Bibliothèque nationale de France

provide many illustrations, but most of them have been adopted,[100] including images of blood vessels.[101]

The neurological images used in the two manuscripts vary significantly or are different. For example, the image on the cauda equina based on Laurentius is only included in the Paris Library Manuscript.[102] It is beyond the scope of this chapter to analyse all sources and examine further details of the *Manchu Anatomy*. Though the text refers to Dionis's work, it would be false to state that the *Manchu Anatomy* is a synthesis of two European anatomical books; rather it compiles the 'best' of European anatomical historical depictions. Even the image of the famous Englishmen and hepatologist Francis (Franziskus) Glisson is included.[103] However, as Martha Hanson states, the prestigious project was never translated into Chinese to be published for a broader audience and most copies ended up in European libraries.[104]

Nevertheless, the Mongolian National Library in Ulaanbaatar exhibits an early twentieth-century translation into the Mongolian language which contains the same images and sequence as the Paris Library Manuscript.[105] It would be interesting to know if there was an attempt to translate the

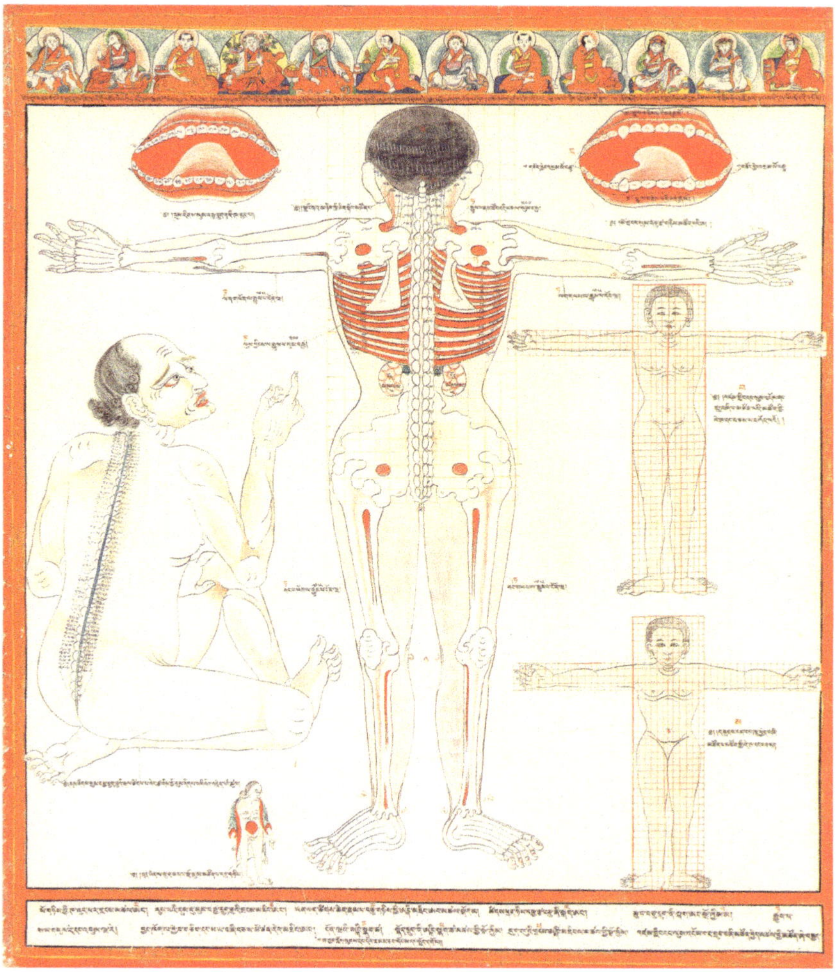

Figure 9.7 Thangka 8 of the illustrations to the Blue Beryl on ideal Body Proportions in Tibetan medicine. Museum of the History of Buryatia, published in Parfionovitch (et al.), *Tibetan Medical Paintings*, 1992, p. 32, London, Serindia. Image credit: Serindia Publications

work into Tibetan, but I could not find any reference to such an endeavour. According to Lobsang Yongdan, several European astronomical texts transmitted by the Jesuits into Manchu were translated first into Mongolian and later into the Tibetan language, whereby authorship of the Catholic foreigners was concealed and the information was 'indigenised'.[106] According to Professor Chang Che-Chia the reorganisation of the sequence of the Paris Library manuscript seems to be an adaption to the Chinese view on internal organs.[107] Although Chinese was the language of the broader population, most of the literati and public officials mastered the Manchu language and had some basic knowledge of Mongolian.[108] The scripts of both languages were very similar and much easier to learn than Chinese characters. There were also Tibetan monks in Beijing who translated texts into Tibetan. This raises the question of the extent to which anatomical texts made their way into Tibetan culture, as Tibet was not as hermetically sealed from outside influences as is often presumed.

However, the *Manchu Anatomy* would have been too late to have any impact on the making of the Blue Beryl or its thangka illustrations because the *Manchu Anatomy* was completed in 1723. With the establishment of Iron Hill Medical College at the end of the seventeenth century, Tibetan anatomical knowledge was consolidated for a long time. What about smaller works that may have reached China's capital through missionaries from other countries? The question remains whether there is a connection between the two representations of the Vitruvian ideal of bodily proportions by Crisóstomo Martínez and Tibetan Medical Thangka number 8. Did a sample of his work make it to Tibet and inspire the local painters, or are the paintings independent expressions of the Roman Vitruvian tradition (Figure 9.7)? It is possible that further research on the transfer of medical knowledge and body ideals from the East Mediterranean region could shed more light on this question (see the essay by Robert Brennan earlier in this volume).

Notes

1 Standaert, 'Ambroise Paré's Anatomy', 1999; Hanson, 'Jesuits and Medicine', 2007, p. 3.
2 Langner, *Johannes Schreck*, 2007, p. 290; Gyatso, *Being Human*, 2015, p. 8.
3 Meyer, 'Golden Century', 2003.
4 Scientific transliteration of the name: Blo-bzang-chos-grags [Dar-mo sman-rams-pa].
5 Czaja, 'Blue Beryl', 2007, pp. 254–255. Classical Tibetan medical texts suggest a form of contagious contact with dried smallpox pustels as a form of prophylactic immunisation: Parfionovitch (et al.), *Illustrations*, 1992, pp. 231–232, no. 84.
6 Byams-pa-phrin-las, 'Gangs ljongs', 2000, pp. 314–315. For more details, see Sabernig, *Visualisierte Heilkunde*, 2017, pp. 48–56.
7 Cf. Zimmel, 'Johann Grueber', 1953.
8 Kidd and Modlin, 'Frederik Ruysch', 1999, p. 69.

9 Graaf's work was published posthumously as *Opera Omnia*, 1705, including many images of the male and female urogenital tract (https://archive.org/details/b30508502_0001/page/n9/mode/2up; accessed 4 November 2023). His image on the pancreas is included in the *Manchu Anatomy*: Graaf, 'Opera Omnia' 1705, p. 388.
10 Kidd and Modlin, 'Frederik Ruysch', 1999, p. 70; Margócsy, 'Philosophy of Wax', 2015, pp. 94–95.
11 Sobiech, 'Nicolaus Steno', 2015, p. 107.
12 Cf. Persaud (et al.), *History*, 2014, p. 252.
13 Valverde, 'Small Parts', 2009, p. 511.
14 Valverde, 'Small Parts', 2009.
15 Valverde, 'Small Parts', 2009, p. 522.
16 Pardo-Tomás and Martínez-Vidal, 'Novator Movement', 2007, pp. 348–349; Valverde, 'Small Parts', 2009, p. 512.
17 Morgado, 'Nuevas Aportaciones', 2012, p. 196.
18 Pardo-Tomás and Martínez-Vidal, 'Novator Movement', 2007, pp. 348–349.
19 Gyatso, *Being Human*, 2015, p. 108.
20 For extensive information: Meyer, 'Golden Century', 2003; Czaja, 'Blue Beryl', 2007; Gyatso, *Being Human*, 2015.
21 For greater detail, see Gyatso, 'Being Human', 2015, pp. 193–208, 251–265. The invisible channels are also known as tantric channels being important for meditation and religious practice. Among the empirically perceptible channels exist 'black vital channels' (*srog rtsa nag po*) which are mainly associated with blood vessels and 'white vital channels' (*srog rtsa dkar po*), identified as nerves or tendons. See Sabernig, *Visualisierte Heilkunde*, 2017, pp. 221–236.
22 Regarding anatomical interpretations: see Gyatso, *Being Human*, 2015, pp. 193–265; Sabernig, 'Anatomical Structures', 2016; *Visualisierte Heilkunde*, 2017, pp. 210–248.
23 Gyatso, 'Experience', 2011, p. 311.
24 Blo-bzang-chos-grags, 'sdong vgrems', 2005.
25 For more details see Sabernig, 'Anatomical Structures', 2016, pp. 25–26.
26 Cf. Kidd and Modlin, 'Frederik Ruysch', 1999, p. 71; Persaud (et al.), *History*, 2014, pp. 109–112.
27 Cf. Kidd and Modlin, 'Frederik Ruysch', 1999, p. 72; Persaud (et al.), *History*, 2014, pp. 92–93; Margócsy, 'Philosophy of Wax', 2015, pp. 99–106.
28 Persaud (et al.), *History*, 2014, pp. 251–252; Sobiech, 'Nicolaus Steno', 2015, p. 117.
29 Valverde, 'Small Parts', 2009, pp. 512–513.
30 Valverde, 'Small Parts', 2009, p. 506.
31 Valverde, 'Small Parts', 2009, p. 514.
32 Morgado, 'Nuevas Aportaciones', 2012, pp. 191–196.
33 Blo-bzang-chos-grags, *levu nyi shu pa*, 2007. See the essay on Tibetan *materia medica:* 'Visual Culture of Tibetan Materia Medica' (pp. 241–252 in this volume).
34 Cf. Schaeffer, 'New Scholarship', 2011, p. 296.
35 Czaja, 'Blue Beryl', 2007, p. 348.
36 Hpheng Ling, *Nationwide*, 2015.
37 For more information, see Taube, *Beiträge*, 1981, pp. 63, 66, 71, 73.
38 Scientific transliteration of the scholars: G.yu-thog Yon-tan-mgon-po, Zur-mkhar Blo-gros-rgyal-po, Sde-srid Sangs-rgyas-rgya-mtsho.
39 Taube, *Beiträge*, 1981, p. 73.
40 Schaeffer, 'Textual Scholarship', 2003, p. 630.
41 For more details on the origin and tradition of medical tree hierarchies, see the source text *Visual Culture of Tibetan Materia Medica* in this volume, or Sabernig, 'Tree of Nosology', 2020, and the murals: Sabernig, *Visualisierte Heilkunde*, 2017, pp. 57–66.

42 More on the Roman architect Vitruv (Marcus Vitruvius Pollio) who lived in the first century BC can be found in this volume's contribution 'I advocate the frequent viewing of [...] green': Ficino, green walls and early modern 'chromotherapy' by Katharine Stahlbuhk.
43 Parfionovitch (et al.), *Illustrations*, 1992, pp. 269–271; scientific transliteration: *Lho-drag sku-skye bstan-vdzin-nor-bu-can*.
44 In detail, see Sabernig, 'Comparison', 2013.
45 Byams-pa-phrin-las, *Gangs ljongs*, 2000, p. 319.
46 Cf. Kidd and Modlin, 'Frederik Ruysch', 1999, p. 76.
47 Cf. Kidd and Modlin, 'Frederik Ruysch', 1999.
48 Artistically exceptional, the images of the atlas were plagiarised by the publication of William Cowper in 1698 who added a more comprehensive and better text: Persaud (et al.), *History*, 2014, p. 197.
49 Valverde, 'Small Parts', 2009, p. 505.
50 Guerrini, 'Duverney's Skeletons', 2003, p. 594.
51 Van de Roemer, 'From Vanitas to Veneration', 2009, p. 1.
52 Margócsy, 'Philosophy of Wax', 2015, p. 107.
53 Kidd and Modlin, 'Frederik Ruysch', 1999, p. 77.
54 Cf. Faller, 'Elemente einer Wissenschaftslehre', 1980; Sobiech, 'Nicolaus Steno', 2015, pp. 110–111.
55 Cf. Sobiech, 'Nicolaus Steno', 2015, pp. 108–109.
56 Valverde, 'Small Parts', 2009, p. 525.
57 Faller, 'Elemente einer Wissenschaftslehre', 1980, p. 186: 'radius seu virga in manu Dei Anatomicus est' (Op. phil. 2.251).
58 Faller, 'Elemente einer Wissenschaftslehre', 1980, p. 172.
59 Morgado, 'Nuevas Aportaciones', 2012, pp. 195–196. Other scholars believe that he had started his work earlier, maybe even before 1680: cf. Valverde, 'Small Parts', 2009, pp. 526–527.
60 Valverde, 'Small Parts', 2009, p. 527. The plates may be viewed in López Piñero, *Crisóstomo Martínez*, 1964.
61 Dionis, *Anatomie de l'Homme*, 1690.
62 López Piñero, *Crisóstomo Martínez*, 1964, pp. 76–78; Valverde, 'Small Parts', 2009, p. 527.
63 Valverde, 'Small Parts', 2009; Morgado, 'Nuevas Aportaciones', 2012, p. 191.
64 Gomez, 'Trabecular Bone', 2002.
65 López Piñero, *Crisóstomo Martínez*, 1964, pp. 76–77; Morgado, 'Nuevas Aportaciones', 2012, p. 192.
66 López Piñero, *Crisóstomo Martínez*, 1964, p. 36; Valverde, 'Small Parts', 2009, p. 528.
67 Langner, *Johannes Schreck*, 2007.
68 Standaert, 'Ambroise Paré's Anatomy', 1999; Hanson, 'Jesuits and Medicine', 2007, p. 3.
69 Langner, *Johannes Schreck*, 2007, p. 28..
70 Lobsang Yongdan, 'Translation', 2015, p. 182.
71 On the extent of European medical texts brought to China by the Jesuits, see Walravens, 'Medical Knowledge', 1996; Hanson, 'Manchu Medical Manuscripts', 2003; Hanson, 'Jesuits and Medicine', 2007; Hanson, 'Significance', 2006; Golvers, 'Jesuits in China', 2011.
72 Asen, 'Manchu Anatomy', 2009, p. 23.
73 Asen, 'Manchu Anatomy', 2009, p. 24.
74 Asen, 'Manchu Anatomy', 2009, pp. 23, 26; Duverney's main anatomical was posthumously published in the middle of the eighteenth century.
75 Asen, 'Manchu Anatomy', 2009, pp. 26–29.
76 Lee, *Körper bilden*, 2019, pp. 167–173.
77 cf. Wung Seok Cha and Hyuk Sang Jung, 'Body Perceptions', 2016.

78 Hanson, 'Jesuits and Medicine', 2007, p. 4.
79 Bartholin, *Bartholinus Anatomy*, 1668. Walravens, 'Medical Knowledge', 1996, pp. 364, 366, and Hanson, 'Significance', 2006, p. 147, write Caspar Bartholin but the revised edition published by his son was used as a template.
80 Asen, 'Manchu Anatomy', 2009, p. 32.
81 Walravens, 'Medical Knowledge', 1996; Hanson, 'Manchu Medical Manuscripts', 2003; Hanson, 'Significance', 2006, pp. 147–148; Hanson, 'Jesuits and Medicine', 2007.
82 Parrenin, *Wargi*, p. 396. In addition, there is another manuscript in the Muséum national d'Histoire naturelle considered to be an earlier version (MS 2009; cf. Walravens, 'Medical Knowledge', 1996, p. 365). Even though the sequence has been organised differently, it contains almost the same illustrations as the Paris National Library manuscript with very few exceptions and according to an informal information of Professor Chang Che-Chia the text is almost identical. See also Sabernig, 'The Manchu Anatomy', forthcoming.
83 http://www5.kb.dk/manus/ortsam/2009/okt/orientalia/object176888/en/#kbOSD-0=page:17 (accessed 8 August 2022).
84 Johnsson, *L'anatomie mandchoue*, 1928.
85 Saunders and Lee, *Historical Origins*, 1981.
86 Walravens, 'Medical Knowledge', 1996, p. 370.
87 The images of Bidloo's atlas engraved by Gerard de Lairesse were plagiarised by the anatomist and surgeon William Copper (1666–1709) resulting in a work better than the original (cf.: Persaud (et al.), *History*, 2014, pp. 197–199).
88 Cf. Parrenin, *Wargi*, p. 396; Bidloo, *Anatomia*, 1685, p. 228, plate 87.
89 Golvers, 'Jesuits in China', 2011, pp. 47–48.
90 Cf. Johnsson, *L'anatomie mandchoue*, 1928, p. 17.
91 Plates 30, 36, and 37.
92 Parrenin, *Wargi*, pp. 355, 367–369; Bidloo, *Anatomia*, 1685, p. 228, plate 87; p. 246, plate 105.
93 cf.: Vesalius, *Fabrica*, 1543, p. 79, plate 57, and Parrenin, *Wargi*, p. 333.
94 Parrenin, *Wargi*, p. 337; Bidloo, *Anatomia*, 1685, p. 234, plate 93 (Figures 6 and 10).
95 Parrenin, *Wargi*, pp. 122–123; Duverney, *Traité*, 1683, plates V, VI, X.
96 Cf. Johnsson, *L'anatomie mandchoue*, 1928, pp. 16–31; Saunders and Lee, *Historical Origins*, 1981, plate 28, 35, 59, 90 (Figures 3–5).
97 Cf. Johnsson, *L'anatomie mandchoue*, 1928, pp. 10–31; Saunders and Lee, *Historical Origins*, 1981, plate 49 (Figure 2), 60 (Figure 2).
98 The images on pages 391–393 (Parrenin, *Wargi*) in the *Manchu Anatomy* correspond with the images of Valverde de Hamusco, *Corpo Humano*, 1560, p. 171, plate 65; p. 173, plate 66; p. 179, plate 69; p. 187, plate 73.
99 Parrenin, *Wargi*, pp. 404–405 in the *Manchu Anatomy* corresponds to Valverde de Hamusco, *Corpo Humano*, 1560, p. 307, plate 133.
100 Cf. Dionis, *Anatomie de l'Homme*, 1690, p. 494, plate 19, and Parrenin, *Wargi*, pp. 375–391.
101 Parrenin, *Wargi*, pp. 66 and 397; Dionis, *Anatomie de l'Homme*, 1690, pp. 494/548: 37–43, 494/548: 44–50.
102 Parrenin, *Wargi*, pp. 349–351; DuLaurens, *Historia Anatomica*, 1600, p. 179.
103 Glisson, *Anatomia Hepatis*, 1665, p. 235.
104 Hanson, 'Jesuits and Medicine', 2007, p. 8.
105 Rinčen, *Dėėrėės togtooson*, 1971.
106 Lobsan Yongdan, 'Translation', 2015, p. 182.
107 Personal communication via e-mail on 21 December 2023.
108 Gimm, 'Zum Geleit', 2013, p. xii.

Source 6

Visual culture of Tibetan materia medica

Katharina Sabernig

Pharmacological treatment is the most essential of the four therapeutic interventions of Tibetan medicine, along with behaviour, nutrition, and external applications. The natural conditions of the Tibetan Plateau provide the conditions for extraordinary fauna and flora with high biodiversity and a rich spectrum of pharmacologically valuable materials. In addition, the import of spices and medical ingredients from neighbouring regions has been well established for centuries. While there exists a longstanding history of textual debates regarding materia medica or how to compile prescriptions, visual presentation of pharmacological knowledge is documented only from the seventeenth century onwards in Tibet; earlier precedents such as Julia Czapla's contribution on Stefan Falimirz' *O ziołach* (1534) are either not attested or have not survived.

The seventeenth century was a time when medicinal substances and spices were already being traded worldwide and European pharmacologists, botanists, and physicians were creating or drawing herbaria in Asia (see Paolo Sanvito's contribution in this volume). Medical illustrations were produced for various reasons, most importantly to illustrate medical knowledge for laypersons and aspiring doctors; another aim was to offer mnemonic aids to facilitate memorising medical content.[1] This essay provides an overview of the visual and textual sources of Tibetan pharmacology.

Pharmacology in the *Four Tantras*

Tibet's central medical book, *Four Tantras* (*Rgyud bzhi*), consists of four parts, each reflecting a distinct perspective on healing: the 'Root Tantra' (*Rtsa rgyud*) is a condensed summary of the core elements of Tibetan medical knowledge, the 'Explanatory Tantra' (*Bshad rgyud*) details preclinical concepts and terminology, the 'Instructional Tantra' (*Man ngag rgyud*) applies the knowledge of diseases, diagnostics, and therapy in clinical practice, and the 'Subsequent Tantra' (*Phyi ma rgyud*) describes special forms of diagnostics and treatment. All four parts deal with pharmacological knowledge in different ways.

The 'Root Tantra' introduces quintessential pharmacological knowledge in three of its six chapters: chapter one describes the ideal place to practise medicine and collect medicinal ingredients; chapter four explains the four therapeutic branches in a nutshell; and chapter six organises the respective knowledge by means of a tree metaphor as a mnemotechnic aid (see Figure S6.1). As regards pharmacological details, three of the thirty-one chapters of the 'Explanatory Tantra' are fundamental for the understanding the essential: chapter nineteen, on 'Taste and Post-digestion' (*ro dang zhu rjes*), describes classical Tibetan pharmacodynamic and pharmacokinetic concepts in theory; chapter twenty, on the 'Effect of Medicines' (*sman gyi nus pa*), lists in detail groups of ingredients including their medical indication such as signs and symptoms or syndromes (Figure S6.4); and chapter twenty-one, on the 'Classification of Medicinal Groups and Method of Application' (*sman gyi sde tshan dang sbyar thabs*), deepens the theoretic knowledge of combining ingredients in a complex formula (Figure S6.5). As for the 'Instructional Tantra', each of its ninety-two chapters deals with a certain group of diseases and syndromes including their classification, aetiology and therapy; in most cases a combination of several medicinal

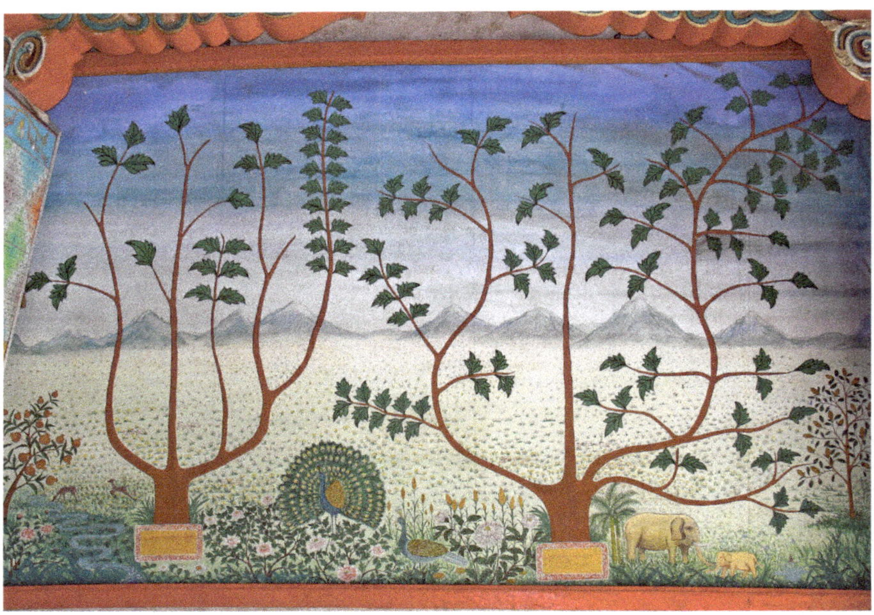

Figure S6.1 Trees of diagnostics and therapy painted by the physician and artist Snying-lcags-byams-zer. Kangtsa Monastery, Gansu Province, 2011. Image credit: Katharina Sabernig

ingredients is named. Of the twenty-five chapters that constitute the 'Subsequent Tantra', these are pharmacologically relevant: ten chapters deal with different groups of 'pacifying' interventions (*zhi byed*), galenic forms of administration such as pills and powders or medicinal butter, ashes or alcoholic solutions; seven chapters treat 'eliminating' methods such as purgatives and emetics as well as nasally applied medicine or enemas (see Figure S6.2). However, being condensed in metrical form, the text is almost incomprehensible if it is not explained by a teacher or a detailed commentary.

The history of Tibetan medicine contains a wealth of explanatory literature, often featuring profound discussions. A seventeenth-century commentary commonly referred to as *Blue Beryl (Vaiḍūrya sngon po)*, authored (or authorised) by Regent Sangye Gyatso (Sde-srid Sangs-rgyas-rgya-mtsho, 1653–1705), is the most famous one, and, in its turn, the textual bedrock of the prestigious visualisation of Tibetan medical knowledge that will be presented in more detail in the next section. Besides commentaries and collections of formulas there is another genre called 'trun-gpe' (*vkhrungs dpe*): literature that lists individual ingredients and explains them according to a variety of Tibetan pharmacodynamic concepts. The twentieth chapter of the 'Explanatory Tantra' is the written core of this text genre.

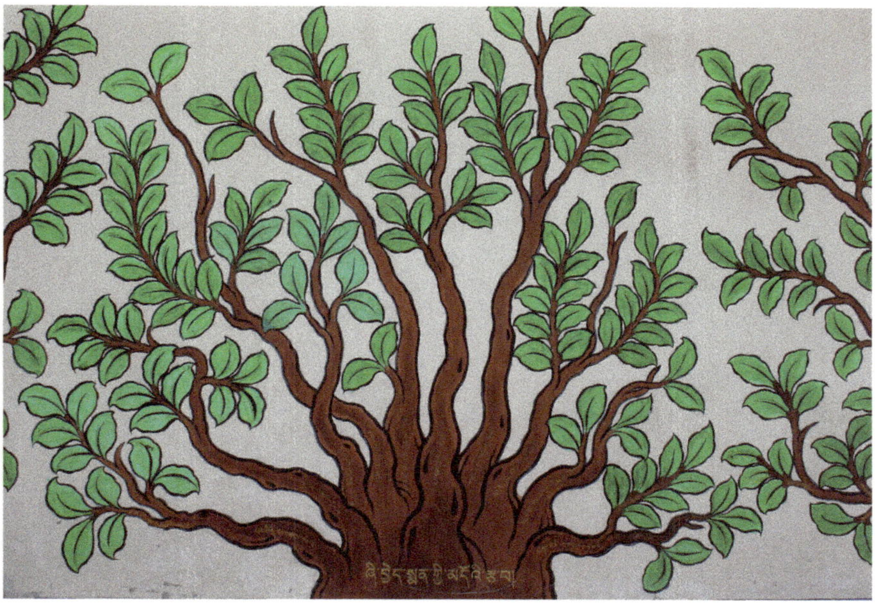

Figure S6.2 Tree depicting ten galenic types of pacifying interventions. Xiahe town, Gansu Province, 2011. Image credit: Katharina Sabernig

The illustrations accompanying the *Blue Beryl*

Visual representations of the materia medica attributed to Sangye Gyatso, transmitted in several versions,[2] are best described, compared, and analysed in two more recent works, an exhibition catalogue on Tibetan Medicine edited by Theresia Hofer as *Bodies in Balance*,[3] and an impressive book on the history of Tibetan medical discussions written by American scholar Janet Gyatso.[4]

During the reign of the V. Dalai Lama (1617–1682) and his Regent (to which position Sangye Gyatso was appointed in 1679), the late seventeenth century became the Golden Age of Tibetan Medicine.[5] A medical college was established at Iron Hill (Chagpori or *Lcags-po-ri*) just opposite the newly constructed Potala palace in Lhasa and a series of painted scrolls (thangkas) were authorised, colourfully and vividly illustrating essential medical content (the exact number varies between seventy-seven and seventy-nine scrolls).[6] The thangka sets preserved today are historical copies of the originals.

The most famous series was probably painted at the beginning of the twentieth century. After the turbulent events of Stalin's purges, the thangkas are now kept in the Museum for the History of Buryatia in Ulan Ude (Buryatia/Russian Federation).[7] The set of images include ten purely anatomical paintings and many thangkas that depict body proportions for external applications or a variety of diagnostic tools (see my contribution '1638 – Bones of Contention' in this book).

Regarding pharmacology, the set includes six thangkas based on chapter twenty, three thangkas on supplementary materia medica and two thangkas illustrating groups of ingredients based on their indication as described in chapter twenty-one. In addition to the list given in the 'Explanatory Tantra', it includes a variety of subspecies. High-value species or cheaper substitutes are presented visually for comparison. Based on the eight major classes listing different ingredients in chapter 20 (57 of inanimate matter, 217 of plant origin and 102 parts of animals), the six thangkas depict 670 ingredients, and almost 400 supplementary materials, thoroughly explained in the Blue Beryl. Two additional thangkas depict the broad variety of medicinal food.

The materials are elaborately drawn in order to be able to discern the qualitative differences between the respective substances. With the exception of spices such as cloves, nutmeg, or cardamom, and fruits such as pears, quinces, or pomegranates, it is usually not clear from the illustrations which part of a plant is to be used.[8] In the case of animal illustrations, however, it is sometimes possible to see which part of the body or tissue is meant. For example, one can see the tongue, certain organs, or the highlighting of blood and fat within the whole body.[9]

When depicting animals, the morphological resemblance to living animals can sometimes only be suspected, especially if these animals are not native to the Tibetan plateau, such as the rhinoceros, which appears more like an antelope or another horned, cloven-hoofed animal.[10] As Janet Gyatso has noted, the images are certainly designed to inspire pleasure and are intended to invite the viewer to let their gaze linger on the illustrations. Various animal figures in the category of nutritive medicine are depicted in lively poses, indicating that the painters had some sense of playful humour.[11]

On thangkas that depict the content of other chapters, one finds sporadic illustrations of medicines and alimentary items; the same applies to illustrations of the 'Root Tantra' and the 'Instructional Tantra'. Several thangkas accompanying the pharmacological chapters of the 'Subsequent Tantra' mainly present manufacturing methods of galenic forms schematically or visualise bodily conditions concerning indications and contraindications of therapeutic interventions.

Textual developments and diffusion to neighbouring countries

Although there is no doubt that there were at least individual precursors to the famous thangka set, almost nothing is known about them. What is well evidenced, however, is a translation of Pedanios Dioscorides' illustrated pharmacopoeia *De Materia medica* into the Persian language (one exists in St Petersburg, Institute of Oriental Manuscripts),[12] and that copies of the illustrations circulated on the Indian subcontinent in the sixteenth century.[13] Even if it is conceivable that they had an influence on the creation of the pharmacological images on the thangkas in Lhasa, no reliable evidence of such a transmission exists. Once the prestigious thangka set was established and authorised – sixty-two items were presented during the enthronement of the VI. Dalai Lama in 1697[14] – several copies were prepared for other institutions in the course of time and sent to places like Beijing or Mongolia; one of the most elaborate even made it to Ulan Ude.[15]

A large part of the thangkas presents medical content in linear order. Like a string of pearls, the materials or other medical topics are presented row by row. This arrangement made it convenient to draw the contents on cards in the traditional oblong book format[16] and use them as mnemonic aids for prospective students. In Mongolia in particular, some of these colourful pharmacological card sets have been preserved, some of which I have seen myself in the Museum for the History of Mongolian Medicine in Ulaanbaatar. In the course of the revival of traditional medicine in recent decades, similar cards have now also been made available in book form.[17] Some of them appear to be copies, if less elaborate, of the original Lhasa template; others appear to be influenced by a nineteenth-century blockprint on Tibeto-Mongolian Materia Medica compiled by Jampal Dorje who flourished in the nineteenth century.

The seventeenth century was not only prosperous with regard to the institutionalisation and visualisation of Tibetan medicine. It was also a time of reformation and clarification of written Tibetan medical knowledge. Concerning materia medica, the development was fuelled by a school dispute that had its origins in the sixteenth century.

The departure point was explanations on materia medica in a commentary on the *Four Tantras* briefly entitled *Transmission of the Elders* (*mes povi zhal lung*) by Zurkhar Lodrö Gyelpo (Zur-mkhar Blo-gros-rgyal-po, 1509–1579). Its lack of practicability was the content of a 'pamphlet' written by Namgyel Dorje from Lhunding (names Lhun-sdings Rnam-rgyal-rdo-rje, life dates unknown) who criticised these explanations. In essence, it was a school dispute between the more theoretically oriented *zur-pa* school based on Buddhist philosophy and the more practically oriented *byang-pa* school.

The Regent Sangye Gyatso, in favour of creating a unified medical standard based on the best views of the varying schools, probably also desired the merging of the two schools as a symbol of political unification of the rival religious groups and family territories.[18] A certain Lobsang Chödrak (Blo-bzang-chos-grags, 1638–1710?, see '1638 – Bones of Contention' in this book) was one of the most important proponents of the *zur-pa* school at that time. Though not responsible for the pharmacological passages in *Transmission of the Elders*, he stood in line of transmission of the *zur-pa* school and completed unfinished sections in the final part of the commentary.

The Regent revealed in his autobiography his deep bond with his teacher Lobsang Chödrak, fifteen years his senior and no less than the personal physician of the V. Dalai Lama. But Sangye Gyatso also wanted to integrate the pharmacological achievements of the rival *byang pa* tradition and, moreover, was not convinced of Lobsang Chödrak's ability to identify plants.[19] This statement, however, should be evaluated within the school dispute and its political implications. It is worth noting, that Lobsang Chödrak also wrote a remarkably comprehensive pharmacopoeia called *The Effects of Medicines in the Twentieth Chapter of the Explanatory Tantra*.[20]

The text, part of the trungpe genre, provides lists of individual medical ingredients from flora, fauna, and inanimate materials consisting of a short summary similar to the 'Explanatory Tantra' and a longer text comprising detailed information. One special feature of Lobsang Chödrak's longer text is the occasional inclusion of corresponding terms in languages such as Sanskrit and other terms and equivalents in North Indian languages. According to Schaeffer he was actually assisted by Indian scholars, especially by Godara, descendent of a Brahmin family, who was employed in the Potala Palace as early as in 1664.[21]

In general, Lobsang Chödrak follows the list of terms in the 'Explanatory Tantra' (with the exceptions of the group of costly gems), but for each substance, in addition to the classical indication, he records not only synonyms in a southern tongue but also taste, other pharmacological qualities and a description of the appearance of the substances. Even though the work represents an impressive contribution to the development of Tibetan medicine, it was not officially given as much prominence.

But pharmacology was only one aspect in the medical career of Lobsang Chödrak, who was later appointed director of the Iron Hill Medical College. Regardless of the conflict mentioned above, it is not so clear what role he played in the making of the *Blue Beryl*; according to Manfred Taube it was Lobsang Chödrak who suggested that the Regent write the commentary.[22]

Many phrases in Lobsang Chödrak's pharmacopoeia can be retrieved in the *Blue Beryl* and its Thangka illustrations. Many of its terms were also adopted in Tibet's most outstanding revised and reorganised pharmacological treatise, a work dating from the early eighteenth century called Crystal Globe and Crystal Rosary (Shel gong Shel phreng) compiled by Deumar Geshe Tendzin Püntsok (Devu-dmar Dge-bshes Bstan-vdzin phuntshogs, 1673–1743), comprising more than nine hundred lemmas and a multitude of sub-terms and synonyms. The morphology of medical ingredients, their effect, and the respective parts of plants and animals to be used are described in a very differentiated manner. Deumar's oeuvre can be regarded as the core treasure of Tibetan pharmacology, a fruitful outcome of the seventeenth-century dispute.[23] No illustrated historical edition is known, but it forms the basis for another work which is considered the culmination of the merging of textual and visual Tibetan pharmacological knowledge.[24]

An Illustrated Tibeto-Mongolian Materia Medica

Based on the pharmacopoeias mentioned, *An Illustrated Tibeto-Mongolian Materia Medica* of Jampal Dorje (Vjam-dpal-rdo-rje, 1792–1855) became an important medical blockprint in the nineteenth century.[25] Although the text did not originally play a predominant role in Tibet itself, it became a significant cultural vehicle for its medicine in those northern regions where Mongolian idioms are mainly spoken. Like the Crystal Globe & Crystal Rosary, Jampal Dorje's work, in addition to materia medica, also presents aliments in condensed form, accompanied by wood carved illustrations. Only slightly more than half of the terms found in the previous works are included, but these are provided in four languages in many cases: Tibetan, Mongolian, Manchurian, and Chinese, the latter in both characters and a phonetic transcription in Tibetan script.[26]

Already fifty years ago, Gene Smith called for comprehensive research into this prestigious pharmacological glossary, unfortunately, without success to date. This highlights the fact that the Tibetan orientation towards the Indian subcontinent changed to an alignment with its north-eastern Mongol neighbour that was united with Tibet within the Manchurian Qing state. In medical terms, this went hand in hand with a shift in focus from an ideal or theory-oriented classification to a more symptom-oriented and differentiated morphological description. The style of the images seems to emulate the illustrations in the *Bencao gangmu* by famous Chinese physician Li Shizhen,[27] but the main text is in Tibetan and follows comprehensive Tibetan features of dietetics and pharmacology. An abridged version of the materia medica blockprint, containing only pictures and lemmas, has also been carved, forming the basis for pharmacological flashcards arranged in a sequence similar to the thangka illustrations. A particularly beautiful edition of such an abridged version with coloured medicinal substances can be found in the Institute for Oriental Manuscripts in St Petersburg.[28]

Visualised tree hierarchies

Thus far, the focus has been on pictorial representations of medical content, predominantly of pharmacologically relevant materials such as plants or animal parts. There is yet another way of visualising pharmacological knowledge that is not representational in the immediate sense, but rather depicts structures in a more abstract way. This final section is about the peculiar Tibetan metaphor of unfolding trees (*sdong vgrems*) that systematically organise concepts of knowledge through hierarchical structures.

The thangka sets already contain three such structural representations of medical content within the illustrations to the sixth chapter of the 'Root Tantra', depicting fundamentals of (1) physiology and pathology, (2) diagnostics, and (3) therapy; the 'tree of therapy' divides into four main branches of which the one representing pharmacology is the largest (see Figure S6.1). These fundamental three didactic pattern can be found everywhere in the sphere of Tibetan medical practice. Figure S6.3 represents the pharmacological branch as described in the 'Root Tantra' in Tibetan script I documented in Ulaanbaatar, Mongolia.

The situation is different with regard to the content of the other tantras. Renovations of exceptional historical images of unfolded trees visualising the content of the 'Explanatory Tantra' can be found in the inner courtyard of the Medical College at Labrang Monastery, situated on the North-Eastern fringe of the Tibetan Plateau. The murals feature no fewer than thirty such tree metaphors, an outstanding elaborate assembly in several respects.[29] Each chapter of the 'Explanatory Tantra' is visualised by means of an individual depiction, based on a seventeenth-century text compiled by Lobsang Chödrak.[30]

An additional chapter, the table of contents, is represented by another mural showing four shrubs with a total of eleven trunks that organise the

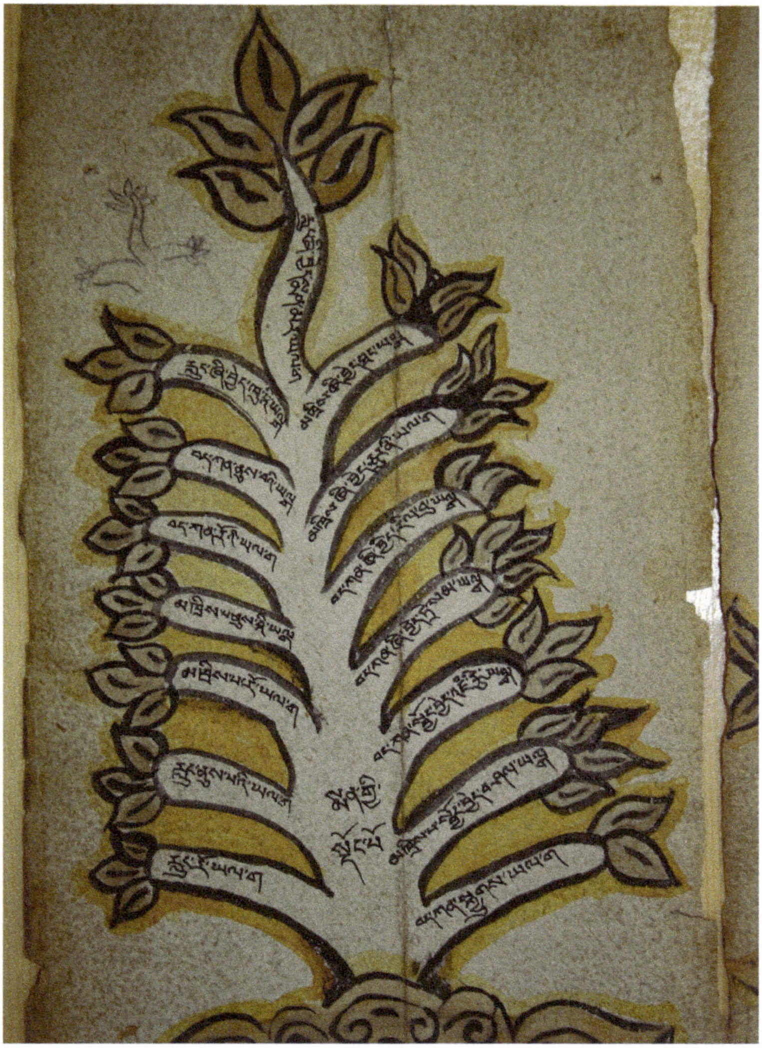

Figure S6.3 Trunk of Pharmacology documented in Mongolia. Ulaanbaatar, Gandan Monastery, 2011. Image credit: Katharina Sabernig

thirty chapters, each represented by a leaf. The experienced teacher thus fulfilled a request of the Regent, who feared that an itemisation of the contents of the 'Explanatory Tantra' by means of tree hierarchies would be too complicated.[31]

In the Labrang representations, the three pharmacological chapters involve eight stems, forty-five twigs or smaller branches, visualising more than six hundred pharmacological ingredients or statements; another tree bears more than two hundred leaves, each symbolising dietary materials

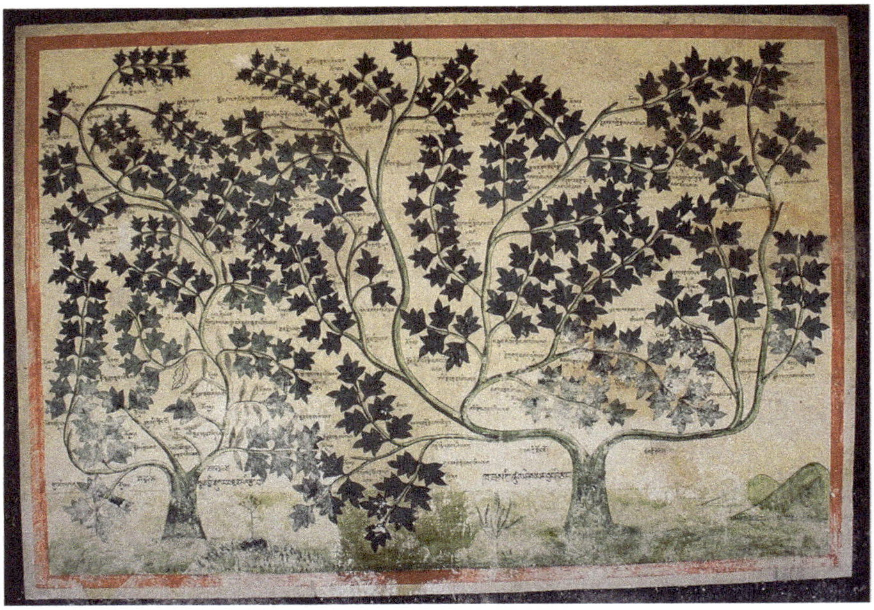

Figure S6.4 Trees of the Explanatory Tantra: chapter 20 on pharmacology on the left side and the chapter 16 on nutrition on the right. Labrang Monestery, Gansu Province 2005. Image credit: Katharina Sabernig

(Figure S6.4). Figure S6.5 presents the knowledge of classification of medicinal groups and methods of application. Notably, the arboreal structures on the murals are only labelled up to the level of the branches.

The more detailed contents of the structure are not listed expressis verbis on the murals, but only symbolised by leaves of varying counts, the intended contents of which the aspiring doctor is required to learn by heart. Here we also see a significant difference between the murals and the thangka images. While the thangkas show in detail the individual materials that are assigned to medical groups, the mural symbolises only the respective group. The rest of the content of the chapter, however, is not further illustrated in the thangka but shown in the mural by two large trunks. In many cases the thangkas and the murals complement each other.[32]

The murals are thus used as mind-maps to help memorise huge amounts of textual knowledge. They can also be used for exams, for example to demonstrate one's grasp and understanding of the content of a chapter by laying out and clarifying its structure. In Labrang Monastery I was shown a set of prepared plastic leaves for the purpose of teaching and for examinations. Even though the textual tradition of the tree metaphor is widespread in the Tibetan cultural area, the visualisation of the whole 'Explanatory Tantra' is a regional peculiarity in the area of Labrang Monastery not documented anywhere else. Several trained doctors have

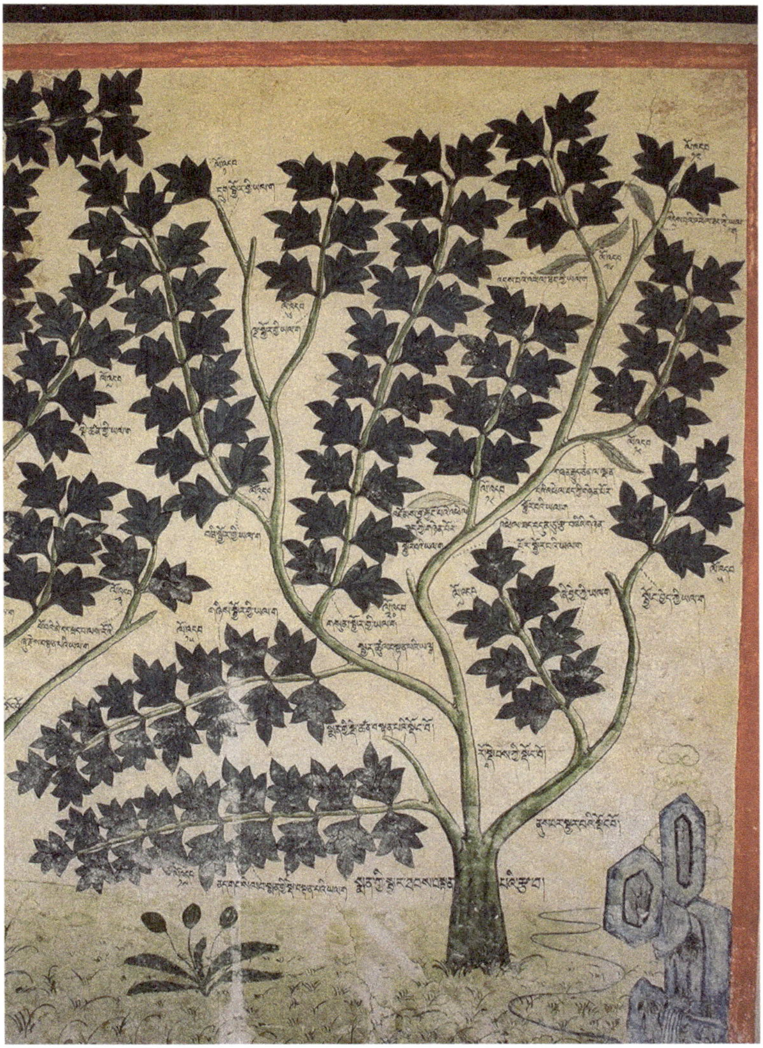

Figure S6.5 Tree on classification of medicinal groups and methods of application, chapter 21. Labrang Monestery, Gansu Province 2005. Image credit: Katharina Sabernig

confirmed to me that they had been encouraged as students to memorise the medical curriculum by using the 'unfolding trees'.

Notes

1 Meyer, 'Introduction', 1992, p. 7.
2 E.g.: Parfionovitch (et al.), *Tibetan Medical Paintings*, 1992; Byams-pa-vphrin-las and Wang Lei, *Tibetan Medical Thangka*, 1994.

3 See in particular Hofer, 'Illustrated Materia Medica', 2014.
4 Gyatso, *Being Human*, 2015.
5 Meyer, 'Golden Century', 2003.
6 The thangka set held in Lhasa includes two more anatomical paintings depicting the human body and superficial blood vessels in crouching position (Byams-pa-vphrin-las and Wang Lei, *Tibetan Medical Thangka*, 1994).
7 Parfionovitch (et al.), *Tibetan Medical Paintings*, 1992.
8 Parfionovitch (et al.), *Tibetan Medical Paintings*, 1992: Thangka 24 nos 46–48, 71, 81–84.
9 Parfionovitch (et al.), *Tibetan Medical Paintings*, 1992: Thangka 28 nos 58–60, 70–78, 81–85.
10 Parfionovitch (et al.), *Tibetan Medical Paintings*, 1992, p. 72 nos 10–12. The word *bse ru* means rhinoceros horn, but in Tibetan practice the material is substituted by yak horn. Read more: Sabernig, 'Substitution of rare ingredients', 2011.
11 Gyatso, *Being Human*, 2015, pp. 25–35.
12 State Hermitage Museum, *Brush and Qalam*, 2018, pp. 139–140.
13 For example, Dekkan, 1595, in the collection of Howard Hodgkin, London. See Liebeskind, 'Die Unani-Medizin', 1997, p. 61.
14 Meyer, 'Introduction', 1992, p. 7.
15 Meyer, 'Introduction', 1992, p. 7.
16 A so-called *dpe-cha* format (Tibetan) or *poti* format (Sanskrit: *pustaka*, meaning book).
17 See Sükhbat and Buyandelger, *Mongolian Medicine*, 2006; Hofer, 'Illustrated Materia Medica', 2014, p. 242.
18 In great length: Gyatso, *Being Human*, 2015, pp. 81–96.
19 Kilty, *Mirror of Beryl*, 2010, p. 333.
20 Blo-bzang-chos-grags, *Bshad pavi rgyud*, 2007.
21 Schaeffer, 'New Scholarship', 2011, pp. 295–296. For more details on his pharmacopoeia see Sabernig, 'Tibetan Materia Medica in Dispute', 2014, and Sabernig, 'Treasure in the History', forthcoming.
22 Taube, *Beiträge*, 1981, p. 73.
23 Sabernig, 'Treasure in the History', forthcoming.
24 A modern edition accompanied by photographic images of respective materials and suggestions of identifications was published in Beijing; it also encloses two versions of the illustrated Tibeto-Mongolian Materia Medica of Vjam-dpal-rdo-rje: Bstan-vdzin-phun-tshogs, *Shel gong Shel phreng*, 2017.
25 Vjam-dpal-rdo-rje, *An Illustrated Tibeto-Mongolian Materia Medica*, 1971.
26 Sabernig, 'Treasure in the History', forthcoming.
27 Hofer, 'Illustrated Materia Medica', 2014, p. 230; Czaja, 'The Use of Insects', 2019, p. 4.
28 State Hermitage Museum, *Brush and Qalam*, 2018, p. 246.
29 Sabernig, *Visualisierte Heilkunde*, 2017, pp. 57–66.
30 Blo-bzang-chos-grags, 'Bshad rgyud kyi sdong vgrems', 2005.
31 Meyer, 'Introduction', 1992, p. 9.
32 See for more details: Sabernig, 'Illustrating the bshad rgyud', 2013.

Afterword

Robert Brennan, Fabian Jonietz, and Romana Sammern

This volume opened with the question: 'Ut pictura medicina?' – 'as in painting, so too in medicine?'. In the past, studies of historical interactions between art and medicine have been confined to a teleologically circumscribed range of comparisons, centred around anatomy and optics. The essays in this volume expanded the range of inquiry into a much wider array of techniques, theoretical sources, and social circumstances that were held in common between the two professions in early modernity. By opening up this expanded view, our aim is not simply to suggest an equivalence between the two professions, as if the question itself – *ut pictura medicina*? – could be resolved with a straightforward 'yes' or 'no'. The aim has rather been to foreground a complex web of entanglements, including both connections and disjunctions, affinities and differences, that could ultimately prove as generative and clarifying, if also irresolvable, as the *ut pictura poesis* analogy itself.

To this end, a primary task of these essays has been to demonstrate the significance and scope of the analogy as a feature of early modern discourses of art and medicine. From Taddeo Alderotti to Pier Antonio Fucini, the essays in this volume have brought to light numerous cases in which visual art and medicine were explicitly analogised in theory, and consciously united in practice. These types of convergence far outstrip the traditional conception of art 'aiding' medicine through anatomical illustration, or medicine 'aiding' art through optical theory, for they extend to some of the most foundational practices within each discipline, aligning artistic techniques with medical procedures, medical criteria of diagnosis with artistic methods of observation, and the theoretical aims of art with medical definitions of health, to name just a few of many examples. Alongside identifying the depth of such analogies as they appear in primary sources, a second, equally important task of the volume has been to draw out their wider implications for current scholarship: that is, to show how they can help to open up new interdisciplinary avenues of analysis for histories of the body, embodied knowledge, and transregional connectivity, among other approaches.

In this afterword, we synthesise several themes that emerged out of the book's essays and suggest possible directions for future research. The account that we offer is far from comprehensive in either of these respects. Readers who engage with the essays will surely recognise many further narratives and methodological cues that the following reflections pass over in silence. This includes some of the most conspicuous and persistent themes not only of the volume, but also of broader currents in art history and medical humanities research, such as the role of colour – in its political and aesthetic, as well as diagnostic and therapeutic valences – as a crucially important, shared concern of both disciplines.[1] We hope that scholars will take up and develop many such themes that are not explicitly mentioned in what follows.

Entangled aims?

The volume begins with essays by Catherine Lawless and Carly B. Boxer, exploring a persistent link between the aims and functions of late medieval art and medicine: the use of votive images in processes of divine healing, which both paralleled and competed with the remedies offered by professional physicians. This link remained in place throughout the early modern period and beyond, but not without generating a number of tensions and ambiguities that proved formative for both professions. Indeed, as Lawless and Boxer show, the cult of ex votos gave rise to pressing questions concerning the relation between the religious and scientific function of images, sacred and secular remedies, physical and mental health, as well as tensions between the economic and ethical dimensions of healing. The practice of 'chromotherapy', explored in Katharina Stahlbuhk's essay, straddles similar boundaries between what in retrospect might be regarded as physiological, psychosomatic, and psychological ailments, while in Robert Brennan's essay, economic interests can be seen to impinge upon and trouble distinctions between norms of health and beauty. In general, however, over the course of these first four essays, it is possible to discern a shift from the cultic and curative functions of the votive image toward more aestheticised modes of interaction between art and medicine, centring on visual pleasure and ocular relief.

It is easy to imagine how this shift could be conceived teleologically as part of a broader narrative toward an increasingly familiar, modern distinction between the therapeutic aims of medicine and the aesthetic aims of art. However, comparable – if not identical – distinctions were already well developed within the Galenic tradition of medicine,[2] and on closer examination, each one of the opening four essays also cuts against the grain of such a narrative in certain respects. This is apparent, for example, in Boxer's emphasis on the ex voto's intersection with late-medieval discourses of portraiture, Lawless' exploration of the psychological functions of images in healing practices, Brennan's comparison of medieval and modern 'beauty industries', and Stahlbuhk's observations concerning the survival of chromotherapy in twentieth-century aesthetic and esoteric traditions. Viewed in this light, these early chapters might suggest something less like a step toward the increasing autonomy of art from medicine, and more like a call for further inquiry into why the shifting boundaries between the aesthetic and the therapeutic have remained so permeable and contested from the later Middle Ages into the modern era.

Entangled predicaments?

Another persistent theme of the volume lies in the overlapping social and intellectual predicament of artists and physicians in early modernity. In Minden's essay, for example, we see how Jacopo Berengario staked his authority as a medical writer on handwork, embodied knowledge, and discourses of 'judgement', 'ingenuity', and 'difficulty' that play prominent roles in early modern theories of visual art. Fabian Jonietz demonstrates how such artistic skills could support medical practice, and vice versa, through direct collaborations between physicians and painters, such as Dominicus de Ragusa and Gentile da Fabriano. Paralleling such direct collaborations, the volume has also documented a wide array of cases in which physicians were regarded as specialised viewers of art, from Filippo Villani's account of Stefano Fiorentino (Brennan) to Cellini's praise of Berengario for his 'great intelligence for design' (Minden), as well as the role of physicians as observers of works by artists such as Raphael and Titian (Jonietz). This role becomes all the more conspicuous in the writings of physician-connoisseurs like Giulio Mancini and his student Sebastiano Vannini, as explored by Frances Gage and Fabrizio Federici.[3]

In many of these cases, the interaction of artists and physicians – whether as collaborators or observers – suggests clear affinities between the two disciplines. And yet as Frances Gage shows, Mancini also went to great lengths to distinguish painting and sculpture from other professions, including his own, on the basis of the physical labours involved, generating analogies with slavery or mercenary service that could both trouble and buttress more ennobling comparisons with the liberal arts. A similar tension is apparent in the relationship between the two seventeenth-century sources introduced by Jana Graul and Fabian Jonietz: whereas Bernardino Ramazzini draws upon his medical knowledge to foreground the vile – indeed, literally poisonous – materiality of the painter's profession, Pier

Antonio Fucini cites medical authorities to make a case for the affinity, interdependence, and shared nobility of the two professions.

These conflicting views suggest a variety of directions for future research into the social and intellectual position of early modern artists and physicians, amongst other 'practitioners of the body':[4] research that might usefully expand beyond cases of direct interaction to encompass connections and comparisons between the educational, economic, and institutional settings of each discipline, as well as the broader dynamics of gender, class, and ethnicity that underpin them.

Entangled geographies?

Already in the introduction we noted shared foundations in Arabic medical discourse that linked Cennino Cennini's *Libro dell'arte* with the Florentine *Ricettario*. The sources introduced by Brennan show that well before Cennini, Arabic medical discourse had already constituted an important source for Florentine knowledge of ancient art, including such canonical works as Polykleitos' *Canon*. The continuing vitality of such exchanges is evident in Jonietz's essay, where the work of medical writers like Rhazes, Isaac Judaeus, and Haly Abbas guided the collaboration between Dominicus de Ragusa and Gentile da Fabriano, just as Lorenzo Ghiberti turned to Rhazes, Avicenna, and Averroes as sources for his own writings on art. Whereas in Eurocentric histories of science, these types of connection have traditionally been thought to end with the Scientific Revolution, Sabernig's essay demonstrates their ongoing importance throughout the transformative developments of the seventeenth century.

Sabernig's essay also marks a fitting end to the volume by returning us to the genre of pharmacological literature with which we began in the analysis of Cennini's *Libro* and the Florentine *Ricettario*. The transregional circulation of knowledge mediated by this genre is evident not only from Sabernig's contributions, but also in Julia Czapla and Paolo Sanvito's overviews of Stefan Falimirz' *O ziołach* and Georgius Josephus Camel's drawings. In all of these cases, pharmacology draws artistic and medical practices together, while at the same connecting a wide range of geographies from Poland and the Czech Republic to Tibet and the Philippines. In these respects, the essays should be read alongside recent work on the Atlantic world, in which the circulation of pharmacological knowledge plays a prominent role in stories of colonial extraction and Afro-diasporic resistance.[5] The potential of pharmacology for the writing of transregional, connected histories of both art and medicine thus seems clear. How the multifaceted layers of connection that we observed at the outset of this volume between Cennini and the *Ricettario* might figure within this wider world of interaction remains an open question.

Reevaluating anatomy and optics

In the case of pharmacology, links between art and medicine are most readily apparent at the level of medical illustration: the artist records the appearances of the natural phenomena that the medical writer seeks to catalogue and study. This is comparable to the sorts of links that have guided traditional approaches to the relation of art and medicine, centred around optics and anatomy. This volume has deliberately looked away from these established areas of study in hopes of charting less readily apparent, but

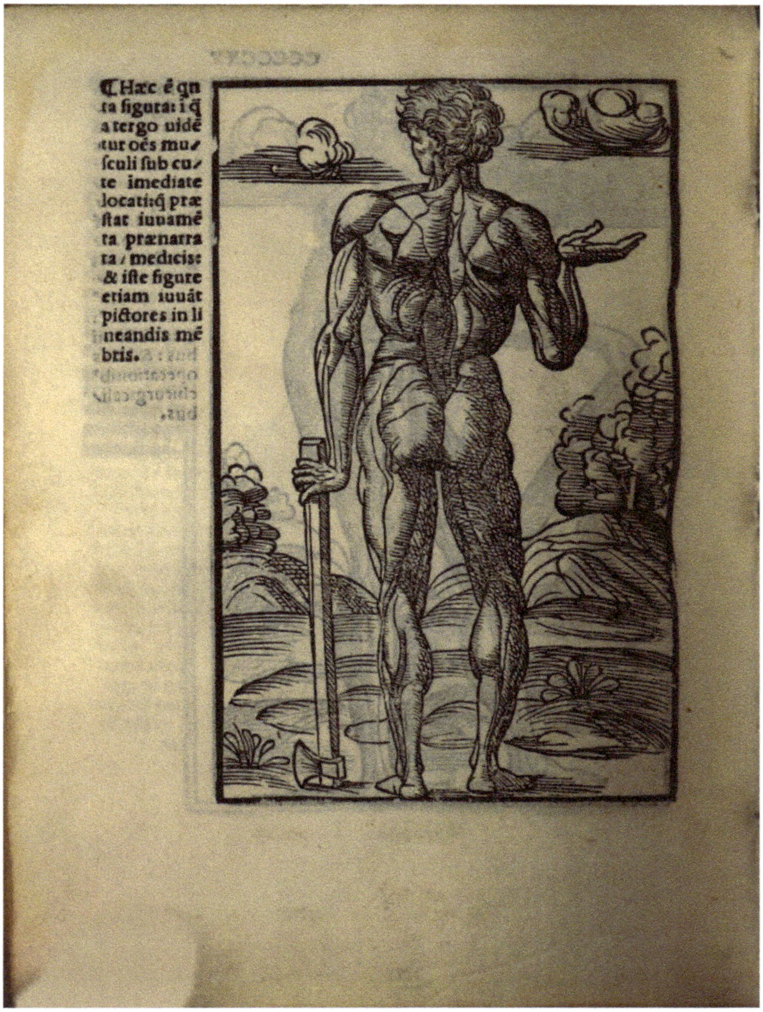

Figure 10.1 Jacopo Berengario da Carpi, Carpi commentaria cum amplissimis additionibus super anatomia Mundini…, Bologna, 1521, fol. 520v. Munich, Bayerische Staatsbibliothek, Res/4 Anat. 38. Image credit: Bayerische Staatsbibliothek

equally crucial modes of exchange. In the future, however, it may become increasingly unnecessary to insist upon such a neat distinction of optics and anatomy from the wider social, epistemological, and political aspects of the relationship between art and medicine.

As Minden noted, for example, Berengario has long stood as a classic figure in studies of art-medicine relations due to the classicising anatomical images that illustrate his treatises, complete with captions that explicitly note how such images 'help painters in delineating the members' (Figure 10.1). However, if we follow Minden's argument and look beyond such explicit points of contact, we find a network of interrelations far more foundational both to Berengario's broader intellectual agenda and to the very craft of art making.

A similar principle can be drawn from other essays as well. In a more traditional paradigm of research, the wax anatomical models noted by Boxer, or the attention that Cimabue and Giotto devote to skeletal and muscular anatomy at the beginning of Brennan's essay, could have stood as the end point of the analysis. Stahlbuhk likewise engages with principles of colour perception that pervade medieval and early modern optical literature, though she scarcely touches upon the concerns with naturalism that have traditionally guided research on the topic in art history.

The same can be said of such canonically important figures as Andreas Vesalius, who surfaces in Jonietz and Sabernig's essays, but without reference to the anatomical illustrations that weigh so heavily in previous art historical scholarship. In all of these cases, the effect has not been to invalidate the mediating role of anatomy and optics, but rather to recast it as the tip of an iceberg, composed of deeper, more pervasive intertwinements that extend far and wide across the early modern world.

Notes

1 For example, Hannah Murphy's important project, *Medicine and the Making of Race, 1440–1720* https://www.mmor.co.uk/ (accessed 6 August 2025).
2 For example, Galen, *Opera omnia*, 1821–1833, vol. 12, 434; Galen, *Opera*, 1490, vol. 1, fol. 198vb.
3 In Italy, this analysis could be extended to figures such as Michele Savonarola, Michelangelo Biondo, Paolo Giovio, and Francesco Scannelli, not to mention other early modern European figures such as Samuel Quiccheberg in Germany or Mayerne and Haydocke in England.
4 Cavallo, *Artisans of the Body*, 2007.
5 Sweet, *Domingos Álvares*, 2011; Gómez, *The Experiential Caribbean*, 2017; Kananoja, *Healing Knowledge in Atlantic Africa*, 2021. For an excellent art historical approach to such issues, see Anna Arabindon-Kesson's project, *Art Hx: Visual and Medical Legacies of British Colonialism* https://artandcolonialmedicine.com/ (accessed 14 January 2025).

Bibliography

Ackerman, James: 'The Involvement of Artists in Renaissance Science', in: *Science and the Arts in the Renaissance*, ed. by John W. Shirley and F. David Hoeniger, Washington 1985, pp. 94–129.

Agosti, Barbara: *Paolo Giovio. Uno storico lombardo nella cultura artistica del Cinquecento*, Florence 2008.

Akopyan, Ovanes and Anastasia Malkova: 'Medicine, Astrology and Self-Censorship: Translating Marsilio Ficino in Muscovy (ca. 1580 – 1620)', in: *Rinascimento* 62 (2022), pp. 165–202.

Alberti, Alessia: 'Dai giardini dipinti alle sale alberate. Precedenti figurative e letterari per la Sala delle Asse', in: *Leonardo da Vinci. All'ombra del Moro. La Sala delle Asse del Castello Sforzesco*, ed. by Claudia Salsi and Alessia Alberti, 2 vols, Milan 2019, vol. II, pp. 108–131.

Alberti, Leon Battista: 'De pictura', in: *Opere volgari*, ed. by Cecil Grayson, 3 vols, Bari 1960–1973, vol. 3, pp. 5–107.

Alberti, Leon Battista: *On Painting*, ed. and transl. by Rocco Sinisgalli, Cambridge 2011.

Albertus Magnus: 'Commentary on Aristotle, On Memory and Recollection', in: *The Medieval Craft of Memory: An Anthology of Texts and Pictures*, ed. by Mary Carruthers and Jan Ziolkowski, Philadelphia 2002, pp. 118–152.

Alce, Venturino and Alfonso d'Amato: *La Biblioteca di S. Domenico in Bologna*, Florence 1961.

Alderotti, Taddeo: *In Galeni micratechnen comentarij*, Naples 1522.

Alderotti, Taddeo: *Expositiones in arduum aphorismorum Ipocratis volume* [...] *In subtilissimum Joannitii Isagogarum libellum*, Venice 1527.

Alderotti, Taddeo: *Libello per conservare la sanità del corpo*, Imola 1852.

Alderotti, Taddeo: *I 'Consilia'*, ed. by Giuseppe Michele Nardi, Turin 1937.

Aldrovandi, Ulisse: *Quadrupedum omnium bisulcorum historia.* [...], Bologna 1621.

Anagnostou, Sabine: 'Missionsmedizin und Missionspharmazie im kolonialen Amerika', in: *Sendung – Eroberung – Begegnung. Franz Xaver, die Gesellschaft Jesu und die katholische Weltkirche im Zeitalter des Barock*, ed. by Johannes Meier (Studien zur Außereuropäischen Christentumsgeschichte [Asien, Afrika, Lateinamerika]. Studies in the History of Christianity in the Non-Western World; 8), Wiesbaden 2005, pp. 261–291.

Antoine, Elizabeth: 'Ex voto', in: *Dictionnaire encyclopédique du Moyen Âge*, ed. by André Vauchez and Catherine Vincent, 2 vols, Paris 1997, vol. 1, p. 564.

Arasse, Daniel: 'Entre devotion et culture: fonctions de l'image religieuse au XVe siècle', in: *Faire croire. Modalités de la diffusion et de la reception des messages religieux du XIIe–XVe siècle*, ed. by André Vauchez, Rome, 1981, pp. 131–146.

Aristotle: *Meteorologica*, transl. by H. D. P. Lee, Cambridge MA 1978.

Aristotle: 'On Marvelous Things Heard', in: *Minor Works*, ed. and transl. by W. S. Hett, Cambridge MA 1980, pp. 238–327.

Aristotle: 'On Plants', in: *Minor Works*, ed. and transl. by W. S. Hett, Cambridge MA 1980, pp. 142–235.

Aristotle: 'On Sense and Sensible Objects', in: *On the Soul – Parva Naturalia – On Breath*, transl. by W. S. Hett, Cambridge MA 1975, pp. 214–286.

Aristotle: *Problems II (Books XXII–XXXVIII)*, transl. by W. S. Hett, Cambridge MA 1965.

Armstrong, Regis J., J. A. Wayne Hellmann, and William J. Short (eds): *The Saint. Vol. I of Francis of Assisi: The Early Documents*, New York 1999.

Armstrong, Regis J., J. A. Wayne Hellmann and William J. Short (eds): *The Founder. Vol. II of Francis of Assisi: The Early Documents*, New York 2000.

Ars medica nelle Gallerie degli Uffizi, ex. cat., ed. by Donatella Lippi (et al.), Florence 2022.

Art of Vesalius, ed. by Robrecht Van Hee and Maurits Biesbrouck, Antwerp (et al.) 2014

Asen, Daniel: '"Manchu Anatomy": Anatomical Knowledge and the Jesuits in Seventeenth- and Eighteenth-Century China', in: *Social History of Medicine* 22:1 (2009), pp. 23–44.

Ash, Eric H.: 'By Any Other Name: Early Modern Expertise and the Problem of Anachronism', in: *History and Technology* 35:1 (2019), pp. 3–30.

À travers le verre du moyen âge à la renaissance, exh. cat., ed. by Danièle Foy and Geneviève Sennequier, Nancy-Maxéville 1989.

Saint Augustine: *The Trinity*, transl. by Stephen McKenna, ed. by The Catholic University of America, Washington 2010.

Azzolini, Monica: 'Leonardo da Vinci's Anatomical Studies in Milan: A Re-examination of Sites and Sources', in: *Visualizing Medieval Medicine and Natural History, 1200–1550*, ed. by Jean A. Givens, Karen M. Reeds and Alain Touwaide, Aldershot 2006, pp. 147–176.

Bacci, Michele: *Il pennello dell'Evangelista. Storia delle immagini sacre attribuite a san Luca*, Pisa 1998.

Bacci, Michele: *Lo spazio dell'anima: vita di una chiesa medievale*, Bari 2005.

Bacci, Michele: 'L'individu en tant prototype dans les ex-voto médiévaux', in: *Degrés – Revue de synthèse à orientation semiologique* 145–146 (2011), pp. 1–14.

Bacci, Michele, 'Italian Ex-Votos and 'Pro-Anima' Images in the Late Middle Ages', in: *Ex-Voto: Votive Giving Across Cultures*, ed. by Ittai Weinryb, New York 2016, pp. 76–105.

Bacon, Roger: *Liber de sensu et sensato. Summa de sophismatibus et distinctionibus*, ed. by Robert Steele, London 1937.

Baglione, Giovanni: *Le vite de' pittori, scultori, et architetti, dal pontificato di Gregorio XIII del 1572 in fino a' tempi di Papa Urbano Ottavo nel 1642*, Rome 1970.

Baldacchini, Lorenzo (ed.): *La Biblioteca Malatestiana di Cesena*, Rome 1992.

Baldasseroni, Alberto and Francesco Carnevale: *Malati di lavoro. Artigiani e lavoratori, medicina e medici da Bernarduni Ramazzini a Luigi Devoto (1700–1900)*, Florence 2015, pp. 35–211.

Baldi, Marialuisa (ed.): *Girolamo Cardano. Le opera, le fonti, la vita*, Milan 1999.

Baldinucci, Filippo: *Notizie de' professori del disegno da Cimabue in qua*, 6 vols, Florence 1681–1728.

Baldinucci, Filippo: *Vita di Gian Lorenzo Bernini con l'inedita vita del Baldinucci scritta dal figlio Francesco Saverio*, ed. by Sergio Samek Ludovici, Milan 1948.

Baldriga, Irene: *L'occhio della lince. I primi Lincei tra arte, scienza e collezionismo (1603–1630)*, Rome 2002.

Bales, Kevin: *Disposable People: New Slavery in the Global Economy*, Berkeley 1999.
Bambach, Carmen: *Leonardo da Vinci: Master Draftsman*, New Haven 2003.
Barkan, Leonard: *Nature's Work of Art: The Human Body as Image of the World*, New Haven 1975.
Baroni, Sandro, Simona Rinaldi, and Paolo Travaglio: 'Formation, Transmission and Genres in the Recipe Books of Art Technology between the Middle Ages and the 18th Century: New Proposals for Analysis and Interpretation', in: *Contribution à une histoire technologique de l'art*, ed. by Claire Betelu, Anne Servais, Cécile Parmentier, actes de journées d'étude de la composante de recherche PBC, Paris 2018, pp. 9–42.
Barr, Helen: 'Alessandro Allori: Schöne Oberfläche und traurig stimmende Knochen (1560er Jahre)', in: *Schönheit – Der Körper als Kunstprodukt*, ed. by Romana Sammern and Julia Saviello, Berlin 2019, pp. 221–230.
Barrett, Anthony A.: *Rome Is Burning: Nero and the Fire that Ended a Dynasty*, Princeton 2022.
Bartholin, Thomas: *Bartholinus Anatomy: Made from the Percepts of His Father, and from the Observation of all Modern Anatomists, Together with His Own*, London 1668.
Bartholomeus Anglicus: *De rerum proprietatibus*, Frankfurt 1601.
Bartisch, Georg: *Οφθαλμοδουλεια. Das ist/Augendienst. [...]*, Dresden 1583.
Baschet, Jérôme: 'Introduction: L'Image-Object', in: *L'image. Fonctions et usages des images dans l'Occident médiéval*. Actes du 6 'International Workshop on Medieval Societies', Centre Ettore Majorana (Erice, Sicile, 17–23 octobre 1992), ed. by Jérôme Baschet and Jean-Claude Schmitt, Paris 1992, pp. 7–28.
Baumann, Helmut and Brigitte Baumann: *Die Mainzer Kräuterbuch-Inkunabeln: 'Herbarius Moguntinus' (1484), 'Gart der Gesundheit' (1485), 'Hortus Sanitatis' (1491). Wissenschaftshistorische Untersuchung der drei Prototypen botanisch-medizinischer Literatur des Spätmittelalters*, Stuttgart 2010.
Baxandall, Michael: 'Bartholomaeus Facius on Painting: A Fifteenth-Century Manuscript of the De Viris Illustribus', in: *Journal of the Warburg and Courtauld Institutes* 27 (1964), pp. 90–107.
Baxandall, Michael: *Giotto and the Orators: Humanist Observers of Painting in Italy and the Discovery of Pictorial Composition, 1350–1450*, Oxford 1971.
Beccadelli, Antonio: *The Hermaphrodite*, ed. by Holt Parker, London 2010.
Beck, Emily: 'Authority, Authorship, and Copying: The *Ricettario Fiorentino* and Manuscript Recipe Culture in Sixteenth-Century Florence', in: *Drugs on the Page*, Pittsburgh 2019, pp. 45–62.
Bedos-Rezak, Brigitte: 'Medieval Identity: A Sign and a Concept', in: *The American Historical Review* 105 (2000), pp. 1489–1533.
Bedos-Rezak, Brigitte: 'Ego, Ordo, Communitas: Seals and the Medieval Semiotics of Personality (1200–1350)', in: *Die Bildlichkeit korporativer Siegel im Mittelalter: Kunstgeschichte und Geschichte im Gespräch*, ed. by M. Spath, Cologne 2009, pp. 47–64.
Bedos-Rezak, Brigitte: *When Ego Was Imago: Signs of Identity in the Middle Ages*, Leiden 2011.
Bell, Adrian R. and Richard S. Dale: 'The Medieval Pilgrimage Business', in: *Enterprise & Society* 12 (2011), pp. 601–627.
Bellori, Giovan Pietro: *Le vite de' pittori scultori e architetti moderni*, 2 vols, ed. by Evelina Borea, Introduction by Giovanni Previtali, Epilogue by Tomaso Montanari, Reprint Turin 2009 (first ed. 1976).
Bellosi, Luciano: 'Giottino e la pittura di filiazione giottesca intorno alla metà del Trecento', in: *Prospettiva* 121/124 (2006), pp. 347–368.
Belting, Hans: *The Image and Its Public in the Middle Ages: Form and Function of Early Paintings of the Passion*, New Rochelle 1990.
Belting, Hans: *Likeness and Presence: A History of the Image Before the Era of Art*, Chicago 1994.

Benvenuto da Imola: *Comentum super Dantis Aldigherij comoediam*, ed. by James Philip Lacaita, Florence 1887.

Berengario da Carpi, Jacopo: *Tractatus de fractura calvae sive cranei*, Bologna 1518.

Berengario da Carpi, Jacopo: *Commentaria cum amplissimis additionibus super anathomia Mundini*, Bologna 1521.

Berengario da Carpi, Jacopo: *Isagoge breves perlucide ac uberrime in anatomiam humani corporis*, Bologna 1522.

Berengario da Carpi, Jacopo: *A Short Introduction to Anatomy*, transl. by L. R. Lind, Chicago 1959.

Bergdolt, Klaus: *Arzt, Krankheit und Therapie bei Petrarca. Die Kritik an Medizin und Naturwissenschaft im italienischen Frühhumanismus*, Weinheim 1992.

Berger, Susanna: 'Georg Bartisch's *Ophthalmodouleia* and His Theory of Painting and Drawing', in: *Early Science and Medicine* 26 (2021), pp. 1–54.

Bernardino Ramazzini, primo medico di lavoro, exh. cat., ed. by Manuela Kahn-Rossi and Tania Previdi, Carpi 2020.

Bernini, Domenico: *Vita di Cavaliere Gio. Lorenzo Bernini*, Rome 1713.

Bernini, Domenico: *The Life of Gian Lorenzo Bernini: A Translation and Critical Edition, with Introduction and Commentary*, ed. by Franco Mormando, University Park 2011.

Bertolotti, Domenico: *Un professore alla Sapienza di Roma nel secolo XVII poco conosciuto*, Rome 1886.

Bettini, Sergio: 'In Biblioteca: Sisto IV, il Platina e l'architettura dipinta nell'affresco di Melozzo da Forlì', in: *Saggi e memorie di storia dell'arte* 34 (2010), pp. 55–66.

Beuzelin, Cécile: 'Jacopo Pontormo: A Scholarly Craftsman', in: *The Artist as Reader: On Education and Non-Education of Early Modern Artists*, ed. by Claus Zittel, Heiko Damm, and Michael Thimann, Leiden 2012, pp. 71–104.

Beyer, Andreas: *Künstler, Leib und Eigensinn. Die vergessene Signatur des Lebens in der Kunst*, Berlin 2022.

Bidloo, Govard: *Anatomia humani corporis: centum & quinque tabvlis per artificiosiss. G. De Lairesse ad vivum delineatis, demonstrata, veterum recentiorumque inventis explicata plurimisque, hactenus non detectis, illvstrata*, Amsterdam 1685.

Biernoff, Suzannah: *Sight and Embodiment in the Middle Ages*, Houndsmill 2002.

Biller, Peter: 'Proto-Racial Thought in Medieval Science', in: *The Origins of Racism in the West*, ed. by Miriam Eliav-Feldon, Benjamin H. Isaac, and Joseph Ziegler, Cambridge 2009, pp. 157–180.

Bindman, David: *Ape to Apollo: Aesthetics and the Idea of Race in the 18th Century*, London 2002.

Bindman, David: *'Race Is Everything': Art and Human Difference*, Chicago 2023.

Bindman, David and Henry Louis Gates, Jr. (eds): *The Image of the Black in Western Art*, 5 vols, Cambridge 2010–2014.

Bisogni, Fabio: 'Ex voto e la scultura in cera nel tardo medioevo', in: *Visions of Holiness: Art and Devotion in Renaissance Italy*, ed. by Andrew Ladis and Shelley E. Zuraw, Athens GA 2001, pp. 66–91.

Black, Christopher: *Early Modern Italy: A Social History*, London 2001.

Blick, Sarah: 'Votives, Images, Interaction and Pilgrimage to the Tomb of and Shrine of St Thomas Becket, Canterbury Cathedral', in: *Push Me, Pull You: Imaginative, Emotional, Physical, and Spatial Interaction in Late Medieval and Renaissance Art*, ed. by Sarah Blick and Laura Gelfand, Leiden 2011, pp. 21–58.

Blo-bzang-chos-grags [Dar-mo sman-rams-pa]: 'Bshad rgyud kyi sdong vgrems legs bshad gser gyi thur ma', in: *Legs bshad gser gyi thur ma bkav phreng mun sel sgron me* (Bod kyi gso ba rig pavi gnav dpe phyogs bsgrigs dpe tshogs), Pe cin 2005, pp. 1–143.

Blo-bzang-chos-grags [Dar-mo sman-rams-pa]: *Bshad pavi rgyud kyi levu nyi shu pa sman gyi nus pa bstan pavi tshig gi don gyi vgrel ba mes povi dgongs rgyan (Bod kyi gso ba rig pavi gnav dpe phyogs bsgrigs dpe tshogs)*, Pe cin 2007, pp. 1–200.

Boenke, Michaela: 'Einleitung', in: Marsilio Ficino, *De vita libri tres – Drei Bücher über das Leben*, transl. and ed. by Michaela Boenke, Munich 2012, pp. 6–32.

Bohde, Daniela: '"Le tinte delle carni": Zur Begrifflichkeit für Haut und Fleisch in italienischen Kunsttraktaten des 15. bis 17. Jahrhunderts', in: *Weder Haut noch Fleisch: Das Inkarnat in der Kunstgeschichte*, ed. by Daniela Bohde and Mechthild Fend, Berlin 2007, pp. 41–63.

Bohn, Babette: *Women Artists, their Patrons, and their Publics in Early Modern Bologna*, University Park 2021.

Bolland, J. and G. Henschen (eds): *Acta sanctorum*, Antwerp, 1643–.

Bolland, J. and G. Henschen (eds): *Acta sanctorum, octobris, tomus IV*, Brussels 1780.

Bolland, J. and G. Henschen (eds): *Acta sanctorum, januarius, tomus III*, Paris 1863.

Bolland, J. and G. Henschen (eds): *Acta sanctorum, aprilis, tomus II*, Paris 1866.

Bolland, J. and G. Henschen (eds): *Acta sanctorum, aprilis, tomus III*, Paris 1866.

Bolland, J. and G. Henschen (eds): *Acta sanctorum, maii, tomus V*, Paris 1866.

Bolland, J. and G. Henschen (eds): *Acta sanctorum, maii, tomus VII*, Paris 1866.

Bonaventura: *Commentaria in quatuor libros sententiarum magistri Petri Lombardi*, Florence 1887.

Bonifacio, Giovanni: *L'arte de' cenni*, Vicenza 1616.

Bonne, Jean-Claude: "Répresentation médiévale et lieu sacré", in: *Luoghi sacri e spazi della santità*, ed. by Sofia Boesch-Gajano and Lucetta Scaraffia, Turin 1990, pp. 565–571.

Bónoli, Fabrizio and Daniela Piliarvu: *I lettori di astronomia presso lo studio di Bologna dal XII al XX secolo*, Bologna 2001.

Bonsanti, Giorgio: '"La pittura non consiste solamente in fare uomini nudi": Considerazioni sul disegno di Raffaello nella Biblioteca Marucelliana', in: *...Per fare notomia*, ed. by Silvia Castelli and Piera Giovanna Tordella, Florence 2021, pp. 56–62.

Boschini, Marco: *Le ricche minere della pittura veneziana*, Venice 1674.

Boureau, Alain: *Théologie, science et censure au XIIIe siècle: le cas de Jean Peckham*, Paris 2008.

Bowles, John P.: 'Blinded by the White: Art History and the Limits of Whiteness', in: *Art Journal* 60:4 (2001), pp. 38–43.

Boxer, Carly B.: 'Uroscopy Diagrams, Judgment, and the Perception of Colour in Late Medieval England', in: *Word & Image* 38:4 (2022), pp. 327–347.

Bracco, Paola, Ottavio Ciappi, and Anna-Marie Hilling: 'La pittura della *Croce* di Ognissanti: letture techniche ed intervento di restauro', in: *L'officina di Giotto: il restauro della Croce di Ognissanti*, ed. by Paola Bracco, Ottavio Ciappi, and Anna-Marie Hilli, Florence 2010, pp. 103–162.

Branca, Vittore (ed.), *Mercanti scrittori: ricordi nella Firenze tra Medioevo e Rinascimento*, Milan 1986.

Brasavola, Antonio Musa: *Index refertissimus in omnes Galeni libros, qui ex Iuntarum tertia editione extant*, Venice 1556.

Bredekamp, Horst: 'Substitutive Image Acts: The Exchange of Body and Image', in: *Image Acts: A Systematic Approach to Visual Agency*, transl. by Elizabeth Clegg, Berlin 2018, pp. 137–192.

Brennan, Robert: *Painting as a Modern Art in Early Renaissance Italy*, London 2019.

Bridget of Sweden: *Revelationes caelestes seraphicae*, Munich 1680.

Britton, Piers: '"Mio malinchonico, o vero...mio pazzo": Michelangelo, Vasari, and the Problem of Artists' Melancholy in Sixteenth-Century Italy', in: *The Sixteenth Century Journal* 34 (2003), pp. 653–675.

Britton, Piers: 'Raphael and the Bad Humours of Painters in Vasari's *Lives of the Artists*', in: *Renaissance Studies* 22 (2008), pp. 174–196.

Bronzini, Giovanni Battista: 'Fenomenologia dell'ex voto', in: *Lares* 44 (1978), pp. 143–176.

Broomhall, Susan: *Women's Medical Work in Early Modern France*, Manchester 2004.

Brucker, Gene: 'Sorcery in Early Renaissance Florence', in: *Studies in the Renaissance* 10 (1963), pp. 7–24.

Bruhn, Matthias: 'Harndruck. Farbskalen zwischen Gestaltung und Diagnostik', in: *Bilder der Präzision. Praktiken der Verfeinerung in Technik, Kunst und Wissenschaft*, ed. by Matthias Bruhn and Sara Hillnhütter, Berlin 2018, pp. 229–235.

Bstan-vdzin-phun-tshogs [18th cent]: *Shel gong shel phreng*. Pe cin 2017, pp. 1–962.

Buck, August: 'Die Medizin im Verständnis des Renaissancehumanismus', in: *Humanismus und Medizin*, ed. by Rudolf Schmitz and Gundolf Keil, Weinheim 1984, pp. 181–198.

Bucklow, Spike: *The Alchemy of Paint: Art, Science and Secrets from the Middle Ages*, London 2009.

Bulang, Tobias: 'Experte oder Scharlatan? Leonhard Thurneysser zum Thurn und seine Uroskopie', in: *Zeitsprünge* 17 (2013), pp. 161–182.

Bułhak, 'Ungler Florian', in: *Drukarze dawnej Polski*, ed. by Alodia Kawecka-Gryczowa, vol. I:1, Wrocław 1983, pp. 307–311.

Bull, George (ed.): *Michelangelo: Life, Letters, and Poetry*, 2nd ed., Oxford 1999 (first 1987).

Burr, David: *Spiritual Franciscans: From Protest to Persecution in the Century after Saint Francis*, University Park 2003.

Byams-pa-vphrin-las and Wang Lei: *Bod lugs gso rig rgyud bzhivi nang don bris cha ngo mtshar mthong ba don ldan = Tibetan Medical Thangka of the Four Medical Tantras*, transl. by Cai Jingfeng, Lha sa 1994.

Byams-pa-phrin-las: *Gangs ljongs gso rig bstan pavi nyin byed rim byon gyi rnam thar phyogs bsgrigs*, Pe cin 2000.

Caciola, Nancy: *Discerning Spirits: Divine and Daemonic Possession in the Middle Ages*, Ithaca 2003.

Camel, Georg Joseph: *Historia Plantarum Species hactenus editas aliasque insuper multas noviter inventas & descriptas complectens* [...], London 1704 (digital version in the Biblioteca – Real Jardín Botánico de Madrid).

Camel, Georg Joseph: *Tractatus de plantis Philippensibus scandentibus*, Philosophical Transactions of the Royal Society 24, 1704, pp. 1707–1722.

Camel, Georg Joseph: *VIII. Georg. Joseph. Camel. De plantis philippensibus scandentibus; pars tertia. ad Jacobum Petiver, S. R. S. nuper transmissa*, London 1705.

Camel, Georg Joseph: 'De quadrupedibus philippensibus tractat. a Reverendo Georg. Jos. Camel, transmissus Jacobo Petiver, pharmacop, & Societ. Regiæ Soc. Londini', in: *Philosophical Transactions of the Royal Society of London*, II, vol. 25, 1706, 2197–2204.

Camel, Georg Joseph: *Herbarum aliarumque stirpium in insulâ Luzone Philippinarum primariâ nascentium icones ab autore delineatæ ineditæ, quarum syllabus in Joann. Raii historiæ plantarum tomo tertio, Katholieke Universiteit Libraries*, Maurits Sabbe Library, Ms. PM0038/V.

Camel, Georg Joseph and John Ray: *Georgii Josephi Camelli, Herbarum aliarumque stirpium in insulâ Luzone Philippinarum primariâ nascentium icones ab autore delineatæ ineditæ, quarum syllabus in Joann. Raii historiæ plantarum tomo tertio*, Leuven, ex coll. Sabbe, Ms. c. 1700.

Campbell, Erin: 'The Art of Aging Gracefully: The Elderly Artist as Courtier in Early Modern Art Theory and Criticism', *The Sixteenth Century Journal* 33 (2002), pp. 321–331.

Campbell, Jean: 'Pier Maria Rossi's Treasure: Love, Knowledge and the Invention of the Source in the Camdera d'Oro at Torrechiara', in: *Emilia and Marche nel Rinascimento. L'identità visiva della 'periferia'*, ed. by Giancarla Periti, Azzano 2005, pp. 63–88.

Campbell, Stephen J.: 'On Renaissance Nonmodernity', in: *I Tatti Studies in the Italian Renaissance* 20:2 (2017), pp. 261–294.

Canali, Ferruccio: 'Brunelleschi, Michelozzo, Alberti e le biblioteche umanistiche: tracce 'michelozziane' tra Firenze e Cesena', in: *Michelozzo. Scultore e architetto (1396–1472)*, ed. by Gabriele Morolli, Florence 1998, pp. 191–202.
Cannon, Joanna: *Religious Poverty, Visual Riches: Art in the Dominican Churches of Central Italy in the Thirteenth and Fourteenth Centuries*, New Haven 2013.
Carbonelli, Giovanni: 'S. Luca medico in una tela di Guglielmo Caccia', in: *Bollettino dell'Istituto Storico Italiano dell'Arte Sanitaria* 8 (1928), pp. 109–113.
Cardano, Girolamo: *De subtilitate*, Nuremberg 1550.
Cardano, Girolamo: *De rerum varietate*, Vicenza 1557.
Cardano, Girolamo: *Opera omnia*, 10 vols, Lyon 1663.
Cardini, Franco: *Le mura di Firenze inargentate. Letture fiorentine*, Palermo 1993.
Caroli, Ernesto (ed.), *Fonti francescane. Nuova edizione*, Padua 2004.
Casserio, Giulio Cesare: *Tabulae anatomicae LXXIIX*, Venice 1627.
Castelli, Silvia and Piera Giovanna Tordella (eds): *…Per fare notomia. Il Cristo anatomico di Raffaello nella Biblioteca Marucelliana di Firenze*, Florence 2021.
Castelnuovo, Enrico: *Un pittore italiano alla corte di Avignone. Matteo Giovanetti e la pittura in Provenza nel secolo XIV*, Turin 1991 (1962).
Cateni, Alessandro: *Giulio Mancini, il viaggio per Roma per vedere le pitture e la riscoperta dei primitivi*, Siena 2021.
Cavallo, Sandra: *Artisans of the Body in Early Modern Italy. Identities, Famlies and Masculinities*, Manchester 2007.
Cavallo, Sandra: 'Conserving Health: The Non-Naturals in Early Modern Culture and Society', in *Conserving Health in Early Modern Culture: Bodies and Environments in Italy and England*, ed. by Sandra Cavallo and Tessa Storey, Manchester 2017, pp. 1–19.
Cavallo, Sandra and Tessa Storey (eds): *Healthy Living in Late Renaissance Italy*, Oxford 2013.
Cavazzini, Patricia: 'La mala fama di Agostino Tassi', in: *Agostino Tassi (1578–1644): Un paesaggista tra immaginario e realtà*, exh. cat. Rome, ed. by Patrizia Cavazzini, Rome 2008, pp. 11–22.
Cavazzini, Patrizia: 'La vita e le opere di Agostino Tassi', in: *Agostino Tassi (1578–1644): Un paesaggista tra immaginario e realtà*, exh. cat. Rome, ed. by Patrizia Cavazzini, Rome 2008, pp. 23–95.
Cavazzini, Patrizia: *Painting as Business in Early Seventeenth-Century Rome*, University Park 2008.
Caviness, Madeline: 'From the Self-Invention of the Whiteman in the Thirteenth Century to *The Good, The Bad, and The Ugly*', in: *Different Visions: A Journal of New Perspectives on Medieval Art* 1 (2008), pp. 1–33.
Cazort, Mimi, Monique Kornell, and Kenneth B. Roberts (eds): *The Ingenious Machine of Nature: Four Centuries of Art and Anatomy*, Ottawa 1996.
Cennini, Cennino: *Il libro dell'arte*, ed. by Fabio Frezzato, Vicenza 2003.
Cennini, Cennino: *Il libro dell'arte*, transl. by Lara Broecke, London 2015.
Chandelier, Joël and Aurélien Robert: 'Nature humaine et complexion du corps chez les médecins italiens de la fine du moyen âge', in: *Revue de synthèse*, 6th series, 134:4 (2013), pp. 474–510.
Charuty, Giordana: 'Le vœu de vivre. Corps morcelés, corps sans âme dans les pèlerinages portugais', *Terrain. Le corps en morceaux*, vol. 18, 1982, at http://terrain.revues.org/3031 (accessed 8 January 2021).
Chastel, André: 'Le dictum Horatii: quidlibet audendi potestas et les artistes (XIIIe–XVIe siècle)', in: *Comptes rendus des séances de l'Académie des Inscriptions et Belles-Lettres* 121:17 (1977), pp. 30–45.
Chave-Mahir, Florence: *L'exorcisme des possédés dans l'Église d'Occident (Xe–XIVe siècle)*, Turnhout 2011.
Chevreau, Urbain: *Histoire du monde. Deuxième edition. Revûe̎, corrigée & augmentée* […], 5 vols, La Haye 1698.

Chojecka, Ewa: 'Krakowska grafika kalendarzowa i astronomiczna XVI wieku', in: *Studia Renesansowe* 3 (1963), pp. 356–357.

Ciatti, Marco: 'The Restoration and the Study of the Crucifix', in: *Giotto: The Santa Maria Novella Crucifix*, ed. by Marco Ciatti and Max Seidel, Florence 2002, pp. 25–64.

Ciuti, Francesco: 'Il Collegio dei fisici e l'Arte dei medici e speziali di Firenze: dalla Repubblica allo Stato mediceo (XIV–XVI secolo)', in: *Archivio Storico Italiano* 170:1, 631 (2012), pp. 3–28.

Clark, John R.: 'Roger Bacon and the Composition of Marsilio Ficino's *De Vita longa* (*De vita*, book II)', in: *Journal of the Warburg and Courtauld Instituties* 49 (1986), pp. 230–233.

Clark, Leah R.: 'Objets croisés: Albarelli as Vessels of Mediation Within and Beyond the Spezieria', in: *Etudes Epistémè: Revue de littérature et de civilisations (XVIe–XVIIIe siècles)* 36 (2019), https://doi.org/10.4000/episteme.6292.

Clines, Robert John: 'Dido and Laura in Carthage: White Purity, Epidermal Race, and Sexual Violence in Petrarch's *Africa*', in: *Postmedieval: A Journal of Medieval Cultural Studies* 14 (2023), pp. 89–118.

Cobet, Carel Gabriel: 'Quinti medici dicta. *γναφεύς – γραφεύς* confusa', in: *Mnemosyne. Bibliotheca Philologica Batava* n.s. 6 (1878), p. 282.

Cobet, Carel Gabriel: 'Ad Galenum', in: *Mnemosyne. Bibliotheca Philologica Batava* n.s. 10 (1882), pp. 251–257.

Cohen, Esther: *The Modulated Scream: Pain in Late Medieval Culture*, Chicago/London 2010.

Compton, Rebekah: 'Green Gardens: Venus' Verdant Virtues', in: *Venus and the Arts of Love in Renaissance Florence*, Cambridge 2021, pp. 129–156.

Condivi, Ascaniano: *Vita di Michelagnolo Buonarroti*, ed. by Giovanni Nencioni, Florence 1998.

Condivi, Ascanio: *The Life of Michelangelo*, ed. by Hellmut Wohl, transl. by Alice Sedgwick Wohl, University Park 1999.

Conserving Health in Early Modern Culture: Bodies and Environments in Italy and England, ed. by Sandra Cavallo and Tessa Storey, Manchester 2017.

Conti, Giordano (ed.): *La Biblioteca Malatestiana*, Bologna 2006.

Cooper, Donal: *'In medio ecclesiae': Screens, Crucifixes, and Shrines in the Franciscan Church Interior in Italy (c. 1230–c. 1400)*, PhD thesis, Courtauld Institute, London, 2000.

Coppens, Christian (Chris): *De vele levens van eeb boek. De 'Fasciculus medicinae' opnieuw bekeken*, Brussels 2009.

Coppens, Christian (Chris): '"For the Benefit of Ordinary People": The Dutch Translation of the *Fasciculus medicinae*, Antwerp 1512', in: *Quærendo* 39 (2009), pp. 168–205.

Copsey, Richard: 'Kenton, Nicholas', in: *Oxford Dictionary of National Biography*, 2008, https://doi.org/10.1093/ref:odnb/15429.

Cornarius, Janus: *Pauli Aeginetae totius rei medicae libri VII.* [...], Basel 1556.

Corradi, Alfonso: *Annali delle epidemie occorse in Italia dalle prime memorie fino al 1850*, 8 vols, Bologna 1865–1894.

Cosmacini, Giorgio: *Storia della medicina del lavoro: da Bernardino Ramazzini a Salvatore Maugeri (1700–1985)*, Milan 2022.

Coulet, Noël: 'Pour l'histoire de l'ex-voto: un prix-fait aixois de 1459', in: *Annales du Midi: revue archéologique, historique et philologique de la France méridionale* 105 (1993), pp. 401–406.

Couleur et soins dans les médecines anciennes aux époques antique et médiévale entre Orient et Occident. Grèce, Rome, Inde, Proche-Orient, ed. by Isabelle Boehm and Laurence Moulinier-Brogi, Toulouse 2021 (*Pallas. Revue d'études antiques* 117 [2021]).

Cousin, Bernard: 'L'ex-voto, document d'histoire, expression d'une société', in: *Archives de sciences sociales des religions* 48 (1979), pp. 107–124.

Cowen, David L. and William H. Helfand: *Pharmacy: An Illustrated History*, New York 1990.
Crispo, Alberto: 'Un inedito *San Luca che risana un fanciullo idropico* di Giovanni Lanfranco', in: *Parma per l'arte* n.s. 15 (2008–2009), pp. 103–104.
Cropper, Elizabeth: *The Domenichino Affair. Novelty, Imitation, and Theft in Seventeenth-Century Rome*, New Haven 2005.
Cuir, Raphaël: *Renaissance de l'anatomie*, Paris 2016.
Cummins, Thomas: 'The Golden Calf in America', in: *The Idol in the Age of Art*, 2009, pp. 77–104.
Czaja, Olaf: 'The Making of the Blue Beryl: Some Remarks on the Textual Sources of the Famous Commentary of Sangye Gyatso (1653–1705)', in: *Soundings in Tibetan Medicine: Anthropological and Historical Perspectives: PIATS 2003: Tibetan Studies: Proceedings of the Tenth Seminar of the International Association for Tibetan Studies, 2003*, ed. by Mona Schrempf, Leiden 2007, pp. 345–371.
Czaja, Olaf: 'The Use of Insects in Tibetan Medicine', in: *Études mongoles et sibérennes, centrasiatiques et tibétaine* 50 (2019), pp. 1–56.
Czapla, Julia: 'Niezwykłe zwierzęta w wyobrażeniach uczonych XVI-wiecznej Rzeczypospolitej. Fauna egzotyczna w traktacie Stefana Falimierza *O ziołach y moczy gich…*', in: *Rocznik Biblioteki Naukowej PAU i PAN w Krakowie* 58 (2013), pp. 357–367.
Czapla, Julia: 'Ikonografia owadów w 'ogrodach zdrowia'. Studium przedstawień owadów na przełomie XV i XVI w.', in: *Owady w literaturze, kulturze, języku i mediach*, ed. by Ewa Borkowska (et al.), Siedlce 2021, pp. 11–35.
Dameron, George W.: *Florence and Its Church in the Age of Dante*, Philadelphia 2005.
Davidsohn, Robert: *Geschichte von Florenz*, 4 vols, Berlin 1896–1927.
de Benedictis, Cristina: '*La vita del cardinale Pietro Stefaneschi* di Sebastiano Vannini', in: *Annali della Scuola Normale Superiore di Pisa* s. III, 6:3 (1976), pp. 955–1016.
de Dominici, Bernardo: *Vite de' pittori, scultori ed architetti napoletani*, ed. by Fiorella Sricchia Santoro and Andrea Zezza, 4 vols, Naples 2003–2014.
DeLancey, Julia A.: '"In the Streets Where They Sell Colors": Placing "vendecolori" in the Urban Fabric of Early Modern Venice', in: *Wallraf-Richartz-Jahrbuch* 72 (2011), pp. 193–232.
del Garbo, Dino: *Expositio super tertia et quarta fen IV libri canonis Avicennae*, Venice 1496.
del Garbo, Tommaso: *Summa medicinalis*, Lyon 1529.
del Serra, Alfio: 'Il restauro', in: *La 'Madonna d'Ognissanti' di Giotto restaurata*, ed. by Annamaria Petrioli Tofani, Florence 1984, pp. 87–96.
Demaitre, Luke: 'Skin and the City: Cosmetic Medicine as an Urban Concern', in: *Between Text and Patient: The Medical Enterprise in Medieval and Early Modern Europe*, ed. by Florence Eliza Glaze and Brian Nance, Florence 2011, pp. 97–120.
Derbes, Anne: *Picturing the Passion in Late Medieval Italy: Narrative Painting, Franciscan Ideologies, and the Levant*, Cambridge 1996.
Der dritte Kommentar Lorenzo Ghibertis. Naturwissenschaften und Medizin in der Kunsttheorie der Frührenaissance, ed. by Klaus Bergdolt, Weinheim 1988.
de Villanova, Arnaldus: 'De cautelis medicorum', in: *Opera*, Lyon 1504, pp. 256v–257v.
Devriese, Lisa: 'Physiognomy in Context: Marginal Annotations in the Manuscripts of the Physiognomonica', in: *Recherches de théologie et philosophie médiévales* 84 (2017), pp. 107–141.
Didi-Huberman, Georges, *Ex-voto: image, organe, temps*, Bayard 2006.
Didi-Huberman, Georges, 'Ex Voto: Image, Organ, Time', in: *L'esprit créateur* (2007), pp. 7–16.
Di Marzo, Gioacchino: *La pittura in Palermo nel Rinascimento. Storia e documenti*, Palermo 1899.
Dionis, Pierre: *L'anatomie de l'homme, suivant la circulation du sang, & les derniéres découverte, démontréé au Jardin-Royal*, Paris 1690.

Disease and Disability in Medieval and Early Modern Art and Literature, ed. by Rinaldo F. Canalis and Massimo Ciavolella, Turnhout 2021.

Dizionario biografico degli Italiani, Rome 1960–[2022].

Drugs on the Page: Pharmacopoeias and Healing Knowledge in the Early Modern Atlantic World, ed. by Mathew Crawford and Joseph Gabriel, Pittsburgh 2019.

Duden, Barbara: *The Woman Beneath the Skin: A Doctor's Patients in Eighteenth-Century Germany*, Cambridge 1991 (first ed. Stuttgart 1987).

Duffy, Eamon: *The Stripping of the Altars: Traditional Religion in England 1400–1580*, New Haven 1992.

DuLaurens, André: *Historia anatomica hvmani corporis et singvlarvm eivs partivm. Mvltis controuersijs & obseruationibus nouis illustrata*, Frankfurt 1600.

Dunlop, Anne: 'On the Origins of European Painting Materials, Real and Imagined' in: *The Matter of Art: Materials, Practices, Cultural Logics, c. 1250–1750*, ed. by Christy Anderson, Anne Dunlop and Pamela H. Smith, Manchester 2014, pp. 68–96.

Durand, Guillaume: *Rationale divinorvm officiorvm, I–IV*, ed. by A. Davril and T. M. Thibodeau, Turnhout 1995.

Durato, Tommaso: *Mai sotto Saturno. Girolamo Manfredi medico e astrologo*, Bologna 2008.

Dürbeck, Helmut: *Zur Charakteristik der griechischen Farbenbezeichnungen*, Bonn 1977.

Durling, Richard J.: 'A Chronological Census of Renaissance Editions and Translations of Galen', in: *Journal of the Warburg and Courtauld Institutes* 24 (1961), pp. 230–305.

Duverney, Joseph-Guichard: *Traité de l'organe de l'ouie, contenant la structure, les usages & les maladies detoutes les parties de l'oreille*, Paris 1683.

Eastaugh, Nicholas (et al.) (eds): *Pigment Compendium. A Dictionary and Optical Microscopy of Historical Pigments*, Oxford 2008.

Edelstein, Bruce: 'The Camera Verde: A Public Center for the Duchess of Florence in the Palazzo Vecchio', in: *Mélanges de l'École française de Rome. Italie et Méditerranée* 115:1 (2003), pp. 51–87.

Eliav-Feldon, Miriam, Benjamin H. Isaac, and Joseph Ziegler (eds): *The Origins of Racism in the West*, Cambridge 2009.

Elkins, James: *What Painting Is: How to Think about Oil Painting, Using the Language of Alchemy*, New York 1999.

Epstein, Steven: *Speaking of Slavery: Color, Ethnicity, and Human Bondage in Italy*, Ithaca 2001.

Falimirz, Stefan: *O ziołach y o moczy gich*, Kraków 1534.

Falimirz, Stefan: *O ziołach y o moczy gich*, ed. by Wiesław Wydra, Poznań 2017.

Faller, Adolf: 'Elemente einer Wissenschaftslehre und einer Wissenschaftskritik in den Schriften von Niels Stensen (1638–1686)', in: *Gesnerus* 37:3/4 (1980), pp. 169–188.

Fancy, Nahyan, Justin Stearns, Sonja Brentjes, A. Tunç Şen, Scott Trigg, Noah Gardiner, Nükhet Varlık, Matthew Melvin-Koushki, and S. Nomanul Haq: 'Current Debates and Emerging Trends in the History of Science in Premodern Islamicate Societies', in: *History of Science* 61:2 (2023), pp. 123–178.

Farago, Claire J.: *Leonardo da Vinci's* Paragone: *A Critical Interpretation with a New Edition of the Text in the* Codex Urbinas, Leiden 1992.

Fechner, Fabian: *Sigismund Aperger (1687–1772) und die Naturbetrachtung in der Jesuitenprovinz Paraguay*, University Tübingen, Magister Thesis, 2008.

Federici, Fabrizio: 'Girolamo Mercuriale e l'"accubitus in coena antiquorum"', in: *Lo sguardo archeologico. I normalisti per Paul Zanker*, ed. by Francesco De Angelis, Pisa 2007, pp. 221–237.

Federici, Fabrizio: '"Bernini artificis prodigiosa manus": il mecenatismo di Urbano VIII nelle rime latine di Sebastiano Vannini', in: *Marburger Jahrbuch für Kunstwissenschaft* 44 (2017), pp. 63–84.

Federici, Fabrizio: 'La riscoperta seicentesca del Medioevo, tra antiquaria e storia dell'arte', in: *Archeologia e Storia dell'arte: contaminazioni, innesti e dissonanze*, ed. by Enrico Parlato, Massimo Pomponi, and Claudia Valeri, Rome 2019, pp. 21–38.

Fehrenbach, Frank: *Quasi Vivo. Lebendigkeit in der italienischen Kunst der Frühen Neuzeit*, Berlin 2021.

Feigenbaum, Gail: '"A likeness in the tomb": Annibale's Self-Portrait Drawing in the J. Paul Getty Museum', in: *Getty Research Journal* 2 (2010), pp. 19–38.

Feingold, Mordechai: *Jesuit Science and the Republic of Letters*, Cambridge MA 2003.

Fend, Mechthild: *Fleshing out Surfaces: Skin in French Art and Medicine, 1650–1850*, Manchester 2016.

Ferrari, Giovanna: 'Public Anatomy Lessons and the Carnival: The Anatomy Theater of Bologna', in: *Past and Present* 117 (1987), pp. 50–106.

Ferrero, Giuseppe Guido (ed.): *Opere di Benvenuto Cellini*, Turin 1971.

Ficino, Marsilio: *Three Books on Life*, ed. by Carol V. Kaske and John R. Klark, Binghamton 1989.

Findlen, Paula and Agostino Scilla: 'A Baroque Painter in Pursuit of Science', in: *Science in the Age of Baroque*, ed. by Ofer Gal and Raz Chen-Morris, Dordrecht 2013, pp. 119–159.

Findlen, Paula and Pamela H. Smith: *Merchants and Marvels: Commerce, Science and Art in Early Modern Europe*, New York 2002.

Finucane, Ronald C.: *Miracles and Pilgrims: Popular Beliefs in Medieval England*, London 1995.

Flesh and Bone: The Art of Anatomy, exh. cat., ed. by Monique Kornell (et al.), Los Angeles 2022.

Flohr, Miko: *The World of the Fullo: Work, Economy, and Society in Roman Italy*, Oxford 2013.

Flora, Holly: *Cimabue and the Franciscans*, London 2018.

Fonseca, Rodrigo: *Del conservare la sanità*, Florence 1603.

Fortuna, Stefania: 'The Latin Editions of Galen's *Opera omnia* (1490–1625) and Their Prefaces', in: *Early Science and Medicine* 17 (2012), pp. 319–412.

Foscati, Alessandra, '"Il mal degli ardenti". Per una storia culturale delle malattie nel Medioevo', in: *Conoscenze mediche sul corpo come tramite di cultura tra Oriente e Occidente. Atti della giornata di studi Palazzo dell'Archiginnasio, Societas Medica Chirirugica Bononiensis, Bologna 20 aprile 2009*, ed. by Andrea Piras and Paolo Delaini, Milan 2010, pp. 49–82.

Freedberg, David: *The Power of Images: Studies in the History and Theory of Response*, Chicago 1989.

French, Roger K.: 'Berengario da Carpi and the Use of Commentary in Anatomical Teaching', in: *The Medical Renaissance of the Sixteenth Century*, ed. by Roger K. French and Iain M. Lonie, Cambridge 1985, pp. 42–74.

Fricke, Beate: '*Artifex* and *Opifex* – The Medieval Artist', in: *A Companion to Medieval Art: Romanesque and Gothic in Northern Europe*, ed. by Conrad Rudolph, New York 2019, pp. 45–70.

Frigo, Alberto: 'Can One Speak of Painting if One Cannot Hold a Brush?: Giulio Mancini, Medicine, and the Birth of the Connoisseur', in: *Journal of the History of Ideas* 73 (2012), pp. 417–436.

Frugoni, Chiara: *Francesco e l'invenzione delle stimmate. Una storia per immagini e parole fino a Bonaventura e a Giotto*, Turin 1993.

Gadebusch Bondio, Mariacarla: 'La carne di fuori: Discorsi medici sulla natura e l'estetica della pelle nel '500', in: *Micrologus* 13 (2005), pp. 537–570.

Gaeta, Marcello: *Giotto und die* croci dipinte *des Trecento: Studien zu Typus, Genese und Rezeption*, Münster 2013.

Gage, Frances: 'Exercise for Mind and Body: Giulio Mancini, Collecting, and the Beholding of Landscape Painting in the Seventeenth Century', in: *Renaissance Quarterly* 61 (2008), pp. 1167–1207.

Gage, Frances: 'New Documents on Giulio Mancini and Guercino', *The Burlington Magazine* 156 (2014), pp. 653–656.

Gage, Frances: *Painting as Medicine in Early Modern Rome: Giulio Mancini and the Efficacy of Art*, University Park 2016.

Gage, Frances: 'Chasing Good Air and Viewing Beautiful Perspectives: Painting and Health Preservation in Seventeenth-Century Rome', in: *Conserving Health in Early Modern Culture: Bodies and Environments in Italy and England*, ed. by Sandra Cavallo and Tessa Storey, Manchester 2017, pp. 237–259.

Gage, Frances: '"It is not so easy to recognize the periode and age of paintings": Visual and Textual Evidence in Giulio Mancini's *Considerazioni sulla pittura* and in Early Modern Connoisseurship', in: *Zeigen – Überzeugen – Beweisen. Methoden der Wissensproduktion in Kunstliteratur, Kennerschaft und Sammlungspraxis der Frühen Neuzeit*, ed. by Elisabeth Oy-Marra and Irina Schmiedel, Merzhausen 2020, pp. 63–87.

Gage, John: *Colour and Culture: Practice and Meaning from Antiquity to Abstraction*, London 1993.

Gal, Ofer: 'Baroque Modes and the Production of Knowledge', in: *Science in the Age of Baroque*, ed. by Ofer Gal and Raz Chen-Morris, Dordrecht 2013, pp. 1–9.

Galen: *Opera*, ed. by Diomedes Bonardus, Venice 1490.

Galen: *Medicorvm omnivm facile principis de sanitate tuenda libri sex, à Thoma Linacro Anglo latinitate donati, & nunc recens annotationibus sane luculentis, & quæ cinnebtarij uice esse poßint, à Leonharto Fuchsio scholæ Tubingensis professore publico, in studiosorum gratiam, illustrati*, 2 vols, Tübingen 1541.

Galen: *Omnia opera*, ed. by Agostino Gadaldini, 2 vols, Venice 1541–1542.

Galen: *Operum omnium*, ed. by Agostino Ricchi, 8 vols, Venice 1541–1545.

Galen: *De sanitate tuenda libri sex*, Lyon 1548.

Galen: *Delli mezzi, che si possono tenere per conservarci la sanità*, Venice 1549.

Galen: *Opera omnia*, ed. by Karl Gottlob Kühn, 20 vols, Leipzig 1821–1833.

Galen: *Sieben Bücher Anatomie. Ανατομικών εγχειρήσεων*, ed. by Max Simon, 2 vols, Leipzig 1906.

Galen: *De sanitate tuenda*, ed. by Konrad Koch, Leipzig 1923.

Galen: *De complexionibus*, transl. by Burgundio of Pisa, ed. by Richard J. Durling, Berlin 1976.

Galen: *De praecognitione*, ed. by Vivian Nutton, Berlin 1979.

Galen: *On the Doctrines of Hippocrates and Plato: Edition, Translation and Commentary, First part: Books I–V*, ed. by Phillip de Lacy, Berlin 1981.

Galen: *On the Constitution of the Art of Medicine, The Art of Medicine, A Method of Medicine to Glaucon*, ed. and transl. by Ian Johnston, Cambridge 2016.

Galen: *Hygiene*, ed. and transl. by Ian Johnston, 2 vols, Cambridge 2018.

Galen: *On Temperaments*, transl. by Ian Johnston, Cambridge 2020.

Galison, Peter: *Image and Logic: A Material Culture of Microphysics*, Chicago 1997.

Gardner, Julian: *Giotto and His Publics: Three Paradigms of Patronage*, Cambridge MA 2011.

Gasparotto, Davide: 'The Power of Invention: Goldsmiths and *Disegno* in the Renaissance', in: *Donatello, Michelangelo, Cellini: Sculptors' Drawings from Renaissance Italy*, ed. by Michael W. Cole, London 2014, pp. 40–55.

Geddes, Leslie: *Watermarks: Leonardo da Vinci and the Mastery of Nature*, Princeton 2020.

Gender, Health, and Healing, 1250–1550, ed. by Sara Ritchey and Sharon Strocchia, Amsterdam 2020.

Gentilcore, David: 'Purging Filth: Plague and Responses to it in Rome, 1656–7', in: *Rome, Pollution, and Propriety: Dirt, Disease, and Hygiene in the Eternal City from Antiquity to Modernity*, ed. by Mark Bradley with Kenneth Stow, Cambridge 2012, pp. 153–168.

Gentile, Luigi: *I codici Palatini della R. Biblioteca Nazionale Centrale di Firenze*, 3 vols, Rome 1889–1950.

Gentile da Fabriano. Studi e ricerche, ed. by Andrea De Marchi, Laura Laureati and Lorenza Mochi Onori, Milan 2006.

Ghiberti, Lorenzo: *I commentarii (Biblioteca Nazionale Centrale di Firenze, II, I, 333)*, ed. by Lorenzo Bartoli, Florence 1998.

Ghiberti teorico. Natura, arte e coscienza storica nel Quattrocento, ed. by Fabian Jonietz, Wolf-Dietrich Löhr and Alessandro Nova, Milan 2019.

Gicklhorn, Josef and Renée Gicklhorn: *Georg Joseph Kamel S. J. (1661–1706), Apotheker, Botaniker, Arzt und Naturforscher der Philippineninseln*, Eutin 1954.

Gimm, Martin: 'Zum Geleit: Die manjurischen Kaiser und die Fremdsprachen', in: *Auf kaiserlichen Befehl erstelltes Wörterbuch des Manjurischen in fünf Sprachen. 'Fünfsprachenspiegel'. Systematisch angeordneter Wortschatz auf Manjurisch, Tibetisch, Mongolisch, Turki und Chinesisch*, ed. by Oliver Corff, (et al.), Wiesbaden 2013.

Ginzburg, Carlo: 'Spie. Radici di un paradigma indiziario', in: *Crisi della ragione. Nuovi modelli nel rapporto tra sapere e attività umane*, ed. by Aldo Gargani (et al.), Turin 1979, pp. 57–106.

Ginzburg Carignani, Silvia: *Annibale Carracci a Roma: gli affreschi di Palazzo Farnese*, Rome 2000.

Giottus Pictor, vol. 1: *Giottos Leben. Mit einer Sammlung der Urkunden und Texte bis Vasari*, ed. by Michael Viktor Schwarz and Pia Theis, Vienna 2004.

Giura, Giovanni: 'Notizie su due cappelle perdute nella basilica di Santa Croce a Firenze', in: *Commentari d'arte* 49:2 (2011), pp. 29–41

Glisson, Franciscus: *Anatomia hepatis*, Amsterdam 1665.

Golvers, Noël: 'The Jesuits in China and the Circulation of Western Books in the Sciences (17th–18th Centuries): The Medical and Pharmaceutical Sections in the SJ Libraries of Peking', in: *EASTM* 34 (2011), pp. 15–85.

Gómez, Pablo F.: *The Experiential Caribbean: Creating Knowledge and Healing in the Early Modern Atlantic*, Chapel Hill 2017.

Gomez, Santiago: 'Crisóstomo Martínez, 1638–1694: The Discoverer of Trabecular Bone', in: *Endocrine* 17:1 (2002), pp. 3–4.

Górnicki, Bolesław: 'Zarys piśmiennictwa pediatrycznego do roku 1600', in: *Archiwum Historii i Filozofii Medycyny oraz Historii Nauk Przyrodniczych* 18 (1939–1947), pp. 47–102.

Graaf, Reinier de: *Opera omnia*, Amsterdam 1705.

Graul, Jana: 'Intrigues, Punches, and a Poisoned Salad: The Dark Side of Artistic Rivalries', in: *Idols and Rivals. Artistic Competition in Antiquity and the Early Modern Era*, exh. cat., ed. by Gudrun Sowboda, Vienna 2022, pp. 152–159.

Graul, Jana: 'Wenn der frühneuzeitliche Künstler erkrankt: Destruktive Kraft mit kreativem Potential', in: *Kunst und Gebrechen*, ed. by Hildgard Fraueneder, Nora Grundtner and Manfred Kern, Vienna 2024, pp. 75–135.

Gregory, Sharon: 'The Unsympathetic Exemplar in Vasari's "Life of Pontormo"', in: *Renaissance Studies* 23:1 (2009), pp. 1–32.

Grmek, Mirko Dražen: 'Život i djela Dinka Dubrovčania srednjevjekovnog liječnika i medicinskog pisca', in: *Anali Historijskog Instituta u Dubrovniku* 2 (1953), pp. 217–233.

Grmek, Mirko Dražen and Danielle Gourevitch: 'L'école médicale de Quintus et de Numisianus', in: *Études de médicine romaine*, ed. by Guy Sabbah, Saint-Étienne 1988 pp. 43–60.

Grmek, Mirko Dražen and Danielle Gourevitch: 'Aux sources de la doctrine médicale de Galien: l'enseignement de Marinus, Quintus et Numisianus', in: *Aufstieg und Niedergang der römischen Welt*, vol. 37: *Philosophie, Wissenschaften, Technik*, vol. 2: *Wissenschaften (Medizin und Biologie [Forts.])*, ed. by Wolfgang Haase, Berlin/New York 1994, pp. 1491–1528.

Groebner, Valentin: '*Complexio*/Complexion: Categorizing Individual Natures, 1250–1600', in: *The Moral Authority of Nature*, ed. by Lorraine Daston and Fernando Vidal, Chicago 2004, 361–383.

Grosshans, Rainald: *Maerten van Heemskerck. Die Gemälde*, Berlin 1980.

Gründler, Hana, Franziska Lampe and Katharine Stahlbuhk: 'Phänomen "Farbe": Ästhetik – Epistemologie – Politik', in: *kritische berichte* 50:1 (2022), pp. 2–11.

Guerrini, Anita: 'Duverney's Skeletons', *Isis* 94 (2003), pp. 577–603.

Gyatso, Janet: 'Experience, Empiricism, and the Fortunes of Authority: Tibetan Medicine and Buddhism on the Eve of Modernity', in: *Forms of Knowledge in Early Modern Asia: Explorations in the Intellectual History of India and Tibet, 1500–1800*, ed. by Sheldon Pollock, Durham 2011, pp. 311–335.

Gyatso, Janet: *Being Human in a Buddhist World: An Intellectual History of Medicine in Early Modern Tibet*, New York 2015.

Habrich, Christa: 'Lukas, der Arzt, als Schutzheiliger von Kunst und Heilkunde. Zu einem Gemälde des 18. Jahrhunderts', in: *Beiträge zur Geschichte der Pharmazie* 24:4 (1972), pp. 25–26.

Hale, John R.: 'The Soldier in Germanic Graphic Art of the Renaissance', in: *The Journal of Interdisciplinary History* 17 (1986), pp. 85–114.

Hanson, Craig Ashley: *The English Virtuoso: Art, Medicine, and Antiquarianism in the Age of Empiricism*, Chicago 2008.

Hanson, Marta: 'On Manchu Medical Manuscripts and Blockprints: An Essay and Bibliographic Survey', in: *Saksaha* 8 (2003), pp. 1–32.

Hanson, Marta: 'The Significance of Manchu Medical Sources in the Qing', in: *Proceedings of the First North American Conference on Manchu Studies 1*, ed. by Wadley Stephen and Carsten Naeher, Tunguso Sibirica, Wiesbaden 2006, pp. 131–175.

Hanson, Marta: 'Jesuits and Medicine in the Kangxi Court (1662–1722)', *Pacific Rim Report* 43 (2007), pp. 1–8.

Hartnell, Jack: 'Wording the Wound Man', in: *British Art Studies* 6 (2017), https://doi.org/10.17658/issn.2058-5462/issue-06/jhartnell

Hasse, Dag Nikolaus: *Success and Suppression: Arabic Sciences and Philosophy in the Renaissance*, Cambridge 2016.

Haviland, Thomas and Lawrence Charles Parish: 'A Brief Account of the Use of Wax Models in the Study of Medicine', in: *Journal of the History of Medicine and Allied Sciences* 25:1 (1970), pp. 52–75.

Harwood, Winifred: 'Trade and Consumption Patterns in Central Southern England: The Supply of Iron and Wax to Winchester College, c. 1400–1560', in: *Southern History* 29, (2008), pp. 1–28.

Helas, Philine: 'Harnglas und Bahrtuch. Die Versorgung der Kranken im Pellegrinaio in Santa Maria della Scala in Siena (1440)', in: *Spitalobjekte. Materielle Kulturen des Spitals in der Vormoderne*, ed. by Artur Dirmeier, Daniel Drascek and Harriet Rudolph, Regensburg 2023, pp. 75–106.

Heng, Geraldine: *The Invention of Race in the European Middle Ages*, Cambridge 2018.

Henri de Mondeville: *Die Chirurgie des Heinrich von Mondeville, nach Berliner, Erfurter, und Pariser Codices*, ed. Julius Leopold Pagel, Berlin 1892.

Hessler, Christiane J.: *Zum Paragone. Malerei, Skulptur und Dichtung in der Rangstreitkultur des Quattrocento*, Berlin 2014.

Hessler, Christiane J.: '"Et ancora dissono questo più filosaphii" – Ghiberti und die Philosophen', in: *Ghiberti teorico*, 2019, pp. 103–113.

Heydenreich, Gunnar: *Lucas Cranach the Elder: Painting Materials, Techniques and Workshop Practice*, Amsterdam 2007.

Hickley, Helen: 'Medical Diagnosis and the Colour Yellow in Early Modern England', in: *E-rea: Revue électronique d'études sur le monde anglophone* 12:2 (2015), pp. 1–17.

Hildegard von Bingen: *Heilkunde. Das Buch von dem Grund und Wesen und der Heilung von Krankheiten*, transl. by Heinrich Schipperges, Salzburg 1957.

Hippocratis Coi, Et Claudii Galeni Pergameni Archiatrōn Opera, 13 vols, Paris 1679–1689.

Hoare, Alexandra: 'Salvator Rosa's allegory of "Philosophy" as "ut pictura rhetorica": Eloquent Gesture and the Pursuit of Artistic Decorum', in: *Art History* 36:5 (2013), pp. 944–967.

Hofer, Theresia: 'Illustrated Materia Medica Prints, Manuscripts and Modern Books', in: *Bodies in Balance – The Art of Tibetan Medicine*, ed. by Theresia Hofer, New York 2014, pp. 226–245.

Hoffmann, Viktoria v.: '*Ingegniosa peritia*. The Languages of Ingenuity in Italian Renaissance Anatomy', in: *Ingenuity in the Making: Matter and Technique in Early Modern Europe*, ed. by Richard J. Oosterhoff, José Ramon Marcaida and Alexander Marr, Pittsburgh 2021, pp. 94–111.

Hoffmann, Viktoria v.: 'Epistemologies of Touch in Early Modern Holy Autopsies', in: *Renaissance Quarterly* 75 (2022), pp. 542–582.

Holmes, Megan: 'Ex-votos: Materiality, Memory, and Cult', in: *The Idol in the Age of Art: Objects, Devotions and the Early Modern World*, ed. by Michael W. Cole and Rebecca Zorach, Farnham, 2007, pp. 165–188.

Holthaus, Bettina: 'La camera d'oro del Castello di Torrechiara: gli affreschi delle pareti e la ricostruzione dello studiolo', in: *Avrea Parma* 75:1 (1991), pp. 3–17.

Hope, Charles: 'Altarpieces and the Requirements of Patrons', in: *Christianity and the Renaissance: Image and Religious Imagination in the Quattrocento*, ed. by Timothy Verdon and John Henderson, Syracuse 1990, pp. 535–571.

Hope Goodchild, Karen: 'Naturalism and Antiquity, Redefined, in Vasari's "Verzure"', in: *Green Worlds in Early Moderny Italy: Art and the Verdant Earth*, ed. by Karen Hope Goodchild, April Oettinger and Leopoldine van Hogendorp Prosperetti, Amsterdam 2019, pp. 109–130.

Hot Dry Men, Cold Wet Women: The Theory of Humors in Western European Art, 1575–1700, exh. Cat. Omaha/Little Rock/Sarasota, ed. by Zirka Zaremba Filipczak, New York 1997.

Hpheng Ling: *Nationwide Collected Ancient Tibetan Medicine Bookname Catalogue*, Beijing 2015.

Hryniewiecki, Bolesław: 'Falimirz, Stefan', in: *Polski Słownik Biograficzny*, Kraków 1948, pp. 354–355.

Hultquist, Aleksondra: 'The Passions', in: *Early Modern Emotions: An Introduction*, ed. by Susan Broomhall, London 2016, pp. 71–73.

Huygens, Constantijn: 'Excerpts from *The Autobiography of Constantijn Huygens, 1629–1631*', transl. by Benjamin Binstock, in: *Art Humanities: Primary Source Reader, Section 7: Rembrandt* http://projects.mcah.columbia.edu/arthumanities/pdfs/arthum_rembrandt_reader.pdf (accessed 8 July 2022).

Huyssen, Heinrich von: *Curieuse und vollständige Reiß-Beschreibung von gantz Italien*, Freiburg 1701.

Iacobone, Damiano: 'La Sala delle Asse nel Castello Sforzesco e la camera del Papa del Palazzo dei Papi di Avignone. Alcune valutazioni iniziali', in: *Rassegna di studi e notizie* 40 (2018/2019), pp. 15–29.

Iannella, Cecilia: 'Malattia e salute nella predicazione di Giordano da Pisa', in: *Rivista di storia e letteratura religiosa* 31:2 (1995), pp. 177–216.

Il corpo e le arti: accademie, disegno, anatomia, ed. by Marco Ciampolini (et al.), Pisa 2016.

Intermedialität von Bild und Musik, ed. by Martin Zenck (et al.), Munich 2017.

Isidore of Seville: *The 'Etymologies'*, ed. by Stephen A. Barney (et al.), Cambridge 2006.

Jacobs, Fredrika H.: '(Dis)assembling: Marsyas, Michelangelo, and the Accademia del Disegno', in: *The Art Bulletin* 84 (2002), pp. 426–448.

Jacobs, Fredrika H.: 'Infirmity in Votive Culture: A Case Study from the Sanctuary of the Madonna dell'Arco, Naples', in: *Representing Infirmity*, London 2021, pp. 191–212.

Jacobsen, Werner: *Die Maler von Florenz zu Beginn der Renaissance*, Munich 2001.

Jacquart, Danielle: 'A la recherche de la peau dans le discours médical de la fin du Moyen Âge', in: *Micrologus* 13 (2005), pp. 494–510.

Jacquart, Danielle: '"Cœur ou cerveau?" Les hesitations médiévales sur l'origine de la sensation et le choix de Turisanus', in: *Micrologus* 11 (2003), pp. 85–108.

Jakobs, Dörthe: 'Restaurierung und Zeitgeschmack: Der Kruzifixus von Cimabue nach der Restaurierung von Umberto Baldini', in: *Zeitschrift für Kunsttechnologie und Konservierung* 2 (1988), pp. 53–67.

Jankowiak, Lucyna: 'Terminologia medyczna w dziele Stefana Falimirza na tle polszczyzny XVI wieku. Próba rekonesansu', in: *Slavia Occidentalis* 57 (2000), pp. 37–50.

Jankowiak, Lucyna: 'Szesnastowieczne słownictwo medyczne na przykładzie zielnika Stefana Falimirza *O ziołach i mocy ich* z 1534 roku', in: *Ad perpetuam rei memoriam. Profesorowi Wojciechowi Ryszardowi Rzepce z okazji 65. urodzin*, ed. by Jolanta Migdał, Poznań 2005, pp. 151–158.

Jankowiak, Lucyna: *Słownictwo medyczne Stefana Falimirza*, 2 vols, Warsaw 2005–2006.

Jankowiak, Lucyna: 'Zapożyczenia w XVI-wiecznym słownictwie medycznym i ich dzisiejsze losy (na materiale zielnika Stefana Falimirza)', in: *Linguistica Copernicana* 4 (2010), pp. 201–213.

Kołodziejczyk, January: 'Das sogenannte Herbarium von Falimirz (1534) und die Quellen dessen botanischmedizinischen Teiles', in: *Acta Societatis Botanicorum Poloniae* 14 (1937), pp. 289–301.

Johnsson, John William Schibby: *L'anatomie mandchoue et les figures de Th. Bartholin: étude d'iconographie comparée*, Copenhagen 1928.

Jonietz, Fabian: 'Die *Scuole delle arti* als Orte der *aemulatio*: Der Fall der Cappella Brancacci', in: *Aemulatio. Kulturen des Wettstreits in Text und Bild (1450–1620)*, ed. by Jan-Dirk Müller (et al.), Berlin 2011, pp. 769–811.

Jonietz, Fabian: 'Ein unbekannter Kunsttraktat des Pier Antonio Fucini und die Florentiner Malerei des frühen Seicento', in: *'Novità'. Neuheitskonzepte in den Bildkünsten um 1600*, ed. by Ulrich Pfisterer and Gabriele Wimböck, Zürich 2011, pp. 133–185.

Jonietz, Fabian: 'Ghiberti *Viator* and the Geography of the *Commentarii*', in: *Ghiberti teorico*, 2019, pp. 117–134.

Jonietz, Fabian: 'Indecent Creativity and the Tropes of Human Excreta', in: *Indecent Bodies in Early Modern Visual Culture*, ed. by Fabian Jonietz, Mandy Richter and Alison G. Stewart, Amsterdam 2023, pp. 197–227.

Jurdjevic, Mark: 'Prophets and Politicians: Marsilio Ficino, Savonarola and the Valori Family', in: *Past & Present* 183 (2004), pp. 41–77.

Kambaskovic, Danijela: 'Love', in: *Early Modern Emotions: An Introduction*, ed. by Susan Broomhall, London 2016, pp. 53–55.

Kananoja, Kalle: *Healing Knowledge in Atlantic Africa: Cross-Cultural Medical Encounters, 1500–1850*, Cambridge 2021.

Kaplan, Paul H. D.: 'Black Africans in Hohenstaufen Iconography', in: *Gesta* 26:1 (1987), pp. 29–36.

Kaye, Joel: *A History of Balance, 1250–1375: The Emergence of a New Model of Equilibrium and Its Impact on Thought*, New York 2014.

Keil, Gundolf: *Der 'kurze Harntraktat' des Breslauer 'Codex Salernitanus' und seine Sippe*, PhD thesis, University of Bonn 1969.

Kemp, Martin: 'From "Mimesis" to "Fantasia". The Quattrocento Vocabulary of Creation, Inspiration and Genius in the Visual Arts', in: *Viator* 8 (1977), pp. 347–298.

Kemp, Martin: *The Science of Art: Optical Themes in Western Art from Brunelleschi to Seurat*, New Haven 1990.

Kemp, Martin: *Leonardo da Vinci: The Marvelous Works of Nature and Man*, Oxford 2006.

Kemp, Martin: 'The Whole in the Parts and the Parts in the Whole: Leonardo and the Unity of Knowledge', in: *Leonardo da Vinci, 1452–1519: The Design of the World*, ed. by Pietro C. Marani and Maria Teresa Fiorio, Milan 2015, pp. 353–367.

Kennedy, Rebecca Futo and Molly Lewis-Jones (eds): *The Routledge Handbook of Identity and the Environment in the Classical and Medieval Worlds*, London 2016.
Kibre, Pearl: 'Hitherto unnoted medical writings of Dominicus of Ragusa (1424–1425 A.D.)', in: *Bulletin of the History of Medicine* 7:4 (1939), pp. 990–995.
Kibre, Pearl: 'Dominicus de Ragusa, bolognese doctor of arts and medicine', in: *Bulletin of the History of Medicine* 45:4 (1971), pp. 383–386.
Kibre, Pearl: *Studies in Medieval Science, Alchemy, Astrology, Mathematics and Medicine*, Trowbridge 1984.
Kidd, Marc and Irvin M. Modlin: 'Frederik Ruysch: master anatomist and depictor of the surreality of death', in: *Journal of Medical Biography* 7 (1999), pp. 69–77.
Kilty, Gavin: *Mirror of Beryl: A Historical Introduction to Tibetan Medicine by Desi Sangye Gyatso*, transl. by Gavin Kilty, The Library of Tibetan Classics, vol. 28, Boston 2010.
Kim, Dorothy: 'The Politics of the Medieval Preracial', in: *Literature Compass* 18:10 (2021), pp. 1–9.
King, Catherine: 'National Gallery 3902 and the Theme of Luke the Evangelist as Artist and Physician', in: *Zeitschrift für Kunstgeschichte* 48 (1985), pp. 249–255.
Kleider machen Bilder. Vormoderne Strategien vestimentärer Bildsprache, ed. by David Ganz and Marius Rimmele, Emsdetten 2012.
Klein, Robert: '"Giudizio" et "Gusto" dans la théorie de l'art au Cinquecento', in: *Rinascimento seconda serie* 1 (1961), pp. 105–118.
Kleinbub, Christian K.: *Michelangelo's Inner Anatomies*, University Park 2020.
Klemm, Tanja: *Bildphysiologie: Wahrnehmung und Körper in Mittelalter und Renaissance*, Berlin 2013.
Klestinec, Cynthia: *Theaters of Anatomy: Students, Teachers, and Traditions of Dissection in Renaissance Venice*, Baltimore 2011.
Klibansky, Raymond, Erwin Panofsky and Fritz Saxl: *Saturn and Melancholy. Studies in the History of Natural Philosophy, Religion and Art*, London 1964.
Koering, Jérémie: *Les iconophages. Une histoire de l'ingestion des images*, Arles 2021.
Kohle, Hubertus: *Ut pictura poesis non erit: Denis Diderots Kunstbegriff*, Hildesheim 1989.
Koopmans, Rachel: 'Visions, Reliquaries, and the Image of "Becket's Shrine" in the Miracle Windows of Canterbury Cathedral', in: *Gesta* 54 (2015), pp. 37–57.
Koos, Marianne: *Haut, Farbe und Medialität: Oberfläche im Werk von Jean-Étienne Liotard (1702–1789)*, Paderborn 2014.
Kornell, Monique: 'Rosso Fiorentino and the Anatomical Text', in: *The Burlington Magazine* 131:1041 (1989), pp. 842–847.
Krafft, Fritz: *Christus ruft in die Himmelsapotheke. Die Verbildlichung des Heilandsrufs durch Christus als Apotheker*, Altomünster 2002.
Krautheimer, Richard und Trude Krautheimer-Hess: *Lorenzo Ghiberti*, Princeton 1982 (first ed. 1956).
Kreytenberg, Gert: *Orcagna, Andrea di Cione: ein universeller Künstler der Gotik in Florenz*, Mainz 2000.
Kriss-Rettenbeck, Lenz, *Das Votivbild*, Munich 1958.
Kriss-Rettenbeck, Lenz, *Ex-voto. Zeichen, Bild und Abbild im voticbrauchtum*, Zurich, 1972.
Kroupa, Šebestián: *Georg Joseph Kamel (1661–1706): A Jesuit Pharmacist at the Frontiers of Colonial Empires*, PhD thesis, Darwin College Department of History and Philosophy of Science, University of Cambridge, 2019.
Krzak-Weiss, Katarzyna: 'Natura w drewnie wyrzezana. O drzeworytach z polskich zielników drukowanych w XVI stuleciu', in: *Obraz natury w kulturze intelektualnej, literackiej i artystycznej doby staropolskiej*, ed. by Elwira Buszewicz (et al.), Warsaw 2020, pp. 198–220.
Krzysztoflik, Małgorzata: 'Elementy astrologicznej koncepcji makro- i mikrokosmosu w traktacie Stefana Falimirza O *nauce gwiazdecznej*', in: *Terminus* 17 (2015), pp. 89–112.

Kuehni, Rolf G. and Andreas Schwarz: *Color Ordered. A Survey of Color Order Systems from Antiquity to the Present*, Oxford 2008.

Kumler, Aden: 'The Multiplication of the Species: Eucharistic Morphology in the Middle Ages', *Res: Anthropology and Aesthetics* 59/60 (2011), pp. 179–191.

Kumler, Aden: '*Periculum* and *Peritia* in the Late Medieval "Ars Market"', in: *Codex Aquilarensis* 35 (2019), pp. 157–178.

La disputa delle arti nel Quattrocento, ed. by Eugenio Garin, Florence 1947.

Lalli, Carlo and Federica Innocenti: 'La Terra Verde: Glauconite o Celadonite? Confronti su casi studio', in: *Paolo Uccello a Santa Maria Novella. Restauro e studi sulla tecnica in terraverde*, ed. by Cecilia Frosinini, Florence 2021, p. 269.

L'anatomia tra arte e medicina: lo studio del corpo nel tardo Rinascimento, ed. by Andrea Carlino, Cinisello Balsamo 2010.

Land, Norman E.: 'From a Painter to a Doctor: A Brief History of a Joke', in: *Source* 37:2 (2018), pp. 78–85.

Landino, Cristoforo: *Comento sopra la Comedia*, vol. 1, ed. by Paolo Procaccioli, Rome 2001.

Langdon, Helen: 'Two Book Illustrations by Salvator Rosa', in: *The Burlington Magazine* 118 (1976), pp. 698–699.

Langner, Rainer: *Kopernikus in der Verbotenen Stadt: Wie der Jesuit Johannes Schreck das Wissen der Ketzer nach China brachte*, Mainz 2007.

Larson, Wendy R.: 'The Role of Patronage and Audience in the Cults of Sts Margaret and Marina of Antioch', in: *Gender and Holiness: Men, Women and Saints in Late Medieval Europe*, ed. by Samantha J. Riches and Sarah Salih, London 2002, pp. 23–35.

L'arte nella medicina e la medicina nell'arte, ed. by Gian Carlo Mandini, Rome 2008.

Laurenza, Domenico: 'In Search of a Phantom: Marcantonio della Torre and Leonardo's Late Anatomical Studies', in: *Leonardo da Vinci's Anatomical World*, ed. by Alessandro Nova and Domenico Laurenza, Venice 2011, pp. 61–77.

Lawless, Catherine: 'Franco Sacchetti on "Modern Saints"', in: *Medieval Italy: Texts in Translation*, ed. by Katherine Jansen, Joanna Drell and Frances Andrews, Philadelphia 2009, pp. 385–389.

Lawless, Catherine: 'Patienthood in Medieval Tuscany: Beliefs and Cures', in: *Medical Humanities* 42 (2016), pp. 76–80.

Lawless, Catherine: '"Make Your House like a Temple": Gender, Space and Domestic Devotion in Medieval Florence', in: *Religions* 11 (2020), pp. 1–21.

Lazzarini, Pietro: *Il Volto Santo di Lucca, 782–1982*, Lucca 1982.

Le corps transparent, ed. by Victor I. Stoichiță, Maria Portman and Dominic-Alain Boariu, Rome 2013.

Lee, Li-chun: *Körper bilden: Körperdarstellungen in der europäischen und chinesischen Medizin*, Bielefeld 2019.

Lee, Rensselaer W.: *Ut pictura poesis: The Humanistic Theory of Painting*, New York 1967.

Le Goff, Jacques: *Il corpo nel Medioevo*, Bari 2007 (original: *Une histoire du corps au Moyen Âge*, Paris 2003).

Leonardo da Vinci: *Trattato della pittura condotto sul cod. Vaticano Urbinate 1270*, Rome 1890.

Leonardo da Vinci's Anatomical World: Language, Context and 'Disegno', ed. by Alessandro Nova and Domenico Laurenza, Venice 2011.

Leonhard, Karin: *The Fertile Ground of Painting: Seventeenth-Century Still Lifes & Nature Pieces*, London 2020.

Le prime farmacopee italiane ed in particolare dei ricettari fiorentini, ed. by Antonio Corradi, Milan 1887.

Lestari, Maria Lad and Gunawan Indrayanto: *Curcumin*, in: *Profiles of drug substances, excipients and related methodology* 39 (2014), pp. 113–204.

Liebeskind, Claudia: 'Die Unani-Medizin des Subkontinents', in: *Orientalische Medizin – ein illustrierter Führer durch die asiatischen Traditionen des Heilens*, transl. by Thomas Geist and Heike Münnich, ed. by Jan van Alphen, Bern 1997, pp. 39–66.

Lichtenstein, Jacqueline: 'Making Up Representation: The Risks of Femininity', in: *Representations* 20 (1987), pp. 77–87.

Lightbown, R. W.: 'Ex-Votos in Gold and Silver: A Forgotten Art', in: *The Burlington Magazine* 121:915 (1979), pp. 352–359.

Lingo, Stuart: *Federico Barocci: Allure and Devotion in Late Renaissance Painting*, New Haven 2008.

Lobsang Yongdan: 'The Translation of European Astronomical Works into Tibetan in the Early Eighteenth Century', in: *Inner Asia* 17 (2015), pp. 175–198.

Locher, Hubert: 'Ut pictura poesis – Malerei und Dichtung', in: *Metzler Lexikon Kunstwissenschaft. Ideen, Methoden Begriffe*, ed. by Ulrich Pfisterer, Stuttgart 2003, pp. 364–638.

Löhr, Wolf-Dietrich: 'Dantes Täfelchen, Cenninis Zeichenkiste: 'ritratto', 'disegno' und "fantasia" als Instrumente der Bilderzeugung im Trecento', in: *Das Mittelalter* 13 (2008), pp. 148–179.

Löhr, Wolf-Dietrich: '"Disegnia sechondo che huoi". Cennino Cennini e la fantasia artistica', in: *Linea I*, ed. by Marzia Faietti and Gerhard Wolf, Venice 2008, pp. 163–190.

Löhr, Wolf-Dietrich: 'Von Gottes "I" zu Giottos "O". Schöpferhand und Künstlerkörper zwischen Mittelalter und Früher Neuzeit', in: *Auge und Hand*, ed. by Johannes Bilstein and Guido Reuter, Oberhausen 2011, pp. 51–76.

Lombartová, Veronika: *Jezuitská kolej v Českém Krumlově na přelomu 16. a 17. století*, Master's Thesis, University of South Bohemia in České Budějovice, 2007 http://www.nusl.cz/ntk/nusl-44206 (accessed 6 August 2025).

Long, Pamela O.: *Artisan/Practioners and the Rise of the New Sciences, 1400–1600*, Corvallis 2011.

Long, Pamela O.: 'Trading Zones in Early Modern Europe', in: *Isis* 106:4 (2015), pp. 840–847.

Lopez-Jantzen, Nicole: 'Historiography, Periodization, and Race: Italy between Antiquity and the Middle Ages, Europe and Africa', in: *New Literary History* 52:3/4 (2021), pp. 469–287.

López Piñero, José María: *El atlas anatómico de Crisóstomo Martínez, grabador y microscopista del siglo XVII / estudio y transcripción de José María López Piñero*, Valencia 1964.

Lower, Richard: *Tractatus de Corde. Item de Motu Colore Sanguinis et Chyli in EUM Transitu*, London 1669.

Lugli, Emanuele: 'Measuring the Bones: On Francesco di Giorgio Martini's Saluzzianus Skeleton', in: *Art History* 38:2 (2015), pp. 346–363.

Lugli, Emanuele: *The Making of Measure and the Promise of Sameness*, Chicago, 2019.

McCall, Taylor: *The Art of Anatomy in Medieval Europe*, Chicago 2023.

Maccherini, Michele: *Caravaggio e i caravaggeschi nel carteggio familiare di Giulio Mancini*, tesi di dottorato, Università degli Studi di Roma 'La Sapienza', A.A. 1993/1994.

Macer, Aemilius: *De herbarium virtutibus*, Kraków 1532.

McHam, Sarah Blake: *Pliny and the Artistic Culture of the Italian Renaissance: The Legacy of the Natural History*, New Haven 2013.

Machiavelli, Bernardo: *Libro di ricordi*, 1954, at http://www.bibliotecaitaliana.it/testo/bibit000830 (accessed 5 October 2022).

McKitterick, David: *Print, Manuscript and the Search for Order, 1450–1830*, Cambridge 2003.

McLean, Ian, *Girolamo Cardano: De libriis propriis. The Editions of 1544, 1557, 1563, with Supplementary Material*, Milan 2004.

McVaugh, Michael: *The Rational Surgery of the Middle Ages*, Florence 2006.

McVaugh, Michael: 'Galen in the Medieval Universities, 1200–1400', in: *Brill's Companion to the Reception of Galen*, ed. by Petros Bouras-Vallinatos and Barbara Zipser, Leiden 2019, pp. 381–392.

Maetzke, Anna Maria: *Cimabue ad Arezzo: il crocifisso restaurato*, Florence 2001.

Magnago Lampugnani, Anna: *Furor. Vorstellungen künstlerischer Eingebung in der Frühen Neuzeit*, Munich 2020.

Magnus, Hugo: *Die Augenheilkunde der Alten*, Norderstedt 2015 (1901).

Malvasia, Carlo Cesare: *Felsina pittrice*, 2 vols, Bologna 1678.

Malvasia, Carlo Cesare: *Vite di pittori bolognesi (appunti inediti)*, ed. by Adriana Arfelli, Bologna 1961.

Manaresi, Antonio: *Il processo di avvelenamento fatto nel 1665–66 in Bologna contro Lucia Tolomelli per la morte di Elisabetta Sirani*, Bologna 1904.

Mancini, Giulio: 'Alcune considerazioni del'honore fatte da Giulio Mancini per suo trattenimento', Biblioteca Apostolica, Barb. Lat. 4314.

Mancini, Giulio: *Considerazioni sulla pittura*, 2 vols, ed. by Adriana Marucchi, Rome 1956–1957.

Manfredi, Girolamo: *Il novo lvme dell'arte ovvero IL PERCHÉ opera copiosa di varie cognitioni*, Venice 1678.

Marconi, Nicoletta: *Edificando Roma barocca: Macchine, apparati, maestranze e cantieri tra XVI e XVIII secolo*, Rome 2004.

Margócsy, Daniel: 'A Philosophy of Wax: The Anatomy of Frederik Ruysch', in: *The Morbid Anatomy Anthology*, ed. by Joanna Ebenstein and Colin Dickey, Brooklyn 2015.

Marijnissen, Roger-Hendrik: *Dégradation, conservation et restauration de l'œuvre d'art*, 2 vols, Brussels 1967.

Marinozzi, Silvia: 'Ramazzini, Bernardino', in: *Dizionario biografico degli Italiani*, vol. 86, Rome 2016, pp. 282–284.

Marks, Richard: 'Wills and Windows: Documentary Evidence for the Commissioning of Stained Glass Windows in Late Medieval England', in: *Glas, Maleri, Forschung: Internationale Studien zu Ehren von Rüdiger Becksmann*, ed. by Ivo Rauch and Daniel Hess, Berlin 2004, pp. 245–252.

Martin, John Rupert: *The Farnese Gallery*, Princeton 1965.

Martin, Meredith and Gillian Weiss: *The Sun King at Sea: Maritime Art and Galley Slavery in Louis XIV's France*, Los Angeles 2022.

Martinelli, Stefano: *L'immagine del Volto Santo di Luca: il successo europeo di un'iconografia medievale*, Pisa 2016.

Matteini, Mauro (et al.): 'Characteristics of the Materials and Techniques', in: *Giotto: The Santa Maria Novella Crucifix*, ed. by Marco Ciatti and Max Seidel, Florence 2002, pp. 387–403.

Mattern, Suzan P.: *The Prince of Medicine: Galen in the Roman Empire*, Oxford 2013.

Mattioli, Andrea, *De i discorsi [...] nelli sei libri di Pedacio Dioscoride Anazarbeo, della materia medicinale*, 2 vols, Venice 1585 [1584].

Maurette, Pablo: 'The Organ of Organs: Vesalius and the Wonders of the Human Hand', in: *Journal of Medieval and Early Modern Studies* 48:1 (2018), pp. 105–124.

Maxwell-Stuart, Peter G.: *Studies in Greek Colour Terminology*, vol. 2: *Χαροπος*, Leiden 1981.

Medicine and the Five Senses, ed. by W. F. Bynum and Roy Porter, Cambridge 1993.

Meier, Christel: 'Die Bedeutung der Farben im Werk Hildegards von Bingen', in: *Frühmittelalterliche Studien* 6 (1972), pp. 245–355.

Meier, Christel: *Gemma spiritualis. Methode und Gebrauch der Edelsteinallegorese vom frühen Christentum bis ins 18. Jahrhundert*, Munich 1977.

Meiss, Millard: *Painting in Florence and Siena after the Black Death*, Princeton 1951.

Mellinkoff, Ruth: 'Judas's Red Hair and the Jews', in: *Journal of Jewish Art* 9 (1982), pp. 31–46.

Mellinkoff, Ruth: *Outcasts: Signs of Otherness in Northern European Art of the Late Middle Ages*, Berkeley 1993.

Mendelsohn, Leatrice: *Paragoni: Benedetto Varchi's 'Due Lezzioni' and Cinquecento Art Theory*, Ann Arbor 1982.

Mercurio, Scipione: *De gli errori popolari d'Italia, libri sette*, Venice 1603.

Merz, Jörg Martin: 'Landscape Drawings by Pietro da Cortona', in: *Metropolitan Museum Journal* 39 (2004), pp. 127–152.

Meydenbach, Jacob: *Hortus sanitatis*, Mainz 1491.

Meyer, Fernand: 'Introduction: The Medical Paintings of Tibet', in: *Tibetan Medical Paintings: Illustrations to the 'Blue Beryl' treatise of Sangs rgyas Rgya mtsho (1653–1705)*, vol. 1, ed. by Parfionovitch Yuri, Gyurme Dorje, and Fernand Meyer, London 1992, pp. 2–13.

Meyer, Fernand: 'The Golden Century of Tibetan Medicine', in: *Lhasa in the Seventeenth Century: The Capital of the Dalai Lamas*, transl. by Howard Solverson, ed. by Francoise Pommaret, Leiden 2003, pp. 99–117.

Michelangelo, Anatomy as Architecture: Drawings by the Master, exh. cat., Williamsburg 2010.

Minni, Francesco: *Arte e chirurgia. Viaggio tra i capolavori artistici ispirati dalla chirurgia attraverso i secoli*, Bologna 2019.

Mitchell, W. J. T.: *Iconology: Image, Text, Ideology*, Chicago 1986.

Mocan, Mira: *La trasparenza e il riflesso: saggio sull'"alta fantasia" tra Cavalcanti e Dante*, Cluj-Napoca 2005.

Moioli, Pietro and Claudio Seccaroni: 'X-ray Fuorescence (XRF) for Analysis of Pigments', in: *Giotto: The Santa Maria Novella Crucifix*, ed. by Marco Ciatti and Max Seidel, Florence 2002, pp. 375–380.

Molino, Paola: *L'impero di carta. Storia di una biblioteca e di un bibliotecario (Vienna, 1575–1608)*, Rome 2017.

Montraville Green, Robert: *A Translation of Galen's Hygiene (De Sanitate Tuenda)*, Springfield 1951.

Moon, Warren G. (ed.): *Polykleitos, the Doryphoros, and Tradition*, Madison 1995.

Moore, Kathryn Blair: 'Kufesque between Pilgrimage and Polemic: Representations of Arabic in Italian Altarpieces, 13th–15th Centuries', in: *Peregrinations* 7:4 (2021), pp. 152–215.

Morgado, Raúl Velasco: 'Nuevas aportaciones documentales sobre el grabador Crisóstomo Martínez y su Atlas de Anatomía', in: *Asclepio. Revista de Historia de la Medicina y de la Ciencia* 64:1 (2012), pp. 189–212.

Morgagni, Giambattista: *Opera postuma*, 3 vols, Rome 1964–1966.

Möseneder, Karl: *Paracelsus und die Bilder: Über Glauben, Magie und Astrologie im Reformationszeitalter*, Tübingen 2009.

Moulinier-Brogi, Laurence: *L'uroscopie au Moyen Âge. 'Lire dans un verre la nature de l'homme'*, Paris 2012.

Moulinier-Brogi, Laurence: 'L'uroscopie en vulgaire dans l'Occident médiéval: un tour d'horizon', in: *Science Translated: Latin and Vernacular Translations of Scientific Treatises in Medieval Europe*, ed. by Michèle Goyens, Pieter De Leemans and An Smets, Leuven 2008, pp. 221–241.

Müller Hofstede, Justus: 'Abraham Janssens. Zur Problematik des flämischen Caravaggismus', in: *Jahrbuch der Berliner Museen* 13 (1971), pp. 208–303.

Murillo Velarde, Pedro: *Historia de la Provincia de Philipinas de la Compañia de Jesus. Segunda parte, que comprehende los progresos de esta provincia desde el año de 1616 hasta el de 1716*, Manila 1749.

Murphy, Hannah: 'Re-Writing Race in Early Modern European Medicine', in: *History Compass* 19:11 (2021), pp. 1–12.

Music in the Art of Renaissance Italy, ed. by Tim Shephard (et al.), London 2020.

M. Valerii Martialis epigrammatvm, medicæ, aut philosophicæ considerationis enarratio, sive de medica Martialis tractatione commentarivs, ed. by Cesare Zarotti, Venice 1657.

Napolitano, Ennio G.: 'Dall'ottone alla tempera: dinamiche transmediali delle iscrizioni arabe nella pittura trecentesca napoletana', in: *Finxit: Dialoghi tra arte e scrittura dal Medioevo all'Età moderna* 1 (2022), pp. 31–60.

Necipoğlu, Gülru: 'The Scrutinizing Gaze in the Aesthetics of Islamic Visual Cultures: Sight, Insight, and Desire', in: *Muqarnas* 32 (2015), pp. 23–61.

Nelson, Jonathan K.: 'Cancer in Michelangelo's Night: An Analytical Framework for Retrospective Diagnoses', in: *Representing Infirmity*, London 2021, pp. 3–27.

Nigro, Salvatore S. (ed.): *Pontormo: il libro mio*, Genoa 1984.

Nova, Alessandro: 'Valore e limiti del metodo analogico nell'opera di Leonardo da Vinci', in: *Leonardo da Vinci: metodi e techniche per la construzione della conoscenza*, ed. by Pietro C. Marani and Rodolfo Maffeis, Busto Arsizio 2016, pp. 25–36.

Nuovo ricettario composto dal Collegio dei Dottori di Firenze, Florence 1498.

Nutton, Vivian: '*De placitis Hippocratis et Platonis* in the Renaissance', in *Le opere psicologiche di Galeno*, ed. by Paola Manuli and Mario Vegetti, Naples 1988, pp. 281–309.

Nutton, Vivian: *Ancient Medicine*, London 2004.

Offner, Richard: 'The Master of the Fogg Pietà', in: *Studies in Florentine Painting: The Fourteenth Century*, New York 1927, pp. 49–58.

Olson, Todd: 'Caravaggio's Coroner: Forensic Medicine in Giulio Mancini's Art Criticism', in: *Oxford Art Journal* 28 (2005), pp. 85–98.

Orlemanski, Julie: *Symptomatic Subjects: Bodies, Medicine, and Causation in the Literature of Late Medieval England*, Philadelphia 2019.

Orsola Maddalena Caccia, exh. cat., ed. by Antonio Barbato, Paola Caretta and Laura Cottino, Savigliano 2012.

Østrem, Eyolf: 'Deus artifex and Homo creator: Art Between the Human and the Divine', in: *Creatorions: Medieval Rituals, the Arts and the Concept of Creation*, ed. by Sven Rune Havsteen, Nils Holger Peterson, Heinrich W. Schwab, and Eyolf Østrem, Turnhout 2007, pp. 15–48.

Ostrow, Steven: 'Pietro Tacca and his *Quattro Mori*: The Beauty and Identity of the Slaves', in: *Artibus et Historiae* 36 (2015), pp. 145–180.

Ottosson, Per-Gunnar: *Scholastic Medicine and Philosophy: A Study of Commentaries on Galen's Tegni (ca. 1300–1450)*, Naples 1984.

O Ziolach tutecznych y zamorskich, Kraków 1542.

O Ziolach tutecznych y zamorskich, Kraków 1556.

Pächt, Otto and Jonathan J. G. Alexander: *Illuminated Manuscripts in the Bodleian Library Oxford*, vol. 3, Oxford: 1973.

Palermo, Francesco: *I manoscritti dell'I. e R. Palatina di Firenze*, 3 vols Florence 1853–1868.

Panazza, Gaetano: *Il convento agostiniano di San Barnaba a Bresca e gli affreschi della libreria*, Brescia 1990.

Panofsky, Erwin: 'Artist, Scientist, Genius: Notes on the "Renaissance-Dämmerung"', in: *The Renaissance: Six Essays*, New York 1962, pp. 121–182.

Panzanelli, Roberta: 'Compelling Presence: Wax Effigies in Renaissance Florence', in: *Ephemeral Bodies: Wax Sculpture and the Human Figure*, ed. by Roberta Panzanelli, Los Angeles 2008, pp. 13–39.

Pardo-Tomás, José and Àlvar Martínez-Vidal: 'Medicine and the Spanish Novator Movement: Ancients vs. Moderns and Beyond', in: *Beyond the Black Legend: Spain and the Scientific Revolution*, València 2007.

Parfionovitch, Yuri; Gyurme Dorje and Meyer Fernand (eds): *Tibetan Medical Paintings: Illustrations to the 'Blue Beryl' treatise of Sangs rgyas Rgya mtsho (1653–1705)*, London 1992.

Park, Katharine: *Doctors and Medicine in Early Renaissance Florence*, Princeton 1985.

Park, Katharine: 'Impressed Images: Reproducing Wonders', in: *Picturing Science, Producing Art*, ed. by Caroline A. Jones and Peter Galison, New York 1998, pp. 254–271.

Park, Katharine: *Secrets of Women: Gender, Generation and the Origins of Human Dissection*, New York 2006.

Parker, Deborah: *Michelangelo and the Art of Letter Writing*, Cambridge 2010.

Parkhurst, Charles: 'Roger Bacon on Color: Sources, Theories & Influence', in: *The Verbal and the Visual: Essays in Honor of William Sebastian Heckscher*, ed. by Karl-Ludwig Selig and Elizabeth Sears, New York 1990, pp. 151–201.

Parrenin, Dominique: *Wargi namu oktosilame niyalma beye giranggi sudala nirugan-i gisun. Xi yi ren shen gu mo tu shuo.* Source gallica.bnf.fr/Bibliothèque nationale de France. Département des manuscrits. Mandchou 289 /FM 191, 1723 (?).

Parrenin, Dominique: *Ge ti ciowan lu bithe*, Source francearchives.gouv.fr/fr/, MS 2009, 1723.

Pasang Yonten: *Dictionary of Tibetan materia medica.* English version of *Bod kyi sman rdzas rig pa'i tshig mdzod g.Yu thog sngo 'bum dgongs rgyan*, transl. by Yonten Gyatso, Delhi 1998.

Pastoureau, Michel: *Green: The History of a Color*, Princeton 2014.

Pastoureau, Michel: *Jaune. Histoire d'une couleur*, Paris 2019.

Patton, Pamela: 'What Did Medieval Slavery Look Like? Color, Race, and Unfreedom in Later Medieval Iberia', in: *Speculum* 97:3 (2022), pp. 649–697.

Pedersen, Jill: 'The Sala delle Asse as Locus amoenus: Revisiting Leonardo da Vinci's Arboreal Imagery in Milan's Castello Sforzesco', in: *Green Worlds in Early Modern Italy. Art and the Verdant Earth*, ed. by Karen Hope Goodchild, April Oettinger and Leopoldine van Hogendorp Prosperetti, Amsterdam 2019, pp. 98–108.

Pericolo, Lorenzo: 'The Liver, the Heart, and the Brain: Francesco Scannelli and the Body of Painting', in: *Res* 71/72 (2019), pp. 178–191.

Perkinson, Stephen: 'Rethinking the Origins of Portraiture', in: *Gesta* 46 (2007), pp. 135–157.

Perkinson, Stephen: *The Likeness of the King: A Prehistory of Portraiture in Medieval France*, Chicago 2009.

Peroni, Adriano: 'La "Maesta" di Ognissanti rivisitata dopo il restauro', in: *La 'Madonna d'Ognissanti' di Giotto restaurata*, ed. by Annamaria Petrioli Tofani, Florence 1984, pp. 17–36.

Persaud T. V. N., Loukas M. Tubbs R. S.: *A History of Human Anatomy*, Springfield 2014.

Petiver, James: *Gazophylacii naturae & artis decades*, London 1702–1706.

Petrarca, Francesco: *De remediis utriusque fortunae*, ed. by Christophe Carraud, Grenoble 2002.

Petrarca, Francesco: *Invectiva contra quendam magni status hominem sed nullius scientie aut virtutis*, ed. by Francesco Bausi, Florence 2005.

Petroni, Alessandro: *Del viver delli romani et di conservar la sanità: dove di tratta del sito di Roma, dell'aria, de' venti, delle stagioni, dell'acque, de' vini, delle carni, de' pesci, de' frutti, delle herbe, e di tutte l'altre cose pertinenti al governo de gli huomini e delle donne d'ogni età, e conditione. Tradotti dalla lingua Latina nella Vogare, dall'Eccelente Medico M. Basilio Paravicino, Da Como.* Rome, 1592.

Pettegree, Andrew and Malcolm Walsby: *French Books III & IV. Books published in France before 1601 in Latin and Languages other than French*, 2 vols, Leiden 2012.

Pfisterer, Ulrich: 'Künstlerische *potestas audendi* und *licentia* im Quattrocento: Benozzo Gozzoli, Andrea Mantegna, Bertoldo di Giovanni', in: *Römisches Jahrbuch der Bibliotheca Hertziana* 31 (1996), pp. 107–148.

Pfisterer, Ulrich: 'Phidias und Polyklet von Dante bis Vasari: Zu Nachruhm und künstlerischer Rezeption antiker Bildhauer in der Renaissance', in: *Marburger Jahrbuch für Kunstwissenschaft* 26 (1996), pp. 69–97.

Pfisterer, Ulrich: *Donatello und die Entdeckung der Stile, 1430–1445*, Munich 2002.

Pierguidi, Stefano: 'Giulio Mancini e la nascita della "connoisseurship"', in: *Zeitschrift für Kunstgeschichte* 79 (2016), pp. 63–71.
Pietz, William: 'The Problem of the Fetish, II: The Origin of the Fetish', in: *Res: Anthropology and Aesthetics* 13 (1987), pp. 23–45.
Platt, Verity: 'Clever Devices and Cognitive Artefacts: Votive Giving in the Ancient World', in: *Agents of Faith: Votive Giving Across Cultures*, ed. by Ittai Weinryb, New York 2018, pp. 141–158.
Pliny: *Natural History, Books 36–37*, transl. by D. E. Eichholz, Cambridge MA 1962.
Pollitt, Jerome Jordan: *The Art of Ancient Greece: Sources and Documents*, Cambridge 1990.
Polzer, Joseph: 'The Figline Master Revisited', in: *Studi di storia dell'arte* 29 (2018), pp. 27–62.
Pontormo, Jacopo da: *Diario*, Florence 2014.
Pouchelle, Marie-Christine: *The Body and Surgery in the Middle Ages*, transl. by Rosemarry Morris, Cambridge 1990.
Powell, Amy: 'A Point "Ceaselessly Pushed Back": The Origin of Early Netherlandish Painting', in: *The Art Bulletin* 88:4 (2006), pp. 707–728.
Preston Blier, Suzanne: 'Capricious Arts: Idols in Renaissance-era Africa and Europe (The Case of Sapi and Kongo)', in: *The Idol in the Age of Art*, 2009, pp. 11–29.
Prudlo, Donald S.: 'Mothers and the Martyr. The Unlikely Patronage of a Medieval Dominican Preacher', in: *Journal of the History of Sexuality* 21 (2012), pp. 313–324.
Pugliatti, Teresa: *Pittura del Cinquecento in Sicilia. La Sicilia occidentale 1484–1557*, Naples 1998.
Putti, Vittorio: *Berengario da Carpi. Saggio biografico e bibliografico seguito dalla traduzione del 'De fractura calve sive cranei'*, Bologna 1937.
Quiviger, François: 'Benedetto Varchi and the Visual Arts', in: *Journal of the Warburg and Courtauld Institutes* 50 (1987), pp. 219–224.
Radford, Ursula M.: 'The Wax Images found in Exeter Cathedral', in: *The Antiquaries Journal* 29 (1949), pp. 164–168.
Ramazzini, Bernardino: *De morbis artificum diatriba*, Modena 1700.
Ramazzini, Bernardino: *De morbis artificum diatriba*, Utrecht 1703.
Ramazzini, Bernardino: *A Treatise on the Diseases of Tradesmen*, London 1705.
Rankin, Alisha: *Panaceia's Daughters: Noblewomen as Healers in Early Modern Germany*, Chicago 2013.
Rawcliffe, Carole: *Medicine & Society in Later Medieval England*, Stroud 1997.
Ray, John: *Historia plantarum: species hactenus editas aliasque insuper multas noviter inventas & descriptas complectens auctore Joanne Raio*, London 1686.
Raynaud, Dominique: *Studies on Binocular Vision: Optics, Vision and Perspective from the Thirteenth to the Seventeenth Centuries*, Cham 2016.
Razzi, Serafino: *Diario di viaggio di un ricercatore (1572)*, Pistoia 1971.
Rebora, Giovanni: *Un manuale di tintoria del Quattrocento*, Milan 1970.
Redig de Campos, Dioclecio: *I palazzi vaticani*, Bologna 1967.
Reinert, Sophus A.: 'Authority and Expertise at the Origins of Macroeconomics', in: *Antonio Serra and the Economics of Good Government*, ed. by Rosario Patalano and Sophus A. Reinert, New York 2016, pp. 112–142.
Representing Infirmity: Diseased Bodies in Renaissance Italy, ed. by John Henderson, Fredrika Jacobs and Jonathan K. Nelson, London 2021.
Resnick, Irven M.: 'Ps.-Albert the Great on the Physiognomy of Jesus and Mary', in: *Medieval Studies* 64 (2002), pp. 217–240.
Rigaux, Dominique: 'Un image pour la route. L'iconographie de Saint Christophe dans les régions alpines (XIIe–XVe siècle)', in: *Voyages et voyageurs au Moyen Âge*, Actes des congrès de la Société des historiens médiévistes de l'enseignement supérieur public, 26 congrès, Aubazine 1996, pp. 235–266.

Rinčen, Bjambyn (ed.): *Dėėrėės togtooson dürs tus bürijg bürtgėsėn bičig*, Corpus Scriptorum Mongolorum Instituti Linguae et Litterarum Academiae Scientarum Republicae Populi Mongolici, tomus XVII, fasciculus I, Ulaanbaatar 1971.

Rinne, Katherine: 'Urban Ablutions: Cleansing Counter-Reformation Rome', in: *Rome, Pollution, and Propriety: Dirt, Disease, and Hygiene in the Eternal City from Antiquity to Modernity*, ed. by Mark Bradley with Kenneth Stow, Cambridge 2012, pp. 182–201.

Robbins, C. Roxanne: 'Scipione Borghese's Acquisition of Paintings and Drawings by Ottavio Leoni', in: *The Burlington Magazine* 138 (1996), pp. 453–458.

Robertson, Clare. 'Late Annibale and His Workshop: Invention, Imitation and Patronage', in: *Mitteilungen des Kunsthistorischen Institutes in Florenz* 54 (2010–2012), pp. 267–294.

Roeske, Wojciech: 'Polskie drzeworyty aptekarskie z 16 i 17 wieku', in: *Farmacja Polska* 36 (1980), pp. 325–329.

Rösslin, Eucharius: *Der Schwangeren Frauen und hebammen Rosengarten*, Strasburg 1528.

Rostafiński, Józef: 'Nasza literatura botaniczna XVI w. oraz jej autorowie lub tłomacze. Sudyjum krytyczne', in: *Pamiętnik Wydziału matematyczno-przyrodniczego Akademii Umiejętności* 14 (1888), pp. 152–207.

Rostafiński, Józef: 'Porównanie tak zwanych zielników Falimirza, Spiczyńskiego i Siennika', in: *Pamiętnik Wydziału matematyczno-przyrodniczego Akademii Umiejętności* 14 (1888), pp. 116–151.

Rostafiński, Józef: *Symbola ad historiam naturalem medii aevi: plantas, animalia, lapides et cetera simplicia medicamenta quae in Polonia adhibebantur inde a XII usque ad XVI saeculum*, vol. I, Kraków 1900.

Russo, Daniel: 'Religion civique et art monumental à Florence au XIVe siècle. La decoration peinte de la salle capitulaire à Sainte-Marie-Nouvelle', in: *La religion civique à l'époque médiévale et moderne (Chrétienté et Islam)*. Actes du Colloque organisé par le Centre de Recherche 'Histoire Sociale et Culturelle de l'Occident, XIIe–XVIIIe Siècle de l'Université de Paris X-Nanterre et l'Institut Universitaire de France (Nanterre, 21–23 juin 1993), Rome 1995, pp. 279–296.

Sabernig, Katharina: 'The Substitution of Rare Ingredients in Traditional Tibetan Medicine on the Basis of Classical Tibetan Texts, their Use in Modern Formularies and a Case Study from Amdo/Qinghai', in: *Curare* 34 (2011), pp. 83–96.

Sabernig, Katharina: 'Tibetan Medical Paintings Illustrating the Bshad rgyud: A Comparison of the Classical thangka set and Murals in the Medical College in Labrang Monastery', in: *ZAS* 42 (2013), pp. 61–82.

Sabernig, Katharina: 'Tibetan Materia Medica in Dispute: Pharmacological Achievements of Dar-mo sman-rams-pa Blo-bzang Chos-grags', in: *Curare* 37:2 (2014), pp. 100–112.

Sabernig, Katharina: 'Anatomical Structures and the Structure of Anatomy in Tibetan Medicine: The Fourth Chapter of the Explanatory Tantra in its Commentaries', in: *Curare* 39:1 (2016), pp. 22–32.

Sabernig, Katharina: *Visualisierte Heilkunde: eine medizinanthropologische Studie zur Identifizierung der Wandbilder der medizinischen Fakultät des Klosters Labrang [Visualised Medicine: a Medical Anthropology Study for the Identification of Murals in the Medical College at Labrang Monastery]*. PhD thesis, University of Vienna, 2017 https://ubdata.univie.ac.at/AC14498862 (accessed 6 August 2025).

Sabernig, Katharina: 'The Tree of Nosology in Tibetan Medicine', in: *Systems of Classification in Premodern Medical Cultures: Sickness, Health, and Local Epistemologies*, ed. by Ulrike Steinert, London 2020, pp. 233–253.

Sabernig, Katharina: 'The Manchu Anatomy – a Revisited Fabric of Bodily Paintings', in: *Studia Uralo Altaica* 58 (forthcoming).

Sabernig, Katharina: 'The Shel gong Shel phreng: a Treasure in the History of Tibetan Pharmacology', in: *Exploring Himalayan Cultural and Textual Heritage: The Legacy and Impact of René Nebesky-Wojkowitz*, ed. by Gaenszle, Martin, Uwe Niebuhr, Markus Viehbeck, and Verena Widorn, Vienna (forthcoming).

Sacchetti, Franco: *Opere*, ed. by Aldo Borlenghi, Milan 1957.

Sacchetti, Franco: *Il Trecentonovelle*, ed. by E. Faccioli, Turin 2000.

De Saint Hilaire: *L'anatomie du corps humain avec ses maladies et les remedès pour les guérir*, 3rd ed., Paris 1739.

Salutati, Coluccio: *Vom Vorrang der Jurisprudenz oder der Medizin. De nobilitate legum et medicinae*, ed. by Peter Michael Schenkel, Munich 1990.

Sammern, Romana: 'Red, White and Black: Colors of Beauty, Tints of Health and Cosmetic Materials in Early Modern English Art Writing', in: *Early Science and Medicine* 20 (2015), pp. 397–427.

Sammern, Romana: 'Treating Bodily Impurities: Skin, Art, and Medicine', in: *Indecent Bodies in Early Modern Visual Culture*, ed. by Fabian Jonietz, Mandy Richter, and Alison G. Stewart, Amsterdam 2023, pp. 109–128.

Sammern, Romana and Julia Saviello: 'Einleitung: Der schöne Körper als Kunstprodukt', in: *Schönheit – Der Körper als Kunstprodukt*, ed. by Romana Sammern and Julia Saviello, Berlin 2019, pp. 9–38.

Sani, Bernardina: *La fatica virtuosa di Ottavio Leoni*, Turin 2005.

San Luca Evangelista testimone della fede che unisce, 3 vols, Padua 2003–2004.

Sapoznik, Alexandra: 'Bees in the Medieval Economy: Religious Observance and the Production, Trade, and Consumption of Wax in England, c. 1300–1555', in: *The Economic History Review* 72:4 (2019), pp. 1152–1174.

Saunders, John B. and Francis R. Lee: *The Manchu Anatomy and its Historical Origins*, Taipei 1981.

Savoia, Paolo: 'Skills, Knowledge, and Status: The Career of An Early Modern Italian Surgeon', in: *Bulletin of the History of Medicine* 93:1 (2019), pp. 27–54.

Savonarola, Girolamo: *Prediche sopra Ruth e Michea*, ed. by Vincenzo Romano, 2 vols, Rome 1962.

Scarullo, Luigi: *Dizionario degli artisti siciliani*, Bd. 2: *Pittura*, Palermo 1993.

Schaeffer, Kurtis: 'Textual Scholarship, Medical Tradition, and Mahayana Buddhist Ideals in Tibet', in: *Journal of Indian Philosophy* 31:5–6 (2003), pp. 621–641.

Schaeffer, Kurtis: 'New Scholarship in Tibet, 1650–1700', in: *Forms of Knowledge in Early Modern Asia: Explorations in the Intellectual History of India and Tibet, 1500–1800*, ed. by Sheldon Pollock, Durham 2011, pp. 291–310.

Schäffner, Almut: *Terra Verde. Entwicklung und Bedeutung der monochromen Wandmalerei der italienischen Renaissance*, Weimar 2009.

Schleusener-Eichholz, Gudrun: *Das Auge im Mittelalter*, 2 vols, Munich 1985.

Schlosser, Julius von: 'The History of Portraiture in Wax', in: *Ephemeral Bodies: Wax Sculpture and the Human Figure*, ed. by Roberta Panzanelli, Santa Monica 2008, pp. 171–246.

Schmidt, Victor M.: 'Tipologie e funzioni della pittura senese su tavola', in: *Duccio: Siena fra tradizione bizantina e mondo gotico*, ed. by Alessandro Bagnoli (et al.), Milan 2003, pp. 531–569.

Schmidt, Victor M.: *Painted Piety: Panel Paintings for Personal Devotion in Tuscany, 1250–1400*, Florence 2005.

Schuchardt, Christian: *Lucas Cranach des Aelteren Leben und Werke*, 3 vols, Leipzig 1850–1871.

Schuchman, Anne M.: 'Life of Umiliana de' Cerchi (1246) Translated from Latin', in: *Medieval Italy: Texts in Translation*, ed. by Katherine Jansen, Joanna Drell and Frances Andrews, Philadelphia 2009, pp. 377–384.

Schulz, Vera-Simone: 'Bild, Ding, Material: Nimben und Goldgründe italienischer Tafelmalerei in transkultureller Perspektive', in: *Zeitschrift für Kunstgeschichte* 79 (2016), pp. 508–541.

Schulz, Vera-Simone: 'Schriftgestöber und geritztes Gold: Orientalisierende Inschriften in der toskanischen Tafelmalerei um 1300', in: *Zeichentragende Artefakte im sakralen Raum: Zwischen Präzenz und UnSichtbarkeit*, ed. by Wilfried E. Keil (et al.), Berlin 2018, pp. 215–243.

Schwarz, Michael Viktor and Pia Theis: *Giottus Pictor*, vol. 1: *Giottos Leben*, Vienna 2004.

Scudieri, Magnolia: 'La Biblioteca di San Marco dalle origini a oggi', in: *La Biblioteca di Michelozzo a San Marco tra recupero e scoperta*, exh. cat. Florence, Museo di San Marco [30.09.–30.12.2000], ed. by Magnolia Scudieri and Giovanna Rasario, Florence 2000, pp. 9–43.

Scudieri, Magnolia and Michele Ciliberto: 'Un'ipotesi per il verde', in: *La Biblioteca di Michelozzo a San Marco tra recupero e scoperta*, exh. cat. Florence, Museo di San Marco [30.09.–30.12.2000], ed. by Magnolia Scudieri and Giovanna Rasario, Florence 2000, pp. 45–48.

Sears, Elizabeth: 'Craft Ethics and the Critical Eye in Medieval Paris', in: *Gesta* 45 (2006), pp. 221–238.

Šedinová, Hana: 'The Symbolism of the Precious Stones in St Weneceslas Chapel', in: *Artibus et historiae* 20/39 (1999), pp. 75–94.

Seiler, Peter: 'Giotto – das unerreichte Vorbild? Elemente antiker *imitatio auctorum*-Lehren in Cennino Cenninis *Libro dell'arte*', in: *Imitatio als Transformation: Theorie und Praxis der Antikennachahmung in der frühen Neuzeit*, ed. by Ursula Rombach and Peter Seiler, Petersberg 2012, pp. 44–88.

Seracini, Maurizio: 'Diagnostica per immagini dell'opera', in: *La 'Madonna d'Ognissanti' di Giotto restaurata*, ed. by Annamaria Petrioli Tofani, Florence 1984, pp. 99–104.

Serafinelli, Guendalina: 'Patronage, Identity and Devotion in Context: The Cases of Carlo Saraceni, Velentin de Boulogne and Guido Reni', in: *Patronage and Devotion*, exh. cat. (Monte Porzio Catone, 26 March–17 July 2022), ed. by Giovan Battista Fidanza and Guendalina Serafinelli, London 2022, pp. 17–71.

Seveso, Raffaella: 'La biblioteca del convento bresciano decorata da Giovan Pietro da Cemmo', in: *Società, cultura, luoghi al tempo di Ambrogio da Calepio*, ed. by Maria Mencaroni Zoppetti and Erminio Gennario, Bergamo 2005, pp. 311–330.

Shaw, James and Evelyn Welch: *Making and Marketing Medicine in Renaissance Florence*, Amsterdam 2011.

Siennik, Marcin: *Herbarz, to jest ziol tutecznych, postronnych y zamorskich opisanie*, Kraków 1568.

Siennik, Marcin: *Lekarstwa doświadczone, które zebrał uczony lekarz pana Jana Pileckiego*, Kraków 1564.

Singer, Charles: 'The Confluence of Humanism, Anatomy and Art', in: *Fritz Saxl 1890–1948: A Volume of Memorial Essays from his Friends in England*, ed. by James Gordon, London 1957, pp. 261–269.

Siraisi, Nancy G.: *Taddeo Alderotti and His Pupils: Two Generations of Italian Medical Learning*, Princeton 1981.

Siraisi, Nancy G.: *Medieval and Early Renaissance Medicine: An Introduction to Knowledge and Practice*, Chicago 1990.

Siraisi, Nancy G.: 'History, Antiquarianism, and Medicine: The Case of Girolamo Mercuriale', in: *Journal of the History of the Ideas* 64:2 (2003), pp. 231–252.

Skaug, Erling S.: *Giotto and the Flood of Florence in 1333: A Study in Catastrophism, Guild Organisation, and Art Technology*, Florence 2013.

Slive, Seymour: *Jacob van Ruisdael: A Complete Catalogue of his Paintings, Drawings and Etchings*, New Haven 2001.

Smith, Janet G.: 'Santa Umiltà of Faenza: Her Florentine Convent and Its Art', in: *Visions of Holiness: Art and Devotion in Renaissance Italy*, ed. by Andrew Ladis and Shelley E. Zuraw, Athens GA 2001, pp. 37–65.

Smith, Pamela H.: *The Body of the Artisan. Art and Experience in the Scientific Revolution*, Chicago 2004.

Snook, Edith: *Women, Beauty and Power in Early Modern England: A Feminist Literary History*, Basingstoke 2011.
Sobiech, Frank: 'Science, Ethos, and Transcendence in the Anatomy of Nicolaus Steno', in: *The National Catholic Bioethics Quarterly* 15:1 (2015), pp. 107–126.
Sohm, Philip: *The Artist Grows Old: The Aging of Art and Artists in Italy, 1500–1800*, New Haven 2007.
Sparti, Donatella Livia: 'Novità su Giulio Mancini: medicina, arte e presunta "connoisseurship"', in: *Mitteilungen des Kunsthistorischen Institutes in Florenz* 52 (2008), pp. 53–72.
Spies-Gans, Paris A.: 'Why Do We Think There Have Been No Great Women Artists? Revisiting Linda Nochlin and the Archive', in: *The Art Bulletin* 104:4 (2022), pp. 70–94.
Stahlbuhk, Katharine: *Oltre il colore. Die farbreduzierte Wandmalerei zwischen Humilitas und Observanzreformen*, Berlin 2021.
Stahlbuhk, Katharine: '"The Mode of Painting with Green Earth [...] in the Monasteries of the Black Monks." Monochrome Wall Paintings and the Santa Giustina Congregation', in: *The Network of Cassinese Arts in Renaissance Italy*, ed. by Giancarla Periti and Alessandro Nova, Rome 2021, pp. 225–242.
Standaert, Nicolas: 'A Chinese Translation of Ambroise Paré's Anatomy', in: *Sino Western Cultural Relation Journal* 21 (1999), pp. 9–33.
State Hermitage Museum: *Brush and Qalam: 200 Years of the Collection of the Institute of Oriental Manuscripts*, exh. cat. [Кисть и калам : 200 лет коллекции Института Восточных Рукописей : каталог выставки], St Petersburg 2018.
Statuti dell'Arte dei medici e speziali, ed. by Raffaele Ciasca, Florence 1922.
Stefanini, Matilde: 'Camelino. Un colore nel Quattro-Cinquecento tra la pittura e la tovaglia (o viceversa?)', in: *Science and Technology for Cultural Heritage* 25 (2015), pp. 61–70.
Steiner, Emily: 'Naming and Allegory in Late Medieval England', in: *The Journal of English and Germanic Philology*, 106:2 (2007), pp. 248–275.
Sticker, Georg: *Abhandlungen aus der Seuchengeschichte und Seuchenlehre*, 2 vols, Gießen 1908–1910.
Stoichita, Victor I. (ed.): *Le corps transparent*, Rome 2013.
Stoichita, Victor I.: *Darker Shades: The Racial Other in Early Modern Art*, Chicago 2019.
Stolberg, Michael: *Uroscopy in Early Modern Europe*, Farnham 2015.
Stolberg, Michael: *Learned Physicians and Everyday Medical Practice in the Renaissance*, Berlin 2022
Strocchia, Sharon T.: *Forgotten Healers: Women and the Pursuit of Health in Late Renaissance Italy*, Cambridge 2020.
Strohmaier, Gotthard: 'Avicenna between Galen and Aristotle', in: *Brill's Companion to the Reception of Galen*, ed. by Petros Bouras-Vallinatos and Barbara Zipser, Leiden 2019, pp. 215–226.
Strozzi, Alessandra: *Lettere di una gentildonna fiorentina del secolo XV*, ed. by Cesare Guasti, Florence 1877.
Sükhbat, Shagdarzhavyn and Gürzhavyn Buyandelger: Mongol anagaakh ukhaan [Mongolian medicine], Ulaanbaatar 2006.
Summers, David: *Michelangelo and the Language of Art*, Princeton 1981.
Summerscale, Anne: *Malvasia's Life of the Carracci: Commentary and Translation*, University Park 2000.
Sweet, James H.: *Domingos Álvares, African Healing, and the Intellectual History of the Atlantic World*, Chapel Hill 2011.
Szostak, Jan: 'Zielnik Stefana Falimirza z roku 1534, cz. I', in: *Ze Skarbca Kultury* 28 (1977), pp. 7–50.
Szostak, Jan: 'Zielnik Stefana Falimirza z roku 1534, cz. II', in: *Ze Skarbca Kultury* 29 (1977), pp. 4–42.

Szymański, Michał: 'Przyczynek do identyfikacji średniowiecznej aparatury destylacyjnej w Polsce', in: *Acta Universitatis Lodziensis. Folia Archaeologica* 30 (2015), pp. 204–223.

Taape, Tillmann: 'Distilling Reliable Remedies: Hieronymus Brunschwig's *Liber de arte distillandi* (1500) Between Alchemical Learning and Craft Practice', in: *Ambix* 61:3 (2014), pp. 236–256.

Taape, Tillmann: 'Common Medicine for the Common Man: Picturing the "Striped Layman" in Early Vernacular Print', in: *Renaissance Quarterly* 74:1 (2021), pp. 1–58.

Tachau, Katherine H.: 'God's Compass and *Vana Curiositas*: Scientific Study in the Old French Bible Moralisée', in: *The Art Bulletin* 80:1 (1998), pp. 7–33.

Take Care. Kunst und Medizin, exh. cat, ed. by Cathérine Hug (et al.), Cologne 2022.

Tartuferi, Angelo: 'Il crocifisso di Santa Croce nel percorso del Maestro di Figline', in: *Città di vita* 2 (2016), pp. 191–206.

Tartuferi, Angelo and Francesco D'Arelli (eds): *L'arte di Francesco: capolavori d'arte italiana e terre d'Asia dal XIII al XV secolo*, Florence 2015.

Tassoni, Alessandro: *De' pensieri diversi, libri dieci*, Venice 1665.

Taube, Manfred: *Beiträge zur Geschichte der medizinischen Literatur Tibets*, Sankt Augustin 1981.

Teja, Ramón and Giorgio Vespignani: 'Gli obelischi di nuovo innalzati e la chiesa "imperiale" romana di papa Sisto V (1585–1590)', in: *Per respirare a due polmoni: chiese e culture cristiane tra Oriente e Occidente. Studi in onore di Enrico Morini*, ed. by Martina Caroli, Angela Maria Mazzanti and Raffaele Savigni, Bologna 2019, pp. 527–538.

The Body Within: Art, Medicine and Visualization, ed. by Robert Zwijnenberg, Leiden 2009.

The 'De Subtilitate' of Girolamo Cardano, ed. by John M. Forrester, 2 vols, Tempe 2013.

The Dome of Uryne: A Reading Edition of Nine Middle English Uroscopies, ed. by Mary Teresa Tavormina, Oxford 2019.

The Holy Face and Paradox of Representation, ed. by Herbert L. Kessler and Gerhard Wolf, Bologna 1998.

The Idol in the Age of Art: Objects, Devotions and the Early Modern World, ed. by Michael W. Cole and Rebecca Zorach, Surrey 2009.

The Letters of Salvator Rosa: An Italian Transcription, English Translation and Critical Edition, ed. by Alexandra Hoare, 2 vols, London 2018.

The Literary Works of Leonardo da Vinci, ed. by Jean Paul Richter, 2 vols, London 1939.

The Materiality of Color: The Production, Circulation, and Application of Dyes and Pigments, 1400–1800, ed. by Andrea Feeser, Maureen Daly Goggin and Beth Fowkes Tobin, Farnham 2012.

Theophrastus: *On Stones*, transl., ed., and comm. by Earle R. Caley and John F. Richards, Columbus 1956.

The Physician's Art: Representations of Art and Medicine, exh. cat., ed. by Julie V. Hansen and Suzanne Porter, Durham 1999.

Thomas Aquinas: *In Aristotelis stagaritae nonnullos libros commentaria*, Parma 1866.

Thomas Aquinas: *Summa theologica*, in: *Opera omnia iussu Leonis XIII P.M.*, vol. 11: *Tertia pars summae theologiae a quaestione 1 ad quaestionem LIX*, Rome 1903.

Thurneysser zum Thurn, Leonhard: *Βεβαίωσις ἀγωνίσμου. Das ist Confirmatio Concertationis* [...], Berlin 1576.

Tordella, Piera Giovanna: 'Raffaello, cemento dell'anatomia e scienza delle cose ultime', in: *... per fare notomia*, ed. by Silvia Castelli and Piera Giovanna Tordella, Florence 2021, pp. 38–47.

Torrigiano, Pietro: *Plus quam commentum in parvam Galeni artem Turisani Florentini Medici Praestantissimi* [...], Venice 1557.

Torrigio, Francesco Maria: *Le sacre grotte vaticane*, Rome 1639.

Townsend, Eleanor: 'Votive Offerings', in: *Gothic: Art for England 1400–1547*, ed. by Richard Marks and Paul Williamson, London 2003, p. 432.

Traffichetti, Bartolomeo: *L'arte di conservare la sanità, tutta intiera trattata in sei libri, per Bartolomeo Traffichetti, da Bertinoro medico in Rimino*, Pesaro 1565.
Travaglio, Paola: 'Il "Liber colorum secundum magistrum Bernardum quomodo debent sitemperari et temperari et confici": un inedito trattato duecentesco di miniature', in: *Quaderni dell'abbazia* 15 (2008), pp. 2–41.
Trexler, Richard C.: *Public Life in Renaissance Florence*, Ithaca 1980.
Trombetti, Anna Laura: 'Manfredi, Girolamo', in: *Dizionario biografico Italiano* 68 (2007), pp. 696–700.
Ullman, Berthold L. and Philip A. Stadter: *The Public Library of Renaissance Florence. Niccolò Niccoli, Cosimo de' Medici and the Library of San Marco*, Padua 1972.
Unglaub, Jonathan: 'Poussin's Reflection', in: *The Art Bulletin* 86 (2004), pp. 505–528.
Utamura, Okihito: 'Revisiting the Exegetical Tradition of Galen's Prologue to the Art of Medicine before Leoniceno: Logic, Teaching, and Didactics in Pietro Torrigiano's *Plusquam commentum*', in: *History and Philosophy of Logic* 41 (2020), pp. 352–375.
Ut musica pictura, ed. by Cristina Samtarelli, Turin 2010.
Ut pictura poesis: dialogue entre les arts à l'époque moderne (XVe–XVIIIe siècles), ed. by Andréane Audy-Trottier (et al.), Paris 2020.
Vagenheim, Ginette: 'Una collaborazione tra antiquario ed erudito: i disegni e le epigrafi di Pirro Ligorio nel *De arte gymnastica* di Girolamo Mercuriale', in: *Girolamo Mercuriale: medicina e cultura nell'Europa del Cinquecento*, ed. by Alessandro Arcangeli and Vivian Nutton, Florence 2008, pp. 127–157.
Valuable Illuminated Manuscripts, Printed Books, Christie's London 6642, 20 November 2002, London 2002.
Valverde, Nuria: 'Small Parts: Crisóstomo Martínez (1638–1694), Bone Histology, and the Visual Making of Body Wholeness', in: *Isis*. 100:3 (2009), pp. 505–36.
Valverde de Hamusco, Giovanni: *Anatomia del corpo humano*, Roma 1560.
van de Roemer, Gijsbert M.: 'From Vanitas to Veneration: The Embellishments in the Anatomical Cabinet of Frederik Ruysch', in: *Journal of the History of Collections* 22 (2009), pp. 169–186.
van der Lugt, Maaike: *Le ver, le demon et la vierge: les theories médiévales de la génératione extraordinaire*, Paris 2004.
van der Lugt, Maaike: 'La peau noire dans la science médiévale', in: *Micrologus* 13 (2005), pp. 439–475.
van der Velden, Hugo: *The Donor's Image: Gerard Loyet and the Votive Portraits of Charles the Bold*, Turnhout 2000.
van Diemerbroeck, Ysbrand: *Anatome corporis humani*, London 1689.
van Foreest, Pieter: *De incerto, fallaci, urinarum iudicio*, Leiden 1589.
Varchi, Benedetto: *Due lezzioni*, Florence 1549.
Vasari, Giorgio: *Le vite de' più eccellenti pittori scultori et architettori*, ed. by Gaetano Milanesi, 9 vols, Florence, 1875–1885 (reprints 1906, 1973).
Vasari, Giorgio: *La vita di Michelangelo nelle redazioni del 1550 e del 1568*, ed. by Paola Barocchi, 5 vols, Milan 1962.
Vasari, Giorgio: *Le vite de' più eccellenti pittori, scultori, e architettori nelle redazioni del 1550 e 1568*, ed. by Rosanna Bettarini and Paola Barocchi, 6 vols, Florence 1966–1987.
Vauchez, André: *La sainteté en Occident aux derniers siècles du Moyen Âge d'après les procès de canonisation et les documents hagiographiques*, Rome 1981.
Veldman, Ilja M.: 'Maarten van Heemskerck and St Luke's Medical Books', in: *Simiolus* 7 (1974), pp. 91–100.
Veldman, Ilja M.: *Maarten van Heemskerck and Dutch Humanism in the Sixteenth Century*, Maarssen 1977.
Vesalius, Andreas: *De humani corporis fabrica libri septem*, Basel 1543.
Villani, Filippo: *De origine civitatis Florentie et de iusdem famosis civibus*, Padua 1997.
Vitruvius: *On Architecture*, transl. by Richard Schofield, introd. by Robert Tavernor, London 2009.

Vittorini Orgeas, Eleonora: 'La tecnica in terraverde nelle fonti storiche e tecniche', in: *Paolo Uccello a Santa Maria Novella. Restauro e studi sulla tecnica in terraverde*, ed. by Cecilia Frosinini, Florence 2021, pp. 139–149.
Vjam-dpal-rdo-rje: *An Illustrated Tibeto-Mongolian Materia Medica of Ayurveda*, ed. by Lokesh Chandra, New Delhi 1971.
Vlcek, Pavel (ed.): *Ceský Krumlov: The Historic Centre*, Praha 2016.
Volpe, Carlo: 'Il lungo percorso del "dipingere dolcissimo e tanto unito"', in: *Storia dell'arte italiana. Dal medioevo al Novecento*, ed. by Giulio Bollati and Paolo Fossati, Turin 1983, part 5, pp. 231–304.
Voragine, Jacobus de: *The Golden Legend: Readings on the Saints*, transl. by William Granger Ryan, Princeton 2012.
Waetzoldt, Stephan: *Die Kopien des 17. Jahrhunderts nach Mosaiken und Wandmalereien in Rom*, Vienna 1964.
Wald, Peter H. and Gregg M. Stave: *Physical and Biological Hazards of the Workplace*, foreword by James P. Hughes, New York 1994.
Wallace, William: *Michelangelo, God's Architect: The Story of His Final Years & Greatest Masterpiece*, Princeton 2019.
Walravens, Hartmut: 'Medical Knowledge of the Manchus and the *Manchu Anatomy*', in: *Études mongoles et sibériennes: Actes de la 37e P.I.A.C. Conférence internationale permanente des études altaïques: Chantilly, 20–24 juin 1994*, ed. by Marie-Dominique Even and Françoise Aubin, Nanterre 1996, pp. 359–374.
Warburg, Aby: *Bildniskunst und florentinisches Bürgertum*, Leipzig 1902.
Warburg, Aby: 'The Art of Portraiture and the Florentine Bourgeoisie: Domenico Ghirlandaio in Santa Trinita: The Portraits of Lorenzo de' Medici and His Household', in: *The Renewal of Pagan Antiquity*, transl. by David Britt, Santa Monica 1999, pp. 184–223.
Webb, Diana: *Medieval European Pilgrimage*, New York 2002.
Webb, Diana: *Pilgrimage in Medieval England*, Basingstoke 2002.
Wecker, Johann Jacob: *De secretis libri XVII*, Basel 1582.
Weddigen, Tristan: *Raffaels Papageienzimmer: Ritual, Raumfunktion und Dekoration im Vatikanpalast der Renaissance*, Emsdetten 2006.
Weeda, Claire: 'Geographical determinism, ethnicity and religion, c. 1100–1300 CE', in: *The Routledge Handbook of Identity and the Environment in the Classical and Medieval Worlds*, ed. by Kennedy, Rebecca Futo, and Molly Lewis-Jone, London 2016, pp. 93–113.
Weinryb, Ittai: 'Votive Materials: Bodies and Beyond', in: *Agents of Faith: Votive Objects in Time and Place*, ed. by Ittai Weinryb, New York 2018, pp. 33–59.
Weissert, Caecilie: 'Ut pictura musica: Frans Floris and Chromatic Music', in: *Simiolus* 40:4 (2018), pp. 270–291.
Wheeler, Susan: *Five Hundred Years of Medicine in Art: An Illustrated Catalogue of Prints and Drawings from the Clements C. Fry Collection in the Harvey Cushing – John Hay Whitney Medical Library at Yale University*, Aldershot 2001.
Whitaker, Cord: *Black Metaphors: How Modern Racism Emerged from Medieval Race-Thinking*, Philadelphia 2019.
Whittington, Karl: 'Picturing Christ as Surgeon and Patient in British Library MS Sloane 1977', in: *Mediaevalia* 35 (2015), pp. 83–115.
Wickersheimer, Ernest, review of: Josef Gicklhorn, and Renée Gicklhorn, *Georg Joseph Kamel S. J. (1661–1706), Apotheker, Botaniker, Arzt und Naturforscher der Philippineninseln*, in: *Revue d'histoire des sciences* 1955, pp. 277–278.
Wilson, Christopher: 'The Arts of the Great Church', in: *Gothic: Art for England, 1400–1547*, ed. by Richard Marks and Paul Williamson, London 2003, pp. 348–352.
Wolf, Gerhard: *Salus populi romani: Die Geschichte römischer Kultbilder im Mittelalter*, Weinheim 1990.
Wonnecke, Johann: *Gart der Gesundheit*, Mainz 1485.

Wood, Christopher S.: 'The Votive Scenario', in: *Res: Anthropology and Aesthetics* 59/60 (2011), pp. 206–227.

Wood, Christopher S.: 'Public and Private Dimensions of Votive Giving', in: *Agents of Faith: Votive Objects in Time and Place*, ed. by Ittai Weinryb, New York 2018, pp. 67–85.

Woods, David: 'Pliny, Nero and the Emerald (NH 37, 64)', in: *Arctos* 40 (2006), pp. 187–196.

Woods-Marsden, Joanna: *Renaissance Self-Portraiture: The Visual Construction of Identity and the Social Status of the Artist*, New Haven 1998.

Wouk, Edward H.: *Frans Floris (1519/20–1570): Imagining a Northern Renaissance*, Leiden 2018.

Wright, Alison: *The Pollaiuolo Brothers: The Arts of Florence and Rome*, New Haven 2005.

Wung Seok Cha and Hyuk Sang Jung [with assistance of Dong Ryul Kim, You Sang Baik and Tae Woo Kim]: 'Body Perceptions in East Asian Culture', in: *Curare* 39:1 (2016), pp. 75–87.

Zagoury, David: 'Minerva in the Forge of Vulcan: *Ingegno*, *Fatica*, and Imagination in Early Florentine Art Theory', in: *Image, Imagination, and Cognition: Medieval and Early Modern Theory and Practice*, ed. by Christoph Lüthy, Claudia Swan, Paul J. J. M. Bakker and Claus Zittel, Leiden 2018, pp. 61–93.

Zagoury, David: *The Wild Brush: 'Fantasia' in Sixteenth-Century Italian Art and Theory (1501–1568)* (forthcoming).

Zanichelli, Giuseppina: 'La committenza dei Rossi: immagini di potere tra sacro e profano', in: *Le signorie dei Rossi di Parma tra XIV e XVI secolo*, ed. by Letizia Arcangeli and Marco Gentile, Florence 2007, pp. 187–212.

Zapf, Volker: 'Pinder, Ulrich', in: *Deutsches Literatur-Lexikon*, ed. by Wolfgang Achnitz, 8 vols, Berlin 2011–2016, vol. 7, pp. 1631–1635.

Zaun, Stefanie and Hans Geisler: 'Die Harnfarbbezeichnungen im *Fasciculus medicine* und ihre italienischen und spanischen Übersetzungen', in: *Farbe im Mittelalter. Materialität – Medialität – Semantik*, ed. by Ingrid Bennewitz and Andrea Schindler, 2 vols, Berlin 2011, vol. 2, pp. 969–985.

Zemanek, Alicja (et al.): 'Selected Foreign Plants in Old Polish Botanical Literature, Customs and Art (*Acorus calamus, Aesculus hippocastanum, Cannabis sativa, Fagopyrum, Helianthus annuus, Iris*)', in: *Plants and Culture: Seeds of the Cultural Heritage of Europe*, ed. by Jean-Paul Morel and Anna Maria Mercuri, Bari 2009, pp. 179–183.

Zerbi, Gabriele: *Über die Kautelen der Ärzte – De cautelis medicorum (ca. 1495)*, ed. by Mariacarla Gadebusch Bondio, Manuel Förg and Christian Kaiser, Stuttgart 2019.

Zglinicki, Friedrich von: *Die Uroskopie in der bildenden Kunst*, Darmstadt 1982.

Zimmel, Bruno: 'Johann Grueber in Lhasa: Ein Österreicher als erster Europäer in der Stadt des Dalai-Lama', in: *Biblios* 2:3/4 (1953) pp. 127–145.

Zuccari, Federico: *L'idea de' pittori, scultori, et architetti*, 2 vols, Turin 1607.

Index

EU authorised representative for GPSR:
Easy Access System Europe, Mustamäe tee 50,
10621 Tallinn, Estonia
gpsr.requests@easproject.com

www.ingramcontent.com/pod-product-compliance
Ingram Content Group UK Ltd.
Pitfield, Milton Keynes, MK11 3LW, UK
UKHW061858100926
8556IPUK00009B/923

* 9 7 8 1 5 2 6 1 8 2 8 7 6 *